ALTE
HEALTH
EM
FOR P

ALTERNATIVES IN
HEALTH CARE DELIVERY:

EMERGING ROLES
FOR PHYSICIAN ASSISTANTS

Edited by
REGINALD D. CARTER, Ph.D., P.A.
HENRY B. PERRY, M.D., Ph.D.
Department of Community and Family Medicine
Duke University Medical Center
Durham, North Carolina
with 85 contributors

WARREN H. GREEN, INC.
St. Louis, Missouri, U.S.A.

Published by

WARREN H. GREEN, INC.
8356 Olive Blvd.
St. Louis, Missouri 63132, U.S.A.

ISBN No. 0-87527-327-0

Printed in the United States of America

LIST OF CONTRIBUTING AUTHORS

Susan M. Anderson, M.L.S.
Information Specialist
American Academy of Physician Assistants
Arlington, Virginia

Peter L. Andrus, M.D., M.P.H.
Assistant Professor of Community Medicine
Baylor College of Medicine
Houston, Texas

Salvatore Barese, SA, PA-C
Department of Surgery
Plastic and Reconstructive Surgery
Yale University School of Medicine
New Haven, Connecticut

Geoffrey A. Beckett, B.S., PA-C
Physician Assistant
Kennebec Valley Medical Center
Gardiner, Maine

Malcolm S. Beinfield, M.D.
Director
Norwalk Hospital/Yale
Physician Assistant
*   Surgical Residency Program*
Westport, Connecticut

Dean F. Blietz, B.S., SA, PA-C
Surgeon Assistant
Thoracic Surgeons Association, P.C.
Grand Rapids, Michigan

Frederick A. Blount, M.D.
Associate Medical Director
Physician Assistant Program
Bowman Gray School of Medicine
Winston-Salem, North Carolina

James A. Boutsellis, SA, PA-C
Surgeon's Assistant
Private Practice
Rome, Georgia

Linda C. Brandt, A.S.
Administrative Director
Norwalk Hospital/Yale
Surgical Physician Assistant
*   Residency Program*
Norwalk, Connecticut

Winton Briggs, M.D.
Department of Medicine,
*   Attending Physician*
Maine Medical Center
Portland, Maine

Kenneth R. Broda, Ph.D.
Associate Director
Pathologist Assistant Program
Duke University Medical Center
Durham, North Carolina

Cynthia Lee Carson, PA-C
Surgical Physician Assistant
Norwalk Hospital/
*   Yale University School of Medicine*
Norwalk, Connecticut

Reginald D. Carter, Ph.D., PA
Associate Director,
*   Physician Assistant Program*
Duke University Medical Center
Durham, North Carolina

James F. Cawley, M.P.H., PA-C
Assistant Professor
Health Care Science
George Washington University
*   Medical Center*
Washington, D.C.

Paul R. Cheney, Jr., M.D., Ph.D.
Chief, Internal Medicine
USAF Hospital
Mt. Home AFB, Idaho

Richard R. Conn, B.A., OPA-C
Instructor/Coordinator
Orthopaedic Physician's Assistant Program
Kirkwood Community College
Cedar Rapids, Iowa

Joseph P. Conrad, B.H.S., PA-C
Physician Assistant
Kennebec Valley Medical Center
Gardiner, Maine

M. I. Culpepper, Jr., LL.B.
University of Alabama in Birmingham
Birmingham, Alabama

Charles B. Cuono, M.D., Ph.D.
Department of Surgery
Plastic and Reconstructive Surgery
Yale University Medical School
New Haven, Connecticut

Joseph G. Daddabbo, B.S., PA-C
Instructor, Allied Health
Physician Assistant Program
Bowman Gray School of Medicine
Winston-Salem, North Carolina

Henry R. Datelle, Ed.D.
Assistant Director
National Commission on Certification
of Physician's Assistants, Inc.
Atlanta, Georgia

Don E. Detmer, M.D.
Professor
Departments of Preventive Medicine
& Surgery
University of Wisconsin
Madison, Wisconsin

Arnold G. Diethelm, M.D.
Department of Surgery
University of Alabama in Birmingham
Birmingham, Alabama

Earl V. Echard, B.H.S., PA-C
Physician Assistant III
Wayne Correctional Center
Goldsboro, North Carolina

Jessie Edwards, M.S.
Program Director
Physician Assistant Program
University of Nebraska Medical Center
Omaha, Nebraska

E. Harvey Estes, Jr., M.D.
Chairman and Professor
Department of Community &
Family Medicine
Duke University Medical Center
Durham, North Carolina

Carl E. Fasser, PA-C
Director, Physician Assistant Program
Baylor College of Medicine
Houston, Texas

Bruce C. Fichandler, PA-C
Co-Director
Physician Assistant
Surgical Residency Program
Yale University School of Medicine
New Haven, Connecticut

T. Guy Fortney, M.D.
Medical Director
Oak Ridge Gaseous Diffusion Plant
Union Carbide Corporation
Oak Ridge, Tennessee

Timothy N. Frary, B.S., PA-C
Physician Assistant
Black Hills Medical Clinic
Newcastle, Wyoming

J. Garber Galbraith, M.D.
Director, Surgeon's Assistant Program
University of Alabama in Birmingham
School of Medicine
Birmingham, Alabama

James F. Gifford, Jr., Ph.D.
Associate Professor,
Community and Family Medicine
(History of Medicine)
Duke University Medical Center
Durham, North Carolina

Suzanne B. Greenberg, M.S.
Director, Physician Assistant Program
Northeastern University
Boston, Massachusetts

Reuben Gull, M.B., M.D.
Medical Director
General Medical Centers Health Plan
Anaheim, California

Jacqueline B. Hall, SA, B.S.
Associate Director,
Surgeon's Assistant Program
University of Alabama in Birmingham
School of Medicine
Birmingham, Alabama

Charles R. Hatcher, Jr., M.D.
Professor of Surgery (Thoracic)
Emory University School of Medicine
Atlanta, Georgia

J. Jeffrey Heinrich, PA-C
Co-Director
Physician Assistant
Surgical Residency Program
Yale University School of Medicine
New Haven, Connecticut

Paul C. Hendrix, PA-C
Physician Associate Coordinator
Department of Surgery
Duke University Medical Center
Durham, North Carolina

Karen G. Holman, M.D.
Medical Director,
Department of Family Practice
University of Oklahoma
Oklahoma City, Oklahoma

Thomas K. Johnstone, III, PA-C
Physician Assistant
Family Practice Clinic
Reidsville, North Carolina

Fran Piazza Kahler, B.A., PA-C
Physician Assistant
Spurwink Internal Medicine Associates, P.A.
Cape Elizabeth, Maine

John W. Kirklin, M.D.
Department of Surgery
University of Alabama in Birmingham
University Hospital
Birmingham, Alabama

Margaret K. Kirklin, M.D.
Department of Surgery
University of Alabama in Birmingham
University Hospital
Birmingham, Alabama

John P. Kopchak, B.M.S., PA-C
Physician Assistant
Emory University Clinic and Hospital
Atlanta, Georgia

James R. Love, R.N., PA-C
Physician Assistant
Wishek Clinic
Wishek, North Dakota

Virginia K. MacFarlane, Ed.M., PA-C
Physician Assistant Training Program
Bowman Gray School of Medicine
Wake Forest University
Winston-Salem, North Carolina

John McElligott, MPH, PA-C
Physician Associate
Oak Ridge Gaseous Diffusion Plant
Union Carbide Corporation
Oak Ridge, Tennessee

Robert J. Meyer, M.D.
Attending Physician Emergency Department
Kennebec Valley Medical Center
Augusta, Maine

Martin Misrack, OPA-C
Orthopedic Physician Assistant
The Corvallis Clinic, P.C.
Physicians and Surgeons
Corvallis, Oregon

Paula Montgomery-Kowalski, PA-C
Assistant Professor,
Department of Family Practice
University of Oklahoma
Oklahoma City, Oklahoma

John C. Mueller, M.D.
Medical Director
Physician Assistant Program
Bowman Gray School of Medicine
Winston-Salem, North Carolina

Holm W. Neuman, M.D., Ph.D.
Private Practice, Orthodedics
The Corvallis Clinic, P.C.
Physicians and Surgeons
Corvallis, Oregon

John E. Ott, M.D.
Professor and Chairman
Department of Community Health Sciences
George Washington University
Medical Center
Washington, D.C.

W. Ward Patrick, MSPH, M.D.
Assistant Professor
Physician Assistant Program
Bowman Gray School of Medicine
Winston-Salem, North Carolina

Henry B. Perry, M.D., Ph.D.
Assistant Clinical Professor
Community and Family Medicine
Duke University Medical Center
Durham, North Carolina

Jimmie L. Pharris, Ph.D.
Director, Physician Assistant Program
Bowman Gray School of Medicine
Winston-Salem, North Carolina

Michael G. Phillips, PA-C
Assistant Director
Alabama Regional Organ Bank
University of Alabama in Birmingham
Birmingham, Alabama

Terence D. Rafferty, M.D., B.Ch.
Associate Professor, Anesthesiology
Yale University School of Medicine
New Haven, Connecticut

Lanny B. Reimer, M.D.
Private Practice
Black Hills Medical Clinic
Newcastle, Wyoming

Harold F. Rheinlander, M.D.
Professor and Vice-Chairman
Department of Surgery
Tufts University School of Medicine
Boston, Massachusetts

Kathleen M. Rooney, B.A., PA-C
Surgical Physician Assistant
Norwalk Hospital/Yale
Westport, Connecticut

Richard G. Rosen, M.D.
Medical Advisor
Postgraduate Surgical
* Physician Assistant Program*
Montefiore Hospital and Medical Center
Albert Einstein College of Medicine
Bronx, New York

Peter D. Rosenstein, M.P.A.
Executive Director
American Academy of Physician Assistants
Arlington, Virginia

Ashutosh Roy, M.D., Ph.D., MS.Ed.
Medical Director,
* Primary Care PA Program*
University of California School of Medicine
Los Angeles, California

Gordon T. Schaedel, B.S., PA-C
Physician Associate
Cardiovascular & Thoracic Surgery
St. Luke's Roosevelt Hospital Center
New York, New York

Bonnie Schmidt, M.S., CHA
Child Health Associate
University of Colorado
* Health Science Center*
Denver, Colorado

Gary R. Scofield, B.S., M.S., PA-C
Primary Care Physician Assistant
General Medical Centers Health Plan
Santa Fe Spring, California

Quentin W. Smith, M.S.
Baylor College of Medicine
Houston, Texas

Richard A. Smith, M.D., M.P.H.
Director,
* Health Manpower Development Staff*
John A. Burns School of Medicine
University of Hawaii
Honolulu, Hawaii

Douglas E. Stackhouse, B.H.S., PA-C
Physician Assistant
USAF Hospital
Mtn. Home AFB, Idaho

Shepard B. Stone, M.P.S., PA-C
Lecturer, Anesthesiology
Yale University School of Medicine
New Haven, Connecticut

David A. Symond, M.D.
Family Practice
Melford Medical, Melford Valley Hospital
Melford, Utah

Sigmund I. Tannenbaum, M.D.
Chief Resident, Division of Urology
Duke University Medical Center
Durham, North Carolina

Rein Tideiksaar, Ph.D., P.A.
Coordinator, Department of Geriatric
  Medical Education
Jewish Institute for Geriatric Care
New Hyde Park, New York

Luis A. Tomatis, M.D.
Private Practice
Thoracic Surgeons Associates, P.C.
Grand Rapids, Michigan

Clara E. Vanderbilt, PA-C
Director
Postgraduate Surgical
  Physician's Assistant Program
Montefiore Medical Center
Bronx, New York

Daniel T. Vetrosky, B.H.S., PA-C
Physician Assistant, Urology
Duke University Medical Center
Durham, North Carolina

David G. Warren, J.D.
Professor of Health Administration
Duke University Medical Center
Durham, North Carolina

Jerry L. Weston, Sc.D.
Senior Research Manager
National Center for

Health Services Research
Department of Health & Human Services
Hyattsville, Maryland

John D. Whelchel, M.D.
Associate Professor of Surgery
University of Alabama in Birmingham
Birmingham, Alabama

Willis H. Williams, M.D.
Associate Professor of Surgery (Thoracic)
Emory University School of Medicine
Atlanta, Georgia

William M. Wilson, M.A., Ph.D.
Program Director, Utah Medex
University of Utah College of Medicine
Salt Lake City, Utah

Mary G. Wiseman, P.A., M.T., R.T.
Medex
Melford Medical, Melford Valley Hospital
Melford, Utah

Lemuel G. Yerby, III, B.S., PA-C
Physician Assistant
Emory University Clinic
Atlanta, Georgia

Harold A. Zintel, M.D., D.Sc.
Director, Department of
  Special Educational Projects
American College of Surgeons
Chicago, Illinois

DEDICATION

To my wife Sherry and our children, Page and Penny
Reginald D. Carter

To my wife Alice and our children, Baker and Luke
Henry B. Perry

For their continuing love, patience, and understanding

And to the memory of
Ashutosh Roy, M.D. (1929–1983)

FOREWORD

This book is written by physicians, physician assistants, and health educators, administrators and policy makers for individuals who are interested in knowing more about physician assistants. Who is more qualified to discuss the education, employment, and role of the physician assistant than those involved daily in the process? Part one focuses on the development, education, and certification of physician assistants. In part two, physicians and physician assistants describe what it is like to practice together in a variety of settings. Current issues are discussed in part three.

We feel this book is urgently needed to draw attention to a concept that has proven to be correct; quality health care can be provided by well-trained assistants under the supervision of physicians. Physician assistants have received wide acceptance nationally and are now working in a variety of settings within both the private and public sectors of the health care industry. There is a need for new leaders who will be sensitive to the role potential of physician assistants and encourage the use of this manpower resource wisely and appropriately to extend health care services where they are most needed.

Originally, we planned to produce two volumes; one on primary care physician assistants, the other on surgical physician assistants. We soon realized, however, that the roles and issues are basically the same. Although most physician assistants are currently working in primary care practice, a growing trend is toward the use of physician assistants in other clinical specialties, especially surgery. This is why we have devoted an equal amount of time to surgery.

There has been and continues to be much controversy about the terms used to describe physician assistants. In earlier literature, an 's was attached to physician to denote the dependent role of the assistant. This no longer is being used by the American Medical Association or by the American Academy of Physician Assistants for graduates of primary care educational programs. However, the 's is still used by graduates of surgeon's assistant programs. Graduates of primary care educational programs who work for surgeons prefer to be called surgical physician assistants. We have tried to maintain the currently accepted terminology and hope that this will not cause too much confusion. We need to remember that a physician assistant is not an abstract concept; but a person devoted to helping others.

Physician assistants are changing the way that health care services are delivered. Change never occurs without fear and controversy. The traditional role of the physician is changing from the provider to the manager of health care services. Can we accept the changes that are taking place? Will we be able to make the transition and educate physicians and their assistants for new health roles? Hopefully, this book will inspire new ideas and ways to redefine health and its delivery.

PREFACE

It was 1966. As a relatively new Dean, I was gradually getting on top of things when Gene Stead dropped in to visit. He was frustrated by the chronic recurring annual shortage of nurses which caused the Duke Hospital to close down beds. He pointed out there were over 25,000 corpsmen discharged each year from the U.S. Armed Services; unlike U.S. Air Force pilots or mechanics they could not transpose their service career to civilian occupations. He was unclear as to exactly what role the former corpsmen could play in Duke Hospital but he was asking permission to sign up three to five individuals whom he would train in a hand-tailored curriculum. He was not seeking to replace hospital nurses; in fact he wanted to avoid the label "nurse" since he would be dealing with men as well as women. He suggested the term "physician's assistant." He was anxious to have me "protect his flanks" from external health professional guilds. He did not want any funding; from his position as Chairman of the Department of Medicine he could attract external resources for a pilot program. I promised my non-monetary support.

Starting small and developing a curriculum almost on a weekly basis, (like a modern TV soap-opera), the impending success of the program was evident. When 1967 rolled around, Gene was planning to relinquish the Chairmanship of the Department of Medicine. He requested that the responsibility from the operation of the program be shifted to the newly created Department of Community Health Sciences and its Chairman, Dr. E. Harvey Estes. Harvey accepted the challenge and gradually built up the program to its present high quality and size.

The Physician Assistant model was copied very quickly by other institutions in the country. Other types of Assistant Programs emerged; some thrived and continue to provide manpower to health services while others have been discontinued.

From the beginning a key feature was that the Physician Assistant would function under supervision of the licensed physician and not as an independent health professional.

What about the future of Physician Assistants as we face a surplus of physicians in the 1990's? My opinion is that we will be producing fewer graduates, but the quality of the programs will continue to improve. The jobs most likely to disappear from the employment opportunities of Physician Assistants are situations in which the PA functioned as an M.D. substitute in an area of physician shortage. The jobs which will continue to do well are those which are truly Assistants to a Physician where the individual performs under the direct supervision of the physician performing routine and regular tasks that do not require four years of medical school and four to eight years of Residency Training. I continue to be highly optimistic about the future role of Physician Assistants as members of the health care team.

W.G. ANLYAN, M.D.
Vice President for Health Affairs
Duke University Medical Center

ACKNOWLEDGMENTS

There are many people involved in the preparation of this book. We would like to express our appreciation to the following people: Dr. E. Harvey Estes, Jr., chairman of the Department of Community and Family Medicine, and Dr. Michael A. Hamilton, director of the Duke Physician Assistant program, for their encouragement and words of wisdom. We owe much to each chapter author for sharing their knowledge and for meeting our deadlines and putting up with our editorial changes. Thank you seems hardly adequate to express our appreciation to Mr. Ed Pope and Ms. Peggy Ray for proofing manuscripts and to Ms. Carolyn Bunn for typing and making revisions. Most of all, we appreciate the efforts of those who have devoted so much to the growth and development of the physician assistant profession.

Reginald D. Carter
Henry B. Perry

CONTENTS

ALTERNATIVES IN
HEALTH CARE DELIVERY:
EMERGING ROLES
FOR PHYSICIAN ASSISTANTS

PART ONE

AN INTRODUCTION TO THE PHYSICIAN ASSISTANT PROFESSION

Chapter 1

THE DEVELOPMENT
OF THE PHYSICIAN ASSISTANT CONCEPT

JAMES F. GIFFORD, JR., Ph.D.

INTRODUCTION

"Physician Assistant" defines a clinically trained professional capable of expanding the services offered to patients by physicians in both primary care and hospital settings. The *origins* of this concept lie in perennial problems of physician supply, medical education and cost of care that have characterized health care delivery in twentieth century America. The *definition* of the concept came between 1965 and 1971 when these problems interacted with the concern for social justice that emerged in the 1960s and with an anticipated crisis in the availability of clinically trained personnel. During this period, a variety of schools and institutions developed programs for the training of physician assistants and, through conferences on common problems and goals, combined their several programs into a movement. The concept was *institutionalized* between 1971 and 1974 when the federal government assumed significant responsibility for funding programs, when graduate physician assistants began to enter the labor force in numbers and when organizations were established to safeguard the standards and promote the future interests of the physician assistant role. The *maturation* of the concept since 1974, when the number of training programs first reached its current level, has seen nationwide acceptance of the roles of the new health professional, expansion of service possibilities for physician assistants and new challenges to the physician assistant movement in the form of reduction, pointing toward elimination, of federal support for training and of difficulty in qualifying the physician assistant within financial reimbursement plans.

ORIGINS

The major trends that shaped the concept of the physician assistant developed gradually in America in the decades prior to 1960. Throughout this century, Americans placed an increasingly higher value on health care, correspondingly increasing demand for services. From the 1920s on, the cost of these services became a matter of national debate. Simultaneously, concern grew that many persons and groups had inadequate access to care because physicians were maldistributed both geographically and in terms of the ratio of specialists to generalists.

In the early 1960s, these general trends combined with new circumstances to produce a crisis. Many Americans came to view adequate care as a right and to insist that such disadvantaged groups as the poor, women, minorities and the elderly be guaranteed appropriate access to the health care marketplace. At the same time, a combination of heavy demands in practice and the expansion of biomedical knowledge made the continuing education needed by physicians harder and harder to schedule. With national surveys projecting a shortage of physicians just as health care facilities and entitlements were expanding, a critical shortage of clinically trained personnel loomed.

In 1961, Dr. Charles L. Hudson, speaking to an American Medical Association conference on medical education, began the process of differentiating the concept of the physician assistant from the more general category of the physician extender. Extenders such as the nurse-midwife in America and the *Feldsher* in Russia were commonly known. He proposed that persons with no previous medical education be prepared to perform such clinical tasks as suturing, intubation and lumbar puncture, thus freeing physicians for more complex tasks or for contact with additional patients. His "assistants to doctors" were to be drawn from the ranks of the medically untrained because of opposition to redefinition of the role of the persons most obviously available for such duties; nurses. As Hudson envisioned it, the assistant would work solely under the supervision of the doctor and not as an independent practitioner (1).

Hudson's proposal received intellectual assent but was nowhere taken up for immediate implementation. In 1965, Dr. Henry Silver and Loretta Ford, R.N., did establish a program at the University of Colorado which trained baccalaureate nurses for clinical functions in child care stations serving impoverished areas. Their program later became the basis both for the nurse practitioner movement and for the Child Health Associate Program which now is a part of the PA movement. Their program depended, however, on a pattern of close cooperation between doctors and nurses not then often found at other schools (2). In 1965, therefore, practical definition of the physician assistant concept awaited establishment of a training program in local circumstances characteristic of more than one institution.

DEFINITION

The Duke University Medical Center developed the program that first gave

formal definition to the physician assistant concept, admitting a first class of
four students, all ex-Navy corpsmen, in the fall of 1965. The local circumstances leading to its establishment included:

1. A charter obligation imposed by James B. Duke, benefactor of the university, that its medical school and hospital contribute directly to the
   improvement of health care throughout the Carolinas, a dominantly
   rural area,
2. Inability of area physicians to avail themselves of continuing education
   programs because of the pressures of practice,
3. Discussions of the problems of health care delivery that accompanied
   implementation of a new medical curriculum in the Duke University
   School of Medicine,
4. Chronic shortages of trained clinical personnel in the Duke Hospital,
5. Limited experience with training firemen, ex-corpsmen and others in
   attempts to meet these shortages, and
6. Awareness of at least one instance in which a local practitioner had successfully trained a young employee to serve as his assistant in office
   practice.

As chairman of Duke's department of medicine, Dr. Eugene A. Stead, Jr.
was simultaneously aware of all of these circumstances. He first attempted to
address them by designing a master's-level clinically oriented program for
nurses, but failed in three attempts to win accreditation for this effort from the
National League for Nursing. As an alternative, he began to consider training
from military service and from other groups outside the nursing profession. As
a member of the study section of the National Heart Institute, he had discussed his ideas informally with its membership. When Dr. Herbert Saltzman
submitted from Duke a request for support for projects in hyperbaric medicine
that included training funds for technicians to assist physicians involved in
these projects, he and Stead agreed to include also a request for funds to train
a more general type of physician assistant. When, in April, 1965, this grant
was approved, the concept of the physician assistant took on a formal definition for the first time.

The Duke curriculum projected the physician assistant as an allied health
professional rather than as an expanded technician. It included nine months
of basic science courses and fifteen months of clinical training. In recognition
of the fact that each graduate would enter a unique set of practice circumstances, it placed emphasis on habits necessary for lifelong learning and post-
poned modifications of the single curriculum track. In preparing for the
program, the Duke faculty sought a ruling from the office of the Attorney
General of North Carolina as to the place of the physician assistant under the
state's Medical Practice Act. The Attorney General ruled that a physician
could assign a broad range of duties to an assistant, but that no independent

authority attached to the role of the physician assistant. This dependent definition has ever since characterized the concept of the physician assistant (3).

Between 1965 and 1971, programs similar to the type established at Duke opened at Bowman Gray School of Medicine and at Oklahoma, Yale, Alabama, George Washington, Emory and Johns Hopkins universities. Other schools and agencies started programs with unique features which broadened the PA concept. Among these:

1. Federal agencies such as the Public Health Service, the Bureau of Prisons, the Department of Defense and the Indian Health Service expanded programs for training adjunct medical personnel to begin training physician assistants to serve their specialized constituencies.

2. The Department of Surgery at the University of Alabama introduced the first specialty physician assistant program in 1967, emphasizing training in general surgery and a variety of surgical subspecialties as preparation for careers in surgically underserved areas of the state.

3. Alderson-Broaddus College in 1968 combined liberal arts education and physician assistant training in the first four year degree program, a pattern soon followed by Northeastern University in Boston and Mercy College in Detroit.

4. In 1969, Dr. Richard Smith at the University of Washington School of Medicine introduced the Medical Extension (MEDEX) Program, featuring a curriculum of three months of classroom instruction followed by twelve months of apprenticeship under the supervision of a physician who presumably would employ the student upon completion of his training. By 1971 five additional Medex programs opened in Los Angeles, Birmingham, Salt Lake City, Hanover, New Hampshire and Grand Forks, North Dakota.

5. Also in 1969, the University of Colorado established its Child Health Associates Program. Admission required two years of college work but not, necessarily, previous medical training. Three years of training prepared graduates for diagnosis, counseling and prescription of medications for children. Students earned a bachelor's degree after the first two years of the program: beginning in the mid-1970s they could also take a master's degree by completing graduate school requirements. Colorado was the first PA program to offer a graduate degree (4).

Transition from the definition stage to the expansion stage of development of the physician assistant movement was made through a series of conferences at Duke University at which faculty and students discussed common goals, emerging issues, curricula and means of establishing the role of the physician assistant nationwide. The first conference, in March of 1968, established mechanisms for communication among the programs, approved the idea that the physician assistant should work under the license of a physician and led to a successful application to the Department of Health, Education and Welfare for funds to draft model legislation governing PA practice. With $35,389 from this source, a series of meetings led by Martha D. Ballenger, J.D., produced draft legislation that significantly influenced the development of laws enacted in the states. The second conference suggested guidelines for the employment of physician assistants in patient care settings, projected how physician assistants would be accepted within the health care system and first began to involve federal officials in planning for the future development of physician assistants. The third conference, in November of 1970, began the task of formally defining national educational and certification standards and included, by invitation, delegates from many of the major health care organizations in the country.

By the time of the fourth conference in April 1972, the definition of the physician assistant concept essentially was complete. At this conference, delegates studied the first significant feedback from physicians who employed physician assistants in their practices. The various training models were examined in detail and programs freely borrowed successful methods from each other. Seed grants from foundations and federal agencies confirmed that the careful process of gradually involving outside professionals in the development of the physician assistant concept had brought widespread acceptance of the new professional in the medical community (5). Only the legal status of the physician assistant remained somewhat unsettled. Some states provided that physician assistants practiced under general authority delegated to physicians under medical practice acts. Others passed enabling legislation specifying that the practice of physician assistants be regulated by the model legislation drafted at the Duke Conferences. By 1972, seven states enacted general delegatory statutes and seventeen passed regulatory statutes. The remaining states had yet to act.

INSTITUTIONALIZATION

Between 1971 and 1974, the availability of federal funding led to a rapid expansion of the number of training programs for physician assistants and the concept itself was incorporated into organizations for certification of individuals, developing and evaluating educational programs, accrediting these programs and focusing the attention of physician assistants on the expansion and development of their professional opportunities. Prior to 1971, funding for those programs not sponsored by government agencies came almost entirely from local resources and seed grants from the Josiah Macy, Jr., Carnegie and Rockefeller foundations and the Commonwealth Fund. In 1967, the National Advisory Council on Health Manpower recommended that the federal government give high priority to university-based experiments in the training of new types of health professionals. By 1971, when the Comprehensive Health Man-power Act provided significant appropriations for this purpose, such agencies as the Office of Economic Opportunity, the Veterans Administration, the Department of Labor, the Department of Defense and the U.S. Public Health Service already were interested in the physician assistant concept (6). With the new funds available the number of training programs rose from 26 in 1972 to 53 in 1974, a level that since has remained essentially constant.

Expansion, however, was but one evidence of the institutionalization of the physician assistant concept. As noted above, one result of the first Duke con-ference was to base the work of the physician assistant on the license of the supervising physician. Accordingly, some means was necessary for certifying the accomplishments of program graduates to prospective employers. In June of 1970, three programs (Duke, Bowman Gray, University of Texas at Galves-ton) banded together to form the American Registry of Physician's Associates. Its original purpose was to test the competence of physician assistants through voluntary examinations and to certify the results. The first examinations were given in 1972 to graduates of eight programs. The next year the testing func-tion was assumed by the National Board of Medical Examiners and its prestige, coupled with the increasing number of graduates from training pro-grams, attracted 880 candidates to its first sitting in December, 1973 (7). Certification by examination remains a cardinal feature of the physician assis-tant movement.

Also a product of the Registry apparatus was the Association of Physician Assistant Programs. Organized in 1972, its national offices opened in Wash-ington, D.C. in 1974 to serve physician assistants training programs much as the Association of American Medical Colleges serves schools of medicine. Its functions include facilitating curriculum development and exchange of infor-mation among programs, preevaluation of programs, promoting continuing education and sharpening the definition and image of the physician assistant both with the profession and before the public (8).

Efforts to develop means of accreditation of training programs antedated formation of the Association. In 1968, Dr. E. Harvey Estes, Jr. and Dr. Robert Howard of the Duke program first approached the American Medical Associ-ation with a request that it develop educational guidelines for the physician as-sistant movement. Although survey results indicated widespread support for the use of physician assistants and nurse practitioners, the A.M.A. took no im-mediate action, preferring to move slowly in developing guidelines for evaluat-ing all types of new health professionals. Estes and Howard were concerned, however, that acceptance of the physician assistants trained without adequate guidelines would be difficult. They next presented the problem to the Board of Medicine of the National Academy of Sciences. The Academy named a panel of seven persons, including four associated either with Duke or the Duke conferences, to study the need for the physician assistant. Noting the favorable response of physicians to the physician associate and nurse practitioner concepts, the academy recommended in 1970 that the American Medical Association, the Association of American Medical Colleges and appropriate government agencies cooperate in developing standards for physician assistants (9). Embodied as "Essentials for the Educational Program for the Assistant to the Primary Care Physician," these standards were adopted by the American Medical Association House of Delegates in 1971. Site visits and program approvals began in 1972 and in 1974 the Joint Review Committee was named by the U.S. Office of Education as the official accrediting agency for physician assistant programs (10).

The remaining step in institutionalization was establishment of a professional organization for physician assistants themselves. First efforts in this direction came from the desire of students to have a say in determining the shape of their education. In 1968, students from Duke first began to publish a student newsletter and to incorporate an organization under the laws of North Carolina. The Duke students soon were joined by students from Emory, Alderson-Broaddus, Oklahoma and, as the number of programs increased after 1971, other programs as well. In 1971, their organization, the Academy of Physician Assistants, began publication of a journal, *Physician's Associate,* to promote research and serve as a forum for the business of the movement. The Academy also enabled physician assistants to contribute to the process of establishing national standards for accreditation and certification and to participate in efforts to pass practice-enabling legislation in the several states. The Academy promoted efforts to develop continuing education programs which, since 1973, have been prerequisites for Academy membership, and also offered members an employment listing service, newsletters, the journal and a lobbying arm to promote the general interests of physician assistants. Membership now is offered to students and graduates of physician assistant, MEDEX, child health associate, surgical assistant and pediatric nurse practitioner programs.

MATURATION

In August of 1974, fourteen organizations cooperated to establish the National Commission on Certification of Physician Assistants. The Commission sets criteria of eligibility for certification of candidates, sets and administers the examination, issues certificates and advises the National Board of Medical Examiners on adoption of national certification standards. Formation of the Commission was itself a verification that the concept of the physician assistant had matured and that the number of assistants nationwide had reached the "critical mass" necessary for survival. Since 1974, the intellectual content of the concept has not changed appreciably, nor have the institutions supporting it. Change has come internally, from the characteristics of applicants to programs to the variety of settings in which graduates practice, and in interesting ways the questions that challenged the concept initially, questions of financial support and professional acceptance, have returned in new forms to challenge the mature movement.

In the 1960s, physician assistant students were overwhelmingly male, a reflection of the availability of a pool of ex-military corpsmen, the rejection of the physician assistant concept by the organized nursing profession and, perhaps, a measure of bias toward the assumption that women were less likely, over the long run, to remain in practice. Today, almost 40 per cent of physician assistants are women and in the most recent years the percentage of female graduates is above 50. The percentage of ex-corpsmen in the most recent (1981) entering class was less than one third, with stable percentages also of persons from nursing and technical backgrounds, an increasing percentage with experience in a variety of other health fields and a smaller but increasing percentage of students with no health care background. Two thirds of 1981-82 graduates completed at least four years of education beyond high school prior to beginning physician assistant training: the corresponding percentage of graduates with no college preparation is less than ten. The increased attractiveness of the physician assistant concept to a wider variety of more highly qualified candidates marks the maturity of the concept.

The original concept projected the physician assistant serving most frequently as the assistant to the primary care physician, less often in specialty practice. Since 1978 the percentage of physician assistants in primary care settings has remained essentially constant at approximately 74% as has the percentage involved in family practice, approximately 53%. Perhaps reflecting the early involvement of surgery in the physician assistant movement, there have always been more physician assistants practicing in surgical specialties than in medical subspecialties outside primary care. The number of those involved in surgical practice continues to increase, however, while the number and the percentage of those involved in medical subspecialty practice is declining. Over the same period, the percentage of physician assistants serving in solo practice or private group practice settings declined significantly, while the percentage of assistants practicing in institutional settings rose appreciably (11).

These two sets of trends bear directly on the triad of external challenges currently facing the physician assistant movement. The concept of the physician assistant originated in significant part as a partial answer to an anticipated shortage of physicians, particularly in primary care areas. Today, a surplus of physicians is projected and the same federal appropriations process that secured the financial footing of the physician assistant movement also has helped to increase the number of physicians in family practice and other primary care specialties. The number of practice opportunities for physician assistants in the areas of service they have already entered may well be decreasing both absolutely and relative to the number of graduates. There will apparently be a need in the years immediately ahead to open new types of practice settings to physician assistants.

The vitality of the original definition of the physician assistant concept was the product of sharing among many institutions, each of which developed its training model to meet local circumstances. Where some schools aimed at production of generalists whose competencies could be channeled to specific needs at the practice site, others sought to train students for specialty practice or service to a specific constituency. Given the need to expand the variety of settings in which the physician assistants practice, the years immediately ahead may well require a similar variety of special emphases within training programs. The challenge to the movement once again will be to increase vitality by incorporating diversity.

The third challenge is fiscal. Where the originators of the physician assistant concept fought for inclusion in practice-enabling legislation, their heirs now must fight for inclusion of physician assistants within physician reimbursement schemes. Simultaneously, training programs must cope with the loss of federal dollars which is the product both of a strained economy and of the maturity of the physician assistant concept itself. Training fund grants always were predicated on the expectation that success of the physician assistant concept would make its institutions self-supporting. What were not foreseen were the stringent economic circumstances in which success would emerge.

Obviously, these challenges are interactive, and the relationship among them cannot be predicted with precision, even over the short run. Planning for the future, therefore, must begin with a look at the accumulated experience of those physician assistants already in practice and the derivation of whatever generalizations and suggestions flow readily from that experience. The remaining chapters of this book are intended to that purpose.

REFERENCES

1. Hudson, E.: Expansion of Medical Professional Services with Nonprofessional Personnel. *JAMA, 176:*95-97, 1961.
2. Silver, H., and L. Ford: The Pediatric Nurse Practitioner at Colorado. *Am. J. Nurs., 67*:1,443-1,444, 1967.

3. Estes, E.H.: The Duke Physician's Assistant Program. *Arch. Environ. Health, 17*:690-91, 1968. Stead, E.A.: Conserving Costly Talents—Providing Physicians' New Assistants. *JAMA, 198*(10): 182-83, December 5, 1966. Stead, E.A.: The Duke Plan For Physician Assistants. *Med. Times, 95*:40-48, 1967.

4. Carter, R. and J. Gifford: The Emergence of the Physician Assistant Profession. In Perry, H. & B. Breitner: *Physician Assistants.* New York, Human Sciences Press, 1982.

5. Documents pertaining to these conferences are among the papers of the Department of Community Health Sciences, Duke University, Durham, North Carolina.

6. U.S. Department of Health, Education and Welfare: Health Resources Administration. Final Report of the Physician Extender Work Group., October, 1975.

7. Glazer, D.: National Commission on Certification of Physician's Assistants: A Precedent in Collaboration. In: *The New Health Professionals,* A. Bliss and E. Cohen (eds.). Germantown, MD., Aspen System Corporation, 1977.

8. Association of Physician Assistant Programs: National Health Practitioner Program Profile 1979-80. Arlington, VA., 1978.

9. Interview with E. Harvey Estes, M.D., September, 1979.

10. Detmer, L.M.: The American Medical Association Council on Medical Education Accreditation Program for the Education of Assistants to the Primary Care Physicians. *Phys. Assoc., 3*:4-8, 1973.

11. Carter, R.D. *et al.*: Preliminary Report: 1981 National Physician Assistant Survey. Draft report cited by permission of author.

Chapter 2

THE PHYSICIAN ASSISTANT'S CONTRIBUTION TO THE DELIVERY OF HEALTH SERVICES

HENRY B. PERRY, M.D., Ph.D.

INTRODUCTION

It has been fifteen years now since the first physician assistant program was established at Duke University under the leadership of Dr. Eugene Stead. During this period there has been a remarkable growth in utilization of these new health professionals in the provision of health care. There has also developed, during this same period, a substantial body of research documenting their effectiveness. In this chapter, we will describe the findings from studies of quality of patient care provided by physician assistants, their productivity and impact on costs, and comparisons with nurse practitioners.

QUALITY OF CARE

A number of studies have assessed the *process* of medical care provided by physician assistants. Direct observation of physician assistants and comparison with physicians yielded no discernable difference between the two groups in diagnostic or therapeutic appropriateness scores (Duttera and Harlan, 1978). Chart reviews have also produced similar findings (System Sciences, 1978), but in one study, physician assistants ordered laboratory tests and prescribed treatments more appropriately in many situations than did physicians (Kane et al., 1976).

Assessments of the clinical performance of physician assistants by supervising physicians have all been quite favorable (System Sciences, 1978; Crovitz et al, 1973; Perry 1977). In one recent national survey of 165 chairmen of departments of surgery in which physician assistants were working, 60% felt that the quality of surgical patient care had improved as a result of the introduction of physician assistants (Perry et al., 1981).

Several studies have compared medical outcomes among comparable ambulatory patients treated either by physician assistants or by physicians. Measures of symptomatic improvement and return to prior functional status were identical for the two provider groups (Kane *et al.*, 1976; Tomkins *et al.*, 1977), except in one small study where the outcomes obtained by physician assistants were superior (Wright *et al.*, 1977). In reviewing their research on quality of care provided by physician assistants and nurse practitioners, Sox concluded that "the major recent development in primary care may be the discovery that appropriately trained non-physicians can do much of the physician's work with apparent safety and patient satisfaction" (Sox, 1979).

PRODUCTIVITY

A number of studies have assessed the productivity of physician assistants in a variety of primary care settings (System Sciences, 1978; Nelson *et al.*, 1975; Miles and Rushing, 1976; Record, 1976; Scheffler, 1977; Scheffler, 1979). These studies indicate that adding one physician assistant to an ambulatory practice setting is equivalent to adding from 0.37 and 0.76 physicians. Scheffler's estimate that physician assistants are 63% as productive as physicians appears to be a good "middle of the road" estimate and is based upon a larger sample size than the other estimates. These productivity gains are due to physician assistants performing more routine, time consuming tasks, managing uncomplicated patients, and assisting in the care of ambulatory patients with more complex problems. There have been concerns that supervising physicians could employ physician assistants primarily to obtain more time off for themselves rather than expand the total volume of patient care services. The available evidence cited above, however, indicates that this is not the case. Record *et al.* (1981) have estimated that up to 75% of the total office visits in primary care and up to 90% of the total office visits in pediatrics are safely delegable to new health practitioners.

IMPACT ON COSTS

The impact of physician assistants on health care costs is a complex one. With respect to private practice settings, it is customary to charge the same fee for the service whether it is given by the physician assistant or the supervising physician. The reason for this is that the level of quality is assumed to be identical and the supervising physician retains medical and legal responsibility for the activities of his assistant. There is some suggestive evidence, however, that the standard office fee in practices using physician assistants is lower than in other practice settings (System Sciences, 1978).

In private practice settings, the cost savings resulting from physician assistant utilization are retained by the supervising physicians. In one study of twelve practice settings, the net profitability of employing a physician assistant was between $8,000 and $14,000 annually, depending on the computational method used (Nelson *et al.*, 1975). In prepaid practice settings, however, such savings are theoretically returned to the consumer in the form of lower rates. In one such setting (the Kaiser-Permanente Program in Portland, Oregon), each physician assistant generated a net savings for the organization of $10,783 per year in comparison to the estimated costs if the same services had been provided by physicians alone (Record, 1976).

It is estimated that the total cost of training a physician assistant is only 20% of that required to train a physician (exclusive of the cost of post graduate physician residency training). Although the federal government's support of physician assistant training amounts to less than 10% of its support for basic medical education, its per capita average contribution to the education of each physician assistant is greater than that for each medical student (Congressional Budget Office, 1979). Schweitzer (1981) has estimated that the training cost for physicians (including opportunity costs) is $112,800 more than that for physician assistants.

There is some evidence that physician assistants tend to be relatively conservative in their medical decision-making and, as a consequence, generate greater costs for laboratory and diagnostic testing than do physicians (Olsen *et al.*, 1978; Kane *et al.*, 1976). Furthermore, some studies have found that prescription costs and rates of hospitalization are greater following physician assistant utilization (Miles and Rushing, 1976; Wright *et al.*, 1977). Whether these findings reflect inappropriately low use of medical resources by physicians beforehand or unnecessary caution on the part of physician assistants cannot be determined from the data. The use of protocols by physician assistants for specific commonly encountered conditions has been shown to be effective in keeping the ancillary costs of diagnosis and treatment at a minimum (Greenfield *et al.*, 1978).

It has been estimated that the hourly cost of employing a physician assistant is approximately one-third to one-half of employing a physician (Congressional Budget Office, 1979). If one assumes that a patient visit generates the same revenue regardless of the provider and that physician assistants see 60% as many patients as the supervising physician, then there is a net savings of between 10% and 30% for each hour of physician assistant utilization. After adding some additional costs associated with greater use of laboratory and diagnostic studies by physician assistants, one can see that the cost savings of physician assistant employment may be modest.

Record (1981) has taken a different approach and examined the potential cost savings of substitution of new health practitioners for physicians in primary care. If full delegation of office visits are assumed (i.e., 75% of adult office visits and 90% of pediatric office visits are provided by new health practitioners), 45% of the total provider costs of producing primary care outpatient visits could be saved. Certainly, in primary care settings in which all providers are employed and in which the ancillary costs of new health practitioners can readily be controlled, the potential cost savings of using physician assistants are quite substantial. These findings have their greatest implications for institutional providers of health services, including hospital-based primary care programs, HMO's, and government administered programs (e.g., the Indian Health Service and the Military).

COMPARISON WITH NURSE PRACTITIONERS

Nurse practitioners are more numerous than physician assistants (13,000 versus 10,000 in 1979), and there are approximately four times more training programs for nurse practitioners than for physician assistants (Congressional Budget Office, 1979; Henry, 1978). The average number of graduates per year is somewhat greater for nurse practitioners (2,000 versus 1,500 for physician assistants) as well (Congressional Budget Office, 1979). Although there is some variation in length and content among physician assistant training programs, this is much more marked among nurse practitioner programs, particularly among certificate programs. Nurse practitioner programs appear to place greater emphasis upon provider-patient communications, counseling, and role development while physician assistant programs emphasize basic medical sciences as well as surgical and emergency care skills to a greater degree (Institute of Medicine, 1978).

Nurse practitioners are more likely to be working in pediatrics and less likely to be working in family practice or surgery than are physician assistants. The number of pediatric nurse practitioner programs declined from 50 in 1974 to 40 in 1977, representing a drop from 38% to 22% of all nurse practitioner programs. Nevertheless, approximately 32% of all nurse practitioners are working primarily in pediatrics in comparison to less than 5% of physician assistants. One-quarter of nurse practitioners, in comparison to 40% of physician assistants, are working outside of Standard Metropolitan Statistical areas. Nurse practitioners are less likely than physician assistants to work in private practice settings but are more likely to work in school settings or in patients' homes. Nurse practitioners and physician assistants are equally as likely to work in hospital or in community-based clinic settings (Perry and Breitner, 1982a).

Rather important differences in productivity of nurse practitioners and physician assistants have been noted. On the average, physician assistants provide 8 to 10 more hours per week of direct patient care and see twice as many patients per day as do nurse practitioners (Systems Sciences, 1978; Henry, 1978). The exact reasons for these differences have not been determined, but they may be due in part to nurse practitioners spending more time to counsel patients about their medical and psychological needs. Some evidence indicates that physician assistants simply work longer hours than nurse practitioners (Perry and Redmond, 1980). Since physician assistants and nurse practitioners earn similar salaries, and since physician assistants appear to be more productive, they may be more cost-effective in the diagnosis and management of acute-limited illnesses. However, this is an area that needs further study.

A number of studies have found that the quality of primary patient care provided by nurse practitioners like that provided by physician assistants is indistinguishable from that provided by physicians (Sackett *et al.*, 1974; Spitzer *et al.*, 1974; Perrin and Goodman, 1978). One study has compared the performance of nurse practitioners and physician assistants in the management of three diseases—urinary tract infections, adult onset diabetes mellitus, and hypertension (System Sciences, 1978). On the basis of chart evaluations, nurse practitioners received statistically significant higher scores for three out of the six measures. For six performance ratings provided directly by supervising physicians, however, the scores for physician assistants were all significantly higher. Of particular note was the higher rating received by physician assistants in the area of "counseling/instructing patients."

Long-term follow-up data are not yet available, but it appears that approximately one-third to one-quarter of graduates of nurse practitioner training programs are no longer working as nurse practitioners in contrast to approximately 13% of graduates of physician assistant programs who are no longer working as physician assistants (Perry, 1983; Bliss, 1979).

One of the most critical issues facing the nurse practitioner movement is a noted drift away from utilizing physicians in the formal instruction of nurse practitioner programs. The trend toward reliance upon nurse practitioners to train other nurse practitioners will most certainly in the long run be detrimental to the quality of training provided.

CONCLUSION

The contributions to patient care made by the physician assistant profession during the first fifteen years of its existence have been quite remarkable. The concept that appropriately trained non-physicians can perform many aspects of patient care traditionally in the physician's realm just as well or better than physicians is gaining increasing acceptance on the basis of personal experience of physicians with physician assistants *and* on the basis of objective studies. The capability of physician assistants to provide primary care services has been well documented. Their contribution to the effectiveness of patient care for hospitalized patients will most certainly be demonstrated during the current decade.

In spite of the continued rapid growth of the physician assistant profession, it is still quite small relative to the medical profession which is approximately thirty times larger. Although currently there is no projected increase in the numbers of programs training physician assistants in the United States, the demand for physician assistants, particularly in the care of hospitalized patients, will probably continue to at least match the growth of the profession. The cost-effectiveness of physician assistants is most apparent in institutional settings and it can be expected that physician assistants will perform a more important role in these settings in the future. In view of the high quality of care provided by physician assistants with appropriate supervision and in view of the potential cost savings associated with their widespread utilization, a long-term manpower policy of gradually expanding their role in health care delivery and reducing the number of physicians would appear to be highly appropriate over the next two decades.

The physician assistant profession could never have reached its current status without the active support of the medical profession. The physician assistant has been a loyal member of the physician's team and has performed this role admirably. As the physician assistant profession matures, one might expect a somewhat more independent stance by physician assistants in the future. In any event, it appears that physician assistants are a very useful manpower resource in enhancing the effectiveness of patient care and increasing its availability. There is every reason to expect that the capable, enthusiastic, and dedicated individuals making up this new group of health professionals will continue this tradition.

REFERENCES

1. Bliss, A,: Critical Issues Confronting Nurse Practitioners. In Sultz. H., Henry, O.M., and Sullivan, J.A., eds.: *Nurse Practitioners USA*. Lexington, Massachusetts, Lexington Books, 1979.
2. Congressional Budget Office: *Physician Extenders: Their Current and Future Role in Medical Care Delivery*. Washington, Government Publishing Office, 1979.
3. Crovitz, E., Huse, M.M., and Lavis, D.E.: Field Ratings of Physician's Assistants. *Physician's Associate*, 19-21, 1973.
4. Duttera, M.J., and Harlan, W.R.: Evaluation of Physician Assistants in Rural Primary Care. *Archives of Internal Medicine*, 138:224-228, 1978.
5. Greenfield, S., Komaroff, A.L., Pas, T.M., Anderson, H., and Nessim, S.: Efficiency and Cost of Primary Care by Nurses and Physician Assistants. *New England Journal of Medicine*, 298:305-309, 1978.
6. Henry, O.M.: Recent Trends in Nurse Practitioner Preparation and Practice. Paper presented at American Public Health Association Annual Meeting, 1978.

7. Institute of Medicine: *A Manpower Policy for Primary Health Care.* Washington: National Academy of Sciences, 1978.
8. Kane, R.L., Olsen, D.M., and Castle, E.H.: Medex and Their Physician Preceptors—Quality of Care. *Journal of the American Medical Association, 236*:2509-2512, 1976.
9. Miles, D.L., and Rushing, W.A.: A Study of Physician's Assistants in a Rural Setting. *Medical Care, 14*:987-995, 1976.
10. Nelson, E.C., Jacobs, A.R., Cordner, K., and Johnson, K.G.: Financial Impact of Physician Assistants on Medical Practice. *New England Journal of Medicine, 293*:527-530, 1975.
11. Olsen, D.M., Kane, R.L., Manson, J., and Newman, J.: Measuring Impact of Medex Using Third-Party Payer Claims. *Inquiry,* 15:160-165, 1978.
12. Perrin, E.C., and Goodman, H.C.: Telephone Management of Acute Pediatric Illnesses. *New England Journal of Medicine, 298*:130-138, 1978.
13. Perry, H.B.: An Analysis of the Professional Performance of Physician's Assistants. *Journal of Medical Education, 52*:639-647, 1977.
14. Perry, H.B.: Career Trends Among Physician Assistants. *Physician Assistant* (in press, 1983).
15. Perry, H.B., and Breitner, B.: The Physician Assistant and the Nurse Practitioner. In: *Physician Assistants: Their Contribution to Health Care.* New York, Human Sciences Press, 96-127, 1982. Perry, H.B., Detmer, D.E., and Redmond, E.L.: The Current and Future Role of Surgical Physician Assistants. *Annals of Surgery, 193*:132-137, 1981.
16. Perry, H.B., and Redmond, E.: New Health Practitioners in Maine: An Assessment of Their Current Role. *Journal of the Maine Medical Association, 71*:208-214, 1980.
17. Record, J.C.: *Cost Effectiveness of Physician's Assistants.* Bethesda, Maryland, Bureau of Health Manpower Contract No 1-MB-44173(P), 1976.
18. Record, J.C.: The Findings and Policy Implications. In: Record, J.C. (eds.) *Staffing Primary Care in 1990: Physician Replacement and Cost Savings.* New York, Springer Publishing Company, 131-153, 1981.
19. Record, J.C., Bloomquist, R.M., and McCabe, M.A.: Delegation in Adult Primary Care: The Generalizability of HMO Data. In: Record, J.C. (ed.) *Staffing Primary Care in 1980; Physician Replacement and Cost Savings.* New York, Springer Publishing Company, 68-84, 1981.
20. Sackett, D.L., Gent, M., Hay, W.I., Vandervlist, I., Chambers, L., and Macpherson, A.: The Burlington Randomized Trial of the Nurse Practitioner: Health Outcomes of Patients. *Annals of Internal Medicine, 80*:137-142, 1974.
21. Scheffler, R.M.: Supply and Demand for New Health Professionals: Physician Assistants and MEDEX. Bethesda, Maryland, Bureau of Health Manpower Contract No. 1-MB-44184, 1977.
22. Scheffler, R.M.: The Productivity of New Health Practitioners: Physician Assistants and Medex. In Scheffler, R.M. (ed.): *Research in Health Economics.* Greenwich, Connecticut, JAI Press, 37-56, 1979.
23. Schweitzer, S.O: The Relative Costs of Physicians and New Health Practitioners. In: Record, J.C. (ed.): *Staffing Primary Care in 1990: Physician's Replacement and Cost Savings.* New York, Springer Publishing Company, 53-67, 1981.
24. Sox, H.C.: Quality of Patient Care by Nurse Practitioners and Physician Assistants. A ten-Year Perspective. *Annals of Internal Medicine, 91*:459-468, 1979.
25. Spitzer, W.O. Sackett, D.L., Sibley, J.C., Roberts, R.S., Gent, M., Kergin, D.J., Hackett, B.C., and Olynich, A.: The Burlington Randomized Trial of the Nurse Practitioner. *New England Journal of Medicine, 290*:251-256, 1974.
26. Systems Sciences, Inc.: *Survey of Evaluation of the Physician Extender Reimbursement Program.* Bethesda, Maryland, DHEW Contract No. SSA-600-76-0167, 1978.
27. Tomkins, R.K., Wood, R.W., Wolcott, B.W., and Walsh, B.T.: The Effectiveness and Cost of Acute Respiratory Illness Medical Care Provided by Physicians and Algorhythm-Assisted Physician's Assistants. *Medical Care, 15*:991-1003, 1977.

28. Wright, D.D., Kane, R.L., Snell, G.F., and Wooley, F.R.: Costs and Outcomes for Different Primary Care Providers. *Journal of the American Medical Association, 238*:46-50, 1977.

Chapter 3

A DESCRIPTION OF PROFESSIONALLY ACTIVE PHYSICIAN ASSISTANTS

REGINALD D. CARTER, Ph.D.
HENRY B. PERRY, M.D., Ph.D.

As of 1982, approximately 15,000 physician assistants have graduated from AMA approved programs or have been informally trained and subsequently obtained formal certification. Current estimates are that 15-20% of physician assistants are now involved in activities other than working as a physician assistant (1). Thus, we would estimate that 12,000-12,750 physician assistants are now actively employed as physician assistants.

Our most recent knowledge of the physician assistant profession is based on the results of a 1981 survey of the physician assistant profession conducted by the Association of Physician Assistant Programs (APAP) with support from the Robert Wood Johnson Foundation. APAP surveyed 10,700 of its graduates whose addresses were known. A 59% response was obtained, yielding 6,121 respondents. The findings of this 1981 survey are the most recent in a series of national physician assistant surveys conducted in 1978 (2), 1976 (3), and 1974 (4).

BACKGROUND CHARACTERISTICS

Thirty-six percent of physician assistants in 1981 were women. In contrast, in 1974, only 14% of physician assistants were women (4). The most commonly encountered health care background in 1981 was still the role of medical corpsman in the military (see Table 3.1). In 1974, a much higher percentage of physician assistants (55%) had worked previously as a medical corpsman (4). Only 8% of physician assistants in 1981 had never attended college prior to their training, and half had attained at least four years of college education (see Table 3.2). The prior academic preparation for physician assistants has been increasing steadily since the 1974 national survey when only 32% of physician assistants had completed four or more years of college or its equivalent (4).

TABLE 3.1

HEALTH CARE BACKGROUND OF PHYSICIAN ASSISTANTS, 1981

	Percentage (n = 6,121)
Corpsman	32.5
Technician/Technologist	18.4
Registered Nurse	12.1
Other health field	23.3
No health background	13.7
	100.0

TABLE 3.2

ACADEMIC BACKGROUND OF PHYSICIAN ASSISTANTS, 1981

Number of Years of College	*Percentage (n = 6,068)*
Four or more years	50.8
One to three years	40.9
No college	8.3
	100.0

PRACTICE CHARACTERISTICS

Of those currently active as physician assistants, 95% are involved primarily in patient care. The specialties of physician assistants are described in Table 3.3. Three quarters are working in primary care specialties, primarily family practice. General internal medicine, general pediatrics, emergency medicine, and obstetrics and gynecology account for the remainder of the primary care specialties. Medical subspecialties account for only 2.9% of active physician assistants while surgical specialties (13%) and other specialties (9.7%) account for the remainder. A notably greater percentage of women than men physician assistants are working in internal medicine, pediatrics, and obstetrics and gynecology.

The major practice settings of physician assistants are shown in Table 3.4. A major practice setting is defined as the one in which a physician assistant spends most of his or her time. Private practice settings (solo or group practice) are the major practice site for only a third of physician assistants. Almost one-third of physician assistants are working primarily in hospitals; one-quarter, in clinics; and almost 10%, in the military.

The regional distribution of physician assistants is essentially identical to that for the U.S. population. California had more physician assistants (513) than any other state, followed by New York with 483. Table 3.5 describes the size of communities where physician assistants are working. One-quarter are in communities of less than 10,000 persons, and just over a third are in communities of 250,000 or more persons.

TABLE 3.3
SPECIALTIES OF THE PHYSICIAN ASSISTANT PROFESSION, IN 1981

Primary Care Specialties	*Percentage* *(n = 4,496)*
Family Practice	53.5
General Internal Medicine	9.6
Emergency Medicine	4.6
General Pediatrics	3.7
Obstetrics and Gynecology	2.6
Subtotal	74.0
Medical Subspecialties	
Cardiology	1.1
Allergy	0.3
Dermatology	0.2
Endocrinology	0.1
Gastroenterology	0.3
Hematology	0.2
Pulmonary Medicine	0.4
Infectious Disease	0.1
Neurology	0.2
Subtotal	2.9
Surgical Specialties	
General Surgery	4.9
Orthopedic Surgery	3.2
Thoracic and Cardiovascular Surgery	2.6
Urology	0.8
Neurology	0.9
Plastic Surgery	0.4
Otolaryngology	0.4
Ophthalmology	0.2
Subtotal	13.4
Other Specialties	
Industrial and Occupational Medicine	3.2
Psychiatry	0.9
Public Health and Preventive Medicine	0.6
Physical Rehabilitation Medicine	0.1
Radiology	0.1
Anesthesiology	0.2
Other	4.6
Subtotal	9.7
Total	100.0

TABLE 3.4

MAJOR PRACTICE SETTINGS OF PHYSICIAN ASSISTANTS, 1981

	Percentage (n = 4,511)
Solo Practice	19.3
Group Practice	16.5
Hospital	29.9
Non-hospital Clinic	24.9
Military	9.4
	100.0

TABLE 3.5

SIZE OF COMMUNITIES IN WHICH PHYSICIAN ASSISTANTS WORK

Community Size	*Percentage (n = 4,381)*
Under 10,000 persons	26.3
10,000 to 50,000	18.5
50,000 to 250,000	16.4
250,000 and over	38.8
	100.0

TABLE 3.6

SALARIES FOR PHYSICIAN ASSISTANTS BY PRIMARY SPECIALTY, 1981

Primary Specialty	*Average Salary*	*Number*
Allergy	$21,555	9
Anesthesiology	23,516	6
Cardiology	23,260	35
Dermatology	21,563	8
Emergency Medicine	22,332	153
Endocrinology	22,000	2
Family Practice	21,845	1557
Gasteroenterology	21,444	9
Hematology	19,333	3
Industrial Medicine	25,088	65
Infectious Disease	27,000	2
Internal Medicine	21,733	321
Neurosurgery	21,973	31
Neurology	26,538	8
Obstetrics and Gynecology	17,949	73
Occupational Medicine	24,996	48
Ophthalmology	22,250	4
Orthopedic Surgery	22,341	111
Otolaryngology	21,000	11
Pediatrics	19,987	129
Physical Medicine	19,250	4
Plastic Surgery	20,515	13
Psychiatry	22,235	29
Public Health/Preventive Medicine	20,000	19
Pulmonary Medicine	18,833	12
Radiology	25,333	3
General Surgery	22,419	163
Thoracic Surgery	26,660	91
Urology	21,503	29

INCOME

The average income for civilian physician assistants working in patient care in 1981 was $22,179. The average income for each specialty and practice setting grouping are shown in Tables 3.6 and 3.7. Among those specialties with more than 10 physician assistants, the range is a low of $17,949 for obstetrics and gynecology to $26,660 for thoracic surgery. In practice settings, the range is from $19,457 for those working in community clinics to $25,409 for those working in industrial clinics.

TABLE 3.7

SALARIES FOR PHYSICIAN ASSISTANTS BY MAJOR PRACTICE SETTINGS, 1981

Practice Setting	*Average Salary*	*Number*
Solo Office	$22,383	633
Single-Specialty Group	22,511	342
Multi-Specialty Group	21,668	230
Health Maintenance Organization (HMO)	21,439	154
Industrial Setting	25,409	106
Community Clinic	19,457	204
Drug and Alcohol Abuse Clinic	20,132	19
Other Specialty Clinic	20,513	111
Non-profit Hospital	22,099	382
Proprietary Hospital	22,011	160
Veterans Administration Hospital	23,201	243
State-supported Hospital	20,378	71
City or County Hospital	22,017	177
Military Hospital	24,333	12
Nursing Home or Extended Care Facility	21,614	26
Federal Prison	21,119	37
City, County or State Prison	21,558	55
Other	20,531	80

TABLE 3.8

MEAN INCOME FOR CIVILIAN PHYSICIAN ASSISTANTS
INVOLVED IN PATIENT CARE BY YEARS OF EXPERIENCE SINCE GRADUATION

Number of years Since Graduation		*Average Income in 1981*
0-1	(n = 613)	$19,100
2-3	(n = 508)	21,700
4-5	(n = 964)	22,900
6-7	(n = 521)	24,800
8+	(n = 230)	24,041

The average income in 1981 for physician assistants increases from $19,100 for those in their first year of employment to $24,000 for those with more than five years of professional experience as a physician assistant. There does not appear to be any significant increment related to experience after five years of employment (see Table 3.8).

CONCLUSION

In relation to the overall panorama of health care delivery in the United States, the physician assistant profession still is hardly more than a speck on a large mural. There are, for instance, thirty times more physicians than physician assistants. Nevertheless, physician assistants are working in specialties and geographic settings where their unique contributions have been sought, especially in smaller communities and in primary care settings.

The physician assistant profession has been changing rapidly since its inception a decade and a half ago, and continuing change can be expected in the near future. Women, persons with college education prior to beginning physician assistant training, and persons with medical backgrounds other than as medical corpsmen are constituting an increasing percentage of the physician assistant profession.

Trends toward employment in institutional settings and less urban settings have been observed (1). What impact this will have in the long run remains to be seen. The major influences on the physician assistant profession will be brought about as a consensus gradually emerges over the next decade among health policy leaders concerning the potential contribution of physician assistants in improving health services and lowering their costs.

REFERENCES

1. Perry, H.B.: Career Trends Among Physician Assistants: A Cohort Analysis. *Physician Assistant,* (in press).
2. Perry, H.B., and D.W. Fisher: The Physician's Assistant Profession: Results of a 1978 Survey of Graduates. *Journal of Medical Education,* 56:839-845, 1981.
3. Fisher, D.W.: Physician Assistant: A Profile of the Profession. In: D.L. Hiestand and M. Ostow, eds.: *Health Manpower Information For Policy Guidance.* Cambridge, MA, Ballinger Publishing Company, 1976.
4. Perry, H.B.: Physician Assistants: An Overview of an Emerging Health Profession. *Medical Care,* 15:982-990, 1977.

Chapter 4

DEFINING PRIMARY CARE

E. HARVEY ESTES, JR., M.D.

Almost all health professionals claim to understand "primary care," a claim which is implicitly contradicted by the large number of published definitions of the term. Most organizations with an interest in this type of care have developed and published their own definition. Many experts have added to the list. Most feature similar descriptions and characteristics, but it is the subtle differences of emphasis and/or the omissions which provide evidence of some important differences of opinion.

Almost all would agree that the term refers to *personal* health and medical services, as opposed to community, environmental, or occupational health services, which are directed at *groups* of individuals. At the same time, primary care services provided to individuals must include an awareness of health risks faced by individuals as residents of a given community, or as employees in a specific work site.

The Citizen's Commission on Graduate Medical Education, in its influential 1966 report, The Graduate Education of Physicians (The Millis Report) (1), addressed the need for the training of a "primary physician," who would provide continuing comprehensive care for patients. This concept of a first contact or "prime contractor" role is central to most definitions of primary care, yet the provision of first contact care clearly is not enough. An emergency room or a minor emergency center would not qualify under most definitions.

Some definitions emphasize the breadth of services provided. For example, some family physician groups have expressed the opinion that a provider should include services to both sexes, and all age groups, from birth to old age, in order to qualify as a primary care provider. Pediatricians, geriatricians and obstetrician-gynecologists obviously disagree. At the other end of this spectrum, some limited health practitioners, such as nurses and dentists, have claimed membership in the primary care group.

In 1978, the Institute of Medicine of the National Academy of Sciences published a report, *A Manpower Policy for Primary Health Care* (2), which included a study of these and other aspects of the definition of primary care. This study included a detailed review of thirty-eight published definitions; and after carefully weighing them all, a new definition evolved, including a checklist, which can be used for evaluation of a given primary care provider site. This chapter draws heavily on this report.

The Institute of Medicine Report concluded that no single provider group and no single training sequence could claim exclusive rights to the provision of, or training for, primary care. There are many possible paths to the same end. There is also no mode or type of practice which can claim to be "best" for providing primary care. Solo physician practices, group multispecialty practices, and physician assistants and/or nurse practitioners working in areas remote from their physician supervisors have all demonstrated the capability to deliver primary care services meeting stringent standards.

At the same time, no single practitioner can provide good primary care services without the help of others. A key concept of the report is that good primary care services must include the responsibility for establishing a *system* of care, providing access to those services which cannot be provided by the primary care practitioner or primary care group.

The most important conclusion of the Institute of Medicine report is that primary care is a series of services, and that any practice unit which can provide this array of services can be classified as a primary care provider. However, the services must meet certain standards regarding their character, their scope and their degree of integration with each other. The array is extensive and formidable!

The first requirement is accessibility. Patients should be able to reach the practitioner or a member of the team at all hours. In addition, the physical access to care and the cost of the care should make it available to its potential patients. It is recognized that a given solo physician would be unable to provide the temporal coverage mandated by this requirement, but such physicians must provide a coverage arrangement, which is well known to the patients, and which will transmit relevant information back to the primary practitioner.

The second requirement is comprehensiveness of services. The primary care practice unit must be willing and able to handle the great majority of the health and illness problems arising within its patient population. The Institute of Medicine report found it acceptable for a primary care practice unit to limit its services to one age group (i.e., pediatrics), or to one sex (i.e., obstetrics and gynecology), but within that group, this unit must care for common acute illnesses, provide for preventive services, provide counseling regarding life style, and all the range of other services expected of the primary care physician.

It is this willingness to handle patient problems without prior screening, and to help the patient in the solution of all of these problems, either directly or by referral to other practitioners, that most clearly distinguishes the primary care practice unit from others.

The third requirement is coordination of services. The practice unit serves as the patient's interface with other needed practitioners, not only aiding in their selection, but in providing relevant information to these practitioners, and interpreting their advice and opinion back to the patient. In addition the primary care unit helps to coordinate the plan of care with the patient's life style, economic resources, and personal preferences.

The fourth requirement is the provision of continuity of care. It is clear that this cannot be achieved without the previous three requirements. An inaccessible practitioner forces the patient to use the emergency room, thus interfering with continuity. Unwillingness to treat commonly encountered problems forces the patient to utilize other practitioners, leading to the same result.

The creation of an organized, accurate, easily interpreted medical record is an essential tool in accomplishing continuity of care over time, particularly in practice settings in which a number of practitioners share the responsibility.

The fifth and final requirement is not unique to primary care, but is considered so important as to be specifically cited. The primary care practice unit must be accountable; for periodic review of the quality of the care given, for periodic review of the effectiveness and acceptability of its procedures and policies, and for review of the accuracy and appropriateness of information provided to its patients.

This accountability also extends to the community, in that the unit must work toward a safer and more secure community through public education, through prompt reporting of infectious diseases and public health hazards, and through appropriate collective action to achieve a better social and physical environment.

The Institute of Medicine report makes the above requirements explicit by providing a checklist which can be used to evaluate the degree to which a given clinical practice unit complies with these stringent standards. This checklist asks such questions as: "Can medically urgent cases be seen within one hour?", "Is the waiting time for most scheduled appointments less than one hour?" and, "Are the practitioners in the unit willing, if appropriate, to visit the patient at home?". The reader is referred to this report and to the checklist for more details.

Having considered the requirement for primary care, are there aspects of the definition which are of special interest to physician assistants? There are several elements which are not well performed in many primary care practices, and in which the physician assistant can be of great service, both to the practice unit and to its patients.

In providing "around the clock" accessibility, most office units rely on a telephone answering service, yet few office units periodically test the reliability of that service, or the quality and accuracy of its information. The physician assistant can perform such a service, and make appropriate recommendations for improvement.

Another opportunity lies in the design and preparation, or selection, of appropriate informational materials for patients. Through knowledge of the frequently asked questions from patients, and knowledge of sources of information on these topics, timesaving and educational handouts can be provided, not only about medical topics, but about office billing procedures, Medicare/ Medicaid coverage, and so forth.

In providing a comprehensive array of services, attention to preventive services is often weak. The physician assistant can assume the responsibility for designing and implementing a *system* for insuring that all who need such services are contacted and urged to receive them. Education in life style modification, such as smoking cessation and weight control, are also areas in which the physician assistant can be very helpful.

Another area of frequent failure in providing comprehensive services is in providing home services. Physician Assistants cannot only visit the patient in the home, but can also provide a written report of pertinent observations for the office chart, making all providers in the unit more aware of the patient's environment. Visits to nursing homes are also useful and frequently needed services which may be appropriate for physician assistants, though Medicare rules frequently make payment for such visits impossible.

In providing coordinated services, many practice units fail to adequately explain the opinions and recommendations of consultants to the patient and family. A physician assistant can provide a very useful service by securing such information from written reports, from conversations with the responsible primary care physician, from reading, and from conversations with the consultant; then contacting the patient and/or family and offering to share relevant information with them.

A major area of potential service in providing continuous care is in telephone followup after office visits for acute illness. A telephone call to the patient the morning after the visit will be both highly appreciated by the patient and very useful to the practitioner group.

Instruction of the patient in self-monitoring of signs and symptoms is another very useful and productive technique. Home blood pressure recordings provide useful information to the physician and patient and, at the same time, conserve both time and money.

The above are only a few examples of areas in which consideration of the *definition* of primary care can lead to more valuable and effective *services* by the physician assistant in behalf of the practice unit. The reader is urged to consider these and other activities in order to make each primary care unit truly deserving of its name.

REFERENCES

1. Millis, J.S. (Chairman): *The Graduate Education of Physicians.* Report of the Citizens Commission on Graduate Medical Education. Chicago, American Medical Association, 1966.
2. Estes, E.H. (Chairman): *A Manpower Policy for Primary Health Care.* Institute of Medicine, National Academy of Sciences, Washington, 1978.

Chapter 5

EDUCATING THE PRIMARY CARE PHYSICIAN ASSISTANT

ASHUTOSH ROY, M.D., Ph.D., MS.ED.

The first educational program to train physician assistants was established by Eugene Stead, M.D., at Duke University in 1965 (1). Dr. Stead was far ahead of his time in regard to the thinking process and the implementation needed to create this new type of professional who would fulfill not only a need but would also upgrade the quality of patient care and be cost-effective at the same time. The Pediatric Nurse Practitioner Program of the University of Colorado was also established in 1965 (2) and the MEDEX program at Seattle in 1969 (3). Naturally, in that decade and even now, some controversies remain as to the ideal educational program to train such important individuals. Since then to date over 50 educational programs have been developed in the United States with various titles including MEDEX, Child Health Associate, Community Health Medic, Family Nurse Practitioner, Physician Assistant, Physician Associate, and Primary Care Associate (4).

Much of the framework and reference for physician assistant educational programs was suggested by the American Medical Association's House of Delegates in December, 1971. The collaborators were the American Academy of Family Physicians, the American Academy of Pediatrics, the American College of Physicians, and the American Society of Internal Medicine. These organizations sponsored the Joint Review Committee on Educational Programs for the Assistant to the Primary Care Physician. The accreditation is now provided by the Committee on Allied Health Education and Accreditation (CAHEA) by the Joint Review Committee on Educational Programs for Physician Assistants under the auspices of the American Medical Association. The House of Delegates of the American Medical Association (AMA) gave the Council on Medical Education the authority to review and adopt "Essentials" on behalf of the AMA (5).

The Essentials were developed and adopted in 1971. They consist of policy statements, and as such constitute minimum standards of quality in educational programs that are recognized and accredited. *The Guidelines for Educational Program Preparing the Assistant to the Primary Care Physician* describes how the Essentials are interpreted, and illustrate their flexible nature, and also accommodates different approaches to the design and conduct of educational programs (6). In an article in 1975, L.M. Detmer states, "In the fall of 1973, the Council on Medical Education and the Joint Review Committee filed for recognition from the United States Office of Education, and in February 1974 received the maximum award of recognition for four years as the national accrediting agency for this type of education" (7). Currently, there is a listing available of the educational programs in the "National Health Practitioner Program Profile" compiled and published by the Association of Physician Assistant Programs (4).

There are subtle and necessary variations in curriculum design from program to program due to the educational needs, student characteristics, student experience in health related fields, and local demand for a particular type of finished product—a graduate. Nevertheless, typical physician assistant training is, on average, a two-year program. As adapted from the National Health Practitioner Program Profile (4), the didactic training usually consists of nine months and the subjects taught include anatomy, physiology, chemistry, and biochemistry, some medical terminology, human behavioral sciences, pharmacology, including clinical pharmacology, electrocardiography, radiology, clinical medicine, microbiology and pathology.

The clinical clerkships and preceptorship training is 15 months; it includes family practice, internal medicine, ambulatory medicine, emergency medicine, obstetrics/gynecology, pediatrics, general surgery, in-patient care, and psychiatry. It should be noted that not all of these disciplines are included within each program. The preceptorship, which may vary from 3 to 9 months of training, is generally carried out in a physician's office who is preferably either in primary care or family practice. The locations of these clinical training sites vary from a large hospital to a remote clinic in an under- served rural or an inner-city area. The organizational sites of these educational programs vary from medical schools, senior colleges and universities in affiliation with an accredited teaching hospital, to medical educational facilities of the federal government and to other institutions with clinical facilities, which are acceptable to the Council on Medical Education of the American Medical Association (6).

It may be observed that larger academic institutions, medical schools and medical centers have the potential of making significant contributions toward the didactic and clinical practicum of the educational programs. However, traditionally, primary care has not been a preferred focus of such medical educational centers until recently. Therefore, physician assistant programs have taken great care and responsibility to make sure of the importance of primary care focus in their own educational efforts. Smaller institutions in general also develop special educational programs to insure that the focus of training and education is in the area of primary care. Each program has a faculty which includes a program director who is "responsible for the organization, administration, periodic review, continued development and general effectiveness of the program" (6). In some programs, the program director has also assumed the function of the medical director. The medical director is responsible for the clinical instruction and developing relationships with other clinical programs. The medical director should be a physician, licensed in the state, experienced in delivery of primary health care, and who maintains a relationship with state medical associations and other practicing physicians.

A typical program faculty consists of a program director and a medical director, who are also responsible for administration. Some programs in addition will also have an assistant program director, a clinical coordinator, and other "core faculty" members to take part in administrative work. The instructional faculty are selected from the institutional faculty and also from the core program faculty. The program faculty are generally physician assistant graduates academically oriented and experienced in teaching, especially in primary care. The bulk of the clinical teaching is ideally conducted by practicing physicians. The clinical preceptorship, as mentioned before, is in the office of a practicing primary care or family practice physician. It is imperative that the entire teaching faculty be familiar with the role of a physician assistant. The core faculty usually consists of a number of physician assistant graduates, who also serve as role-models to the students. An Advisory Committee is appointed by each program to assist the program director in continuing program development, faculty coordination and administrative function, and also for future planning.

Evaluation is an integral and an important facet of every phase of each educational program. Although evaluation methods may vary, it is the main reference of a program for making curricular or administrative changes. As a matter of fact, self-analysis or self-evaluation for each program is mandatory for maintaining CAHEA accreditation. The accrediting body suggests that in establishing a curriculum, one should follow "a model unit of primary medical care such as the models used in departments of family practice in medical schools and in family practice residencies" (6).

An exemplary model unit of primary medical care could be adapted from the 1971 edition of a Guide for Residency Programs in Family Practice, published by the Residency Review Committee for Family Practice. Many of the programs have designed their curricula on the above basis and also have instituted joint team training with family practice residents, medical students opt-ing for family practice experience, and other allied health professionals. The accrediting body in the guidelines have also set up some basic direction on instructional methodologies. Appropriate instructional materials should be available to meet the student needs in several forms, e.g., classroom presentations, small group discussions, practical demonstrations, and supervised clinical demonstrations. Students are required to take examinations, tests, and quizzes related to didactic and clinical sessions of the educational program. Programs have the responsibility of setting up pass/fail scores and have academic review committees to assess student performance and to provide guidance and counselling to students who are in need.

The length of educational programs are variable, from as short as 12 months to as long as 48 months. The duration depends on the student's background, both clinical and didactic, abilities, maturity and the ability to function and perform the tasks as implied in the "Description of the Occupation" (6). It would be useful now to pick some items from Table 5.1, which need explanation or expansion for the benefit of the reader.

I. APPLICANT POOL

(i) Motivation, Desire, Goal and Attitude Toward Profession

Most of the applicants have high motivation, a desire for service to humanity and the community, and have a very positive attitude toward the profession in spite of the controversies surrounding it. They have the desire to face challenges. There is probably no profession without some negative issues. The applicants are willing to meet the demand of medical care consumers for more time and personal contact. Their desire is also to provide high quality patient care and be cost-effective at the same time. A large number of the applicants have already had some schooling in the biological sciences and have a great deal of interest in it. Some have also been in the health care profession in one role or another, and see this transition as a career opportunity and a chance to achieve their goals. They are highly dedicated and believe in altruism generally. They understand that their wish is to be a "dependent practitioner," teaming up with a physician and other health professionals, and to provide primary care in areas of unmet need — inner city or rural areas. They are interested in patient contact on a one-to-one basis and would like to be involved in patient counselling and patient education, believing strongly in continuity of patient care. They are conscientious and like the idea of promoting and supporting growth of the physician assistant profession. All of the applicants are adults who are eager to learn about medicine. They have the desire for continuing their medical education as a life-long learning process and are willing to follow some of the concepts of adult learning — especially the analogy of Knowles (8).

TABLE 5.1
THE PA EDUCATIONAL PROGRAM PROCESS AND OUTCOME
MAY BE SCHEMATICALLY DIAGRAMMED AS FOLLOWS:

I Applicant Pool	II Selection Process	III Selected Students (PA-S)	IV Educational Program	V Educational Process	VI Outcome
(i) Motivation desired goal and attitude toward profession	(i) Admissions Committee	(i) Acceptance and Registration	(i) Administration	(i) Length of program	(i) Educational program evaluation
(ii) Entry Prerequisites	(ii) Acceptable Number	(ii) Fees and other living expenses (Financial Aid)	(ii) Faculty	(ii) Curriculum design	(ii) Graduation (PA-C)
(iii) Choice of geographical locations	(iii) Acceptance of candidates	(iii) Attending instructional sessions	(iii) Facilities educational and clinical	(iii) Instructional design	(iii) Graduate deployment
(iv) Sound physical and mental health		(iv) Learning	(iv) Funds	(iv) Faculty	(iv) Impact on health care delivery system
(v) Financial considerations and planning		(v) Performance record	(v) Advisory Committee	(v) Teacher/Learner interaction	
(vi) Career opportunities		(vi) Student counseling	(vi) Accreditation (CAHEA)	(vi) Research	
		(vii) Student health record	(vii) Association Membership (APAP)	(vii) CME	
		(viii) Program graduation	(viii) Public education		
		(ix) Passing NCCPA exam (PA-C)	(ix) Obtain State Board of Medical Quality Assurance Accreditation		

In summary, therefore, we find a group of adult learners interested in a life-long career in the science and art of medicine, serving humanity in areas of unmet need. They also satisfy most of the characteristics of a profession as defined by some sociologists, according to S. Abrahamson in a chapter entitled "Education for Health Professions: Problems and Prospects" (9).

(ii) Entry Prerequisites

As has been mentioned before, these vary from program to program, but schooling in biological sciences and an experience in any of the health professions is highly desirable (4).

(iii) Choice of Geographical Locations

The educational programs for physician assistants are widespread throughout the United States. There are approximately 27 states offering one or more programs for such training. Many applicants select a training program to apply to because of their wish to locate in the same general area after completing their training. This is risky, since in many programs the ratio of applicants to positions in the educational program may be around 5:1 or greater. However, there is greater mobility for a person after graduation and certification. Therefore it is recommended that applications be made to programs in more than one geographic area.

(iv) Sound Physical and Mental Health

It is necessary for an applicant to submit evidence of good health as mentioned in the Guidelines for Educational Programs for the Assistant to the Primary Care Physician (5). When students are in the clinical setting, they are required to be up-to-date with their own immunizations and other checkups necessary for working in that particular setting. In addition, balanced mental health is critical for such students. There is a tremendous amount of pressure on the student from various sources—element of time in which to learn medicine, financial burdens, family concerns, and other human stress that is involved for one to remain interested and involved in the health care field. Such day-to-day issues as trying to explain to patients and others what a physician assistant is add a great deal to the amount of stress. On top of this, there is peer pressure for better performance and educational program pressure for becoming an ideal physician assistant. It is believed that coping with stress effectively is a must in this profession and other health related professions.

(v) Financial Considerations and Planning

Candidates planning to enter an educational program to become a physician assistant must plan very carefully in choosing a program which will suit their personal needs, depending on their educational and clinical backgrounds. They should consider their emotional needs and those of their family. As mentioned before, the stress during the training will mount considerably to the point of interfering with the learning situation if emotional needs are not considered prior to entry into an educational program. Considerations should also be given not only to personal physical and mental health, but also to that of family members.

The above two factors plus lack of financial planning are major causes of attrition. Although students' financial aids are becoming difficult to obtain, some assistance is still available in different types of state and federal aids. There are not as many sources to turn to as there are for medical students. Since education costs have risen sharply over the last few years, many students have also had to work during their training to obtain additional financial support. However, too many hours of such work take time away from the time required to complete an educational program successfully. Consequently, grades may drop when students resort to working for too many hours. Personal and family financial support, program tuition, fees, equipment and textbooks, NCCPA exam fees, and travel expenses to and from school should be taken into account as a part of the total financial planning.

(vi) Career Opportunities

These should be considered as part of planning by an applicant with specific desire for a particular geographic location and type of practice that will satisfy the needs of one's own ego. Currently, there is a lot of flexibility in making the right choice.

II. SELECTION PROCESS

(i) Admissions Committee

As a general rule, admissions committees are set up by educational programs for the selection of students. The process and the number of members of the committees vary. Some programs may require the candidate to take admission tests (to be used as pre-tests or for entry level tests), both written and oral. Despite all the grading systems and point scores awarded to the candidate based on performance in these tests, "gut level" feeling plays an important role in the final selection. The members of admission committees are conscientious, are looking for the best fit to their educational programs, and therefore seldom do any major complaints arise about the selection process. Most programs will select a number of students depending on the number of available slots and put a number of students on an alternate list, so that the number of available slots can be filled in case there are withdrawals by candidates after final selection.

(ii) Acceptable Number

Guidance is obtained from the Guidelines for Educational Programs (6) to determine the number of candidates that is acceptable. Enrollment of students should be conducive to the most effective learning through various teaching techniques. The learner/teacher ratio should be commensurate with acceptable educational practices especially for teaching in clinical areas, where often a 1:1 ratio may be preferred so that individual learning can be accomplished to meet the defined learning objectives. Group instruction should also be encouraged. On August 7, 1981, 58 CAHEA approved educational programs had 3,448 enrolled students for 1979–1980 with 1,463 students graduating (10).

(iii) Acceptance of Candidates

Candidates are duly notified if they are accepted, classified as alternates, or rejected by each educational program; providing ample time to the candidates to make any necessary planning. It is the policy of the Association of Physician Assistant Programs that the member program notify applicants of their status on or before April 15. This policy is followed by 30 programs (4).

III. SELECTED PHYSICIAN ASSISTANT STUDENTS (PA-S)

(i) Acceptance and Regulations

Each selected candidate who wishes to enroll in an educational program must notify the program as soon as possible, and not later than one month after receipt of the letter of acceptance. Formal registration should be completed with the program, and students should obtain a copy of rules and regulations, list of textbooks, list of equipment, schedules, identification badge (noting that they are in a student status), prescribed uniform, and take care of other necessary details as determined by the educational program commensurate with the policies of the institution where the program is housed.

(ii) Fees and Other Living Expenses

It will be worthwhile here to present a table as published in the National Health Practitioner Program Profile (4) Table 5.2.

TABLE 5.2
ESTIMATED FIRST-YEAR STUDENT EXPENSES*

Expense Item	Range	Average	Median
Tuition and Fees			
Resident	$20–5,200	$2,329	$2,590
Non-resident	$400–6,236	$3,370	$2,918
Room & Board (minimum)	$900–4,000	$2,700	$1,550

*Figures based on data provided in Spring, 1980 (4).

(iii) Attending Instructional Sessions

It seems that a more motivated student does not want to miss any of the instructional sessions (didactic or clinical). More and more educational programs are providing students with programmed instruction and self-learning programs. Students are also encouraged to form study groups for facilitation of learning. However, sometimes the number of instructional hours is so overwhelming that students, if they know a subject very well or have had some clinical experience in a specialty, may wish to take some time off, after proving their capabilities and expertise, which has to be agreed upon by the instructor. It has also been evidenced that students would naturally like to stay away from an instructor where very little learning is taking place. In this event, most educational programs offer other remedial sessions. Educational programs in general distribute full semesters, quarter, or annual schedules of all the didactic and clinical sessions to the students, so that they can budget their time, which becomes a scarce commodity.

(iv) Learning

Documented factors affecting learning: "The question of how learning takes place can be approached from many ways, but here we are concerned about the learning process which includes such factors as perception, memory, cognitive function and so forth" (Cross, 1980) (11). Typically, such literature emphasizes measurement of mental ability, perception and sensation, memory and cognitive function. Tough (1971) (12) raised the issue of self-directed learning, when adults plan their own learning, how they choose to learn, and what problems they encounter. Many famous researchers have written about the learning process, such as William James, John Dewey, Edward Thorndike, Kurt Lewin, B.V. Skinner, and Jean Piaget as mentioned by K. Patricia Cross in her book *Adults as Learners,* (1980) (11). Birren and Schaie (1979) (13), Kidd (1973) (14), Horn (1970) (15), and Schaie & Schaie (1980) (16) have currently written on learning psychology. Kidd (1973) (14) talks about three factors affecting learning in older adults—decreased reaction time, decreased vision and decreased hearing. There are several references of intellectual functioning starting with Wechsler (1948) (17), who claimed that most human abilities decline progressively after 18 and 25 years of age. However, Arenberg and Robertson-Tchabo (1977) (18) take the opposite view that intellectual functioning depends on kinds of abilities, research design, tests, and conditions under which intelligence is measured. Horn (1970) (15) proposes the idea of nature vs. mature controversy. He says there are "bullish" and "bearish" stances. "Bullish" implies that intelligence is a product of learning and should increase from infancy to old age. The "bearish" stance implies the biological approach and compares intelligence to growth in stature. Intelligence grows up to late teens or twenties, remains stable until late years and then decreases.

Schaie and Schaie (1980) claimed that older people compensate loss of quickness by experience and wisdom. Harry L. Miller (1967) (19) came up with the idea of Field Force Analysis showing how socioeconomic status directly influences participation in adult learning. His social class theory is based on the "needs hierarchy" of Maslow (1954) (20). Allen Tough (1979) (21) is a leading proponent of the theory of self-directed learning. His model consists of five stages, (i) engaging in a learning activity, (ii) retaining knowledge or skill, (iii) applying the knowledge, (iv) gaining material reward, and (v) gaining a symbolic reward. At each stage, personal feelings such as pleasure, self-esteem and other factors are the benefits derived from such actions.

"Self-directed Learning" approach as advocated by Knowles (22) in 1975 may be quite appropriate to assume by a learner as there is a defined goal, and the assumptions about learners fits in with the students in most of the educational programs. He has also suggested several specific strategies about self-directed learning.

(v) Performance Record

Student performance records are maintained by all of the educational programs and the students receive feedback on all of their didactic and clinical performance. The affiliated institutions also maintain copies of such records and provide official transcripts. The required number of credits are added up on a cumulative basis and degrees or certificates are awarded based on successful student performance. These records are confidential in nature.

(vi) Student Counselling

Basically, the educational programs provide two types of counselling, one for guidance during the learning phase, and the other one for placement after graduation. Guidance is provided on a one-to-one basis on educational principles, learning materials, clinical performance skills and also for maintaining a well-balanced mental health. Financial counselling is also provided by the programs. In case of physical illness or need for immunizations, medical support is provided. Most educational programs provide counselling for placement and maintain a record of available job openings. A list of different types of counsellors are also available and the students utilize their services as necessary.

(vii) Student Health Record

A record of each student's health is maintained by the educational program. When a student is in a clinical setting or a hospital, these clinical settings should provide protection for the student's health. If necessary, physical examination, chest x-rays, immunizations, and necessary lab data are obtained and steps are taken to maintain a student's health.

(viii) Program Graduation

Usually, this is a function of the students who are about to graduate. They form committees with a few program staff/faculty members to plan for this event. Graduation expenses are totally provided by some programs, while others will provide partial support.

(ix) Passing the NCCPA Examination (PA-C)

This is not only a very important objective for the students but it is also a responsibility of the individual programs. In 1972, the National Board of Medical Examiners (NBME) accepted the responsibility of developing a national certifying examination for insuring that individuals have achieved minimum standards of proficiency in delivery of primary health care (4). The NBME assumed such responsibility because the certification of physician assistant graduates is closely aligned to physicians. The American Medical Association (AMA) agreed with this concept and collaborated with NBME in the development, maintenance and administration of a national examination for certifying physician assistants.

The National Certifying Examination for Physician Assistants in Primary Care was administered by NBME for two years — 1973 and 1974. The National Commission on Certification of Physician Assistants (NCCPA) assumed this responsibility in 1975. It is interesting to note that by February, 1980, which is the month when the results are posted, the NCCPA had certified over 8,000 PA's.

The Board of Directors of the NCCPA is comprised of representatives from the following organizations: American Academy of Family Physicians, American Academy of Pediatrics, American Academy of Physician Assistants, American College of Physicians, American College of Surgeons, American Hospital Association, American Medical Association, American Nurses Association, American Society of Internal Medicine, Association of American Medical Colleges, Association of Physician Assistant Programs, Federation of State Medical Boards of United States Department of Defense (4).

The NCCPA has accepted responsibilities including the setting of eligibility criteria, registration of candidates, administration of the exam, setting of standards, issue and verification of certificates, re-registration of certificates every two years by CME credits accumulated, and re-certification of PA-C's every six years by exam.

IV. EDUCATION PROGRAM

(iv) Funds

The availability of funds remains as the number one factor for maintaining and operating an educational program. A few programs have been forced to close down due to lack of funds. Funds are obtained by the educational programs from a variety of sources which include the Federal Government, the States, private foundations, program fees collected from the selected students' "home base" institutions, and alumni associations of the past PA graduates. As with every educational program, due to the current financial status of the country, fund raising has become a special concern for all. Unless federal support is continued, more programs may have to be closed. CAHEA accreditation for educational programs requires that sufficient financial resources are available for continued operation and should be assured for each class of students enrolled. Although in years past, some PA students received stipends or did not pay program fees, many programs now have instituted fees to meet the financial requirements. However, none of the programs are charging excessive student fees. A listing of the fees of different educational programs is published in the National Health Practitioner Program Profile; estimated student expenses will be found in Table 5.2 (4).

(vi) Accreditation

The AMA, in collaboration with 45 allied health and medical specialty societies, has developed 26 allied health professions or occupations for which it accredits 2,995 allied health educational programs (5). The CAHEA is responsible for accreditation of the educational programs for primary care physician assistants. It is also responsible for development of the "Essentials" (6). "A further implication of the assessment of the reliability and validity of the "Essentials" is that the feasibility of establishing a relative value for each essential requirement for program evaluation makes it possible to differentiate between those standards that are viewed as indispensable requirements and those that are viewed as merely desirable." The above statement was made in the section of AMA's Allied Health Education and Accreditation (5). Furthermore, in 1981 the CAHEA was very seriously considering a self-analysis and self-study reporting system for educational programs. Experiments will be carried out to determine the feasibility of such a system on a pilot basis, to determine its efficiency and cost-effectiveness. Site visitor's workshops prepare the evaluators to conduct such visits for accreditation. Joint site visits are also in the offing as a total of 28 joint site visits have been arranged for 1982 to 1983 for some allied health programs (5). A post-survey questionnaire is also used by CAHEA evaluating accreditation. A letter is sent to the Program Directors shortly after a site visit including such questions as: (1) the arrangement for the site visit, (2) the activities of team members, (3) the extent and depth of personnel participation in institutions and, (4) suggestions for improving the overall program review process (5). The duration of accreditation varies for each PA educational program.

(vii) Membership in the Association of Physician Assistant Programs (APAP)

The APAP was formed in 1972 to foster the concept of physician assistants. Among its activities are: (a) participation in training program accreditation, (b) program curriculum development, (c) evaluation, (d) Continuing Medical Education (CME).

Virtually all of the CAHEA approved educational programs are members of the APAP. The other functions of APAP include: attempt to maximize PA service to the public and establish links between member programs through the Newsletter publication, and through semi-annual and annual meetings. APAP also informs federal officials and members of the Congress and their staff about physician assistant education and training. It also provides information to potential physician assistant candidates and others about the profession. Additional pertinent information regarding physician assistants and the various physician assistant programs is provided by APAP through the National Health Practitioner Program Profile, which is updated every year. The benefits to the members are substantial by keeping every educational program constantly informed about the latest developments in funding, in regulation, and in the educational process.

(viii) Public Education

Public education is a critical factor for the physician assistant profession. There are several bodies that are currently involved in this important sector. APAP has recognized this and in many ways helps to promote such activity. The American Academy of Physician Assistant (AAPA) which was formed by graduate physician assistants in 1968, facilitates public education through publications, displays and the use of different types of public communications media. Many educational programs are also involved in these activities in conjunction with alumni associations of the past graduates.

(ix) State Board of Medical Quality Assurance Accreditation

Although state licensure boards may have different names, educational programs obtain accreditation from such bodies in addition to CAHEA accreditation. This accreditation helps in obtaining certification for physician assistant graduates.

V. EDUCATIONAL PROCESS

(ii) Curriculum Design

The curriculum design has some subtle differences from one educational program to another, but the objectives are well-defined in the "Essentials" (6). The objectives include achievement-oriented general courses and topics of study which provide graduates with the necessary knowledge, skills, and abilities to accurately and reliably perform tasks, functions, and duties implied in the "Description of the Occupation" (6). Another objective is that "the curriculum should be broad enough to provide the assistant to the primary care physician with the technical capabilities, behavioral characteristics, and judgement necessary to perform in a professional capacity..." The curriculum design often reflects the modified Kemp model (23) these include the following: (a) topics and general purposes such as assumptions, objectives and areas to cover, (b) student characteristics such as background, achievement, and understanding, (c) learning objectives including who, what, by when, and how well, (d) subject content such as textbooks, clinical experience, faculty expertise, (e) pre-test, which can be used as a component of evaluation and reflects achievements of students, in order to determine what needs to be presented, (f) support services for teaching and learning activities, e.g., budget, personnel, schedules, facilities, audio-visual equipment, models, and (g) evaluation which provides the measurement of pupil progress.

The items from (c) through (g) are utilized to revise, refine and make the curriculum flexible and fit into the learning objectives. Curriculum design obviously needs a lot of time and careful planning. One also has to consider the role of tradition in medical education, resistance to change, the effort required, budgetary considerations, and number of full-time faculty hours needed.

(iii) Instructional Design

In educational programs, the instructional design usually depends upon the individual instructor. However, through in-program faculty development, certain generalized instructional designs are implemented. The basic premise is, of course, to provide and facilitate learning experiences for the students. Basic assumptions include "that every human being is educable within his or her capabilities." It is also assumed that no two humans are exactly alike when it comes to learning. In a sound educational process, the student is influenced and motivated by the teacher. It should also be considered that the ultimate objective of every activity is to promote the student's learning relevant to the practice of the profession. There are three main categories of objectives as defined by Benjamin Bloom in 1956 (24), and Krathwohl in 1964 (25), in the Taxonomy of *Educational Objectives*. The Taxonomy is divided into three parts: (1) the cognitive domain, (2) the affective domain and, (3) the psychomotor domain. The cognitive domain includes objectives such as knowledge, understanding, and thinking skills. The affective domain includes objectives which emphasize feelings, attitudes, emotion, interests, appreciation and methods of adjustment. The psychomotor domain includes objectives which emphasize motor skills. An individual instructional model may be adapted by an instructor as suggested by R.M. Gagne, 1970 (26). This model suggests several steps to gain and control attention, inform the learner of the expected outcomes, stimulate recall, present stimuli inherent in learning, offer guidance for learning, provide feedback, and appraise performance. For students to develop clinical skills, specific strategies as suggested by Goldstein may be followed (27). This strategy includes defining a goal with specific behavioral skills. Some specific strategies suggested are remodeling, role-playing, social reinforcement, patient education and performance feedback. All of the above are given consideration in educational programs.

(iv) Teacher/Learner Interaction

This is a very important part of learning and one must determine the most efficient and effective method. Again, faculty development programs within an educational program can be most helpful in this area. Most instructors should be able to learn how to determine the objectives, list learner characteristics, determine content of instruction and also develop evaluation methods (23). There are many ways to learn, but interaction between teacher and student by means of discussion on an individual or group basis is very important. Students are also encouraged to work individually by reading texts, solving problems, writing reports, working in labs or clinical areas, utilizing various audio and audiovisual materials. In educational programs, in general, the instructors are highly motivated and always strive for achieving a very healthy teacher/learner relationship.

(vi) Research

Almost all the educational programs are involved in research of one sort or another. The programs understand that in educational settings, research is one of the most important functions. Researchers have the opportunity, at least twice a year, to report their research activities in the semi-annual and annual meetings of the APAP and to publish their work in different peer journals.

(vii) Continuing Medical Education (CME)

Many programs are involved in providing CME credits to the past graduates. Formats vary and include week-long seminars as well as once a week sessions spread over several months.

VI. OUTCOME

(i) Educational Program Evaluation

It is recognized that in many respects contemporary evaluation methodologies are not fully adequate. Nevertheless, educational programs must develop and implement evaluation of all phases of training within the best means available (6). Usually, three different groups are involved in the process of evaluation—the student, the graduate and the faculty in an educational program. The student is not only evaluated by the faculty on performance of the cognitive affective, and psychomotor areas of the training, but also on the effect of the program and its overall educational process, and the program. The graduate evaluation is again two-fold.

The current clinical performance of the graduate is evaluated by the employing physician; who in turn evaluates the overall educational program in regard to unfulfilled needs and areas where more time or emphasis should have been placed. Each program also objectively evaluates its component in great detail. Usually, the following steps are involved for the purpose of evaluation: The formulation of objectives includes behavioral objectives, criteria development, selection and construction of instruments, establishment of evaluation design, conduct of assessment and measurement, collection of data, and interpretation of data. The diagram below illustrates some traditional approaches to assessment and measurement:

	Oral Test
Knowledge (Tests)	Essay type-test
(Cognitive domain)	Objective tests
	Behavior
Attitudes (Inference)	Interview
(Affective domain)	Inventories
	Rating scales
Skills (observation)	Check lists
(Psychomotor domain)	Records

At this point, the time-honored qualities of measurement principles for tests must be considered: (a) *Validity*—does it measure what it is constructed to measure? One has to appreciate that it is criterion related. It should be predictive and a good indicator of a specific outcome; (b) *Reliability*—How representative is the measurement? Is it consistent: does the measurement vary with time or repeated administrations? Does it measure what it is supposed to measure?; (c) *Objectivity*—Do independent scorers agree? Is it easy to construct, administer, score and interpret? According to the guidelines as provided in the "Essentials" (6), each educational program should develop a mechanism for self-evaluation. The CAHEA accrediting body expects every educational program to provide objective determination of the reliability and validity of educational standards. Thus, having developed a device for evaluation, every program has the opportunity of improving its educational program through feedback.

(iv) Impact on Health Care Delivery System

Certainly, the long and comprehensive planning and implementation necessary to produce a new type of health care practitioner has become very productive. The description of a physician assistant and the tasks performed by this professional fit snugly with what was expected of them. Thus, the efforts and the expenses, the hard toil of the educational programs, have not been in vain.

In summary, the physician assistant concept, in contrast to other established health careers, has progressed rapidly toward ensuring the American public of receiving only the highest quality of health care at a reduced cost by its rapid and organized approach to programmatic accreditation, certification of graduate competency, and participatory continuing medical education.

REFERENCES

1. Stead, E.A.: Conserving Costly Talents—Providing Physicians New Assistants. *JAMA, 198*:1108–1109, 1966.
2. Silver, H.K., Ford, L.C., and Stearly, S.: A Program to Increase Health Care for Children: The Pediatric Nurse Practitioner Program. *Pediatrics, 39*:756–760, 1967,
3. Smith, R.A.: MEDEX, *JAMA, 211*:1843–1845, 1970. Sidel, V.W.: Feldshers and Feldsherism: *New Engl J Med, 278*:981–992, 1968.
4. National Health Practitioner Program Profile, 5th Ed. Preface, page iii, 1981 to 1982.
5. 81st Annual Report on Medical Education in the U.S., 1980–1981: *JAMA, 246*:No. 25, Dec. 25, 1981.
6. Guidelines for Educational Programs for the Assistant to the Primary Care Physician— American Medical Association—Division of Medical Education—Department of Allied Medical Professions and Services, February, 1974.
7. Detmer, L.M.: *J. of the Amer. Dietetic Assn, 66*:269–274, 1975.
8. Knowles, M.S.: The Modern Practice of Adult Education: Andragogy Versus Pedagogy. New York Association Press, 1970.
9. Abrahamson, S.: Education for Health Professions: Problems and Prospects. Editor: M. Goaz in: Issues in Higher Education and the Professions in the 1980's. Libraries Unlimited, Inc. Littleton, Colorado, 1981.
10. National Academy of Sciences, Board on Medicine. New Members of the Physician's Health Team: Physician's Assistants. Report of the Ad Hoc Panel of New Members of the Physician's Health Team. Washington, DC; National Academy of Sciences, 1970.
11. K. Patricia Cross: Adults as Learners. Berkley, Educational Testing Service, 1980.
12. Tough, A.: The Adult's Learning Projects: A Fresh Approach to Theory and Practice in Adult Learning. Research in Education Series No. 1. Toronto, The Ontario Institute for Studies in Education, 1971.
13. Birren, J.E., and Schaie, K.A. (eds): *Handbook of the Psychology of Aging.* New York, Van Nostrand Reinhold Company, 1977.
14. Kidd, J.R.: How Adults Learn. New York, Association Press, 1973.
15. Horn, J.L.: Organization of Data on Life-Span Development of Human Abilities. In: L.R.

Goulut, and P.B. Baltes (eds.): Life Span Developmental Psychology: Research and Theory. New York, Academy Press, 1970.

16. Schaie, K.W., and Schaie, J.P.: Intellectual Development. In A.W. Chickering and Associates. *The Modern-American College*. San Francisco, CA, Josey-Hass, 1980. 1970.

17. Wechsler, D.: The Measurement and Appraisal of Adult Intelligence, 4th Ed. Baltimore, Williams and Wilkins Company, 1958.

18. Arenberg, D., and Robertson-Tchabo, E.A.: Learning and Aging. In: J.E. Birren and K.W. Schaie (eds.): *Handbook of the Psychology of Aging*. New York, Van Nostrand Reinhold Company, 1977.

19. Miller, H.L.: Participation of Adults in Education: A Force-Field Analysis. Boston Center for the Study of Liberal Education for Adults at Boston University, Occasional Papers No. 14, 1967.

20. Maslow, A.H.: Motivation and Personality. New York, Harper & Row, 1954.

21. Touch, A.: Choosing to Learn. Unpublished manuscript, June 1979. Cited in Reference No. 15.

22. Knowles, M.: Self-Directed Hearing: A Guide for Learners and Teachers. New York, Association Press, 1975.

23. Kemp, J.E.: Instructional Design, 2nd Edition. Fearon-Pitman Publishers, Inc., Belmont, California, 1977.

24. Bloom, B.S., *et al.*: Cognitive Domain: 1977. Taxonomy of Educational Objectives, Handbook 1. New York, D. McKay, 1956.

25. Krathwohl, D.R., *et al.*: Affective Domain Taxonomy of Educational Objectives: Handbook 2. New York, D. McKay, 1964.

26. R.M. Gagne: The Conditions of Learning. New York, Holt, Rinehart and Winston, 1970.

27. A. Goldstein: Skill Training for Community Living: Applying Structured Learning Therapy. New York, Pergamon Press, 1976.

Chapter 6

TRAINING PROGRAMS FOR MILITARY PHYSICIAN ASSISTANTS, ORTHOPEDIC PHYSICIAN ASSISTANTS, AND PATHOLOGIST ASSISTANTS

JESSIE EDWARDS, M.S.
RICHARD R. CONN, OPA-C
KENNETH R. BRODA, PH.D.

I. MILITARY PHYSICIAN ASSISTANT PROGRAMS

A. Historical Perspective

The role of nonphysicians in the provision of primary care to members of the military services spans two centuries. The very nature of the structure and deployment of combat military units generates a need for supporting medical manpower unlike the civilian community. It simply is not feasible from a supply side or economic viewpoint to staff relatively small, highly mobile, and widely dispersed military units with physicians. During the 1960s and early 1970s, the conscription of physicians under the selective service system provided a reasonable number of doctors for the three services. However, in the mid 1960s personnel planners, anticipating the end of the doctor draft, became increasingly concerned about a projected shortage of physicians, especially primary care doctors. It was only natural that their attention was attracted to the physician assistant concept which was beginning to be embraced by many prestigious academic health centers, and by the American Medical Association. These observations led the Department of Defense to endorse the training of physician assistants by the three military services.

B. The Army Program

The U.S. Army's Academy of Health Care Sciences operates the Army PA Program. It is located at Fort Sam Houston, Texas, and began in early 1972. Students are Army, medical, enlisted personnel who have at least three years of clinical experience, which is defined as personal contact with patients sufficient to develop an understanding of the physical and psychological needs of a sick or injured person. In addition to clinical experience, successful applicants must satisfy certain educational, biographical, and physical qualifications.

The curriculum is divided into two phases. The didactic phase, Phase I, is 39 weeks in duration and is conducted at Fort Sam Houston, Texas. Phase II, the clinical phase, is 52 weeks in duration and is conducted at selected Army medical facilities throughout the continental United States.

The material presented in the didactic phase is arranged essentially in block fashion by systems considering the clinical anatomy, physiology, pharmacology, and pathology applicable to each system. Concurrent with classroom instruction, application of the material presented is taught in a local major Army medical center.

During the twelve month clinical phase, students spend time with physician preceptors in ambulatory clinics, inpatient areas, and other settings. Emphasis is placed on the student perfecting his ability to solicit a good medical history, perform physical examinations, and manage common medical problems. Student progress is monitored by oral and written examinations and a comprehensive final examination.

The Army uses physician assistants in a variety of military health care facilities ranging from field aid stations to community hospitals to large medical centers. Projections include the use of physician assistants in specialty areas such as orthopedics, emergency medicine, aviation medicine, and occupational medicine.

C. The Navy Program

In late 1971, the Navy accepted its first group of enlisted persons to begin training as primary care physician assistants. Until last year, two programs were operated by the Navy, one at Portsmouth, Virginia, and one at San Diego, California. Only the Portsmouth program is currently operational.

The curriculum includes 700 hours of lectures during a 20-week didactic phase followed by 32 weeks of clinical clerkships at various Navy medical facilities. The classroom portion includes instruction in the basic medical sciences including anatomy, physiology, microbiology, and biochemistry with extensive practical experience in physical examination techniques. The clinical clerkships are based on the traditional medical preceptor model of education.

The Navy PAs function much like their civilian counterparts in that they collect a data base, perform thorough physical examinations, order diagnostic and laboratory tests, and manage common medical problems. Initially, most Navy PAs were assigned to large regional medical centers where they worked in outpatient clinics, emergency rooms, and in remote clinics. Later, assignment policies were modified to include utilization on aircraft carriers and to other Navy operational units.

D. The Air Force Program

The Air Force established its primary care physician assistant program in the summer of 1971 at its School of Health Care Sciences, Sheppard Air Force Base, Texas. Currently, it provides training only for Air Force PA students; however, at one time, it also served the PA training needs of the Army and Navy.

Students are selected from enlisted persons with a minimum of two, and not more than thirteen, years of military service. Applicants must have at least one year of health care experience, meet certain mental and physical requirements, and receive a favorable evaluation from local medical authorities. Persons with at least two years of college work are given preference in the selection process.

The curriculum is divided into two phases. Phase I is three trimesters, and includes about 1400 hours of instruction. Material presented is similar to that taught in medical school and is about as complex. Heavy emphasis is given to anatomy, physiology, and pharmacology. A large number of lectures covering topics of a clinical nature are presented, and several of the courses are behavior oriented. Students learn patient evaluation techniques at a local Air Force hospital.

The clinical year, Phase II, consists of physician supervised clinical practicums at several Air Force hospitals. Each student spends varying amounts of time on ten clinical services with emphasis given to the internal medicine service, and to the pediatric service.

The Air Force utilizes PAs extensively in family practice clinics and in their walk-in clinics. Although supervised by physicians, they were initially given a greater role in primary care than many of their civilian counterparts and exercise considerable autonomy in the management of patients with minor and self-limiting medical problems.

E. General Observations

The physician assistant programs operated by the military services are similar in many respects, yet quite different in others. Each incorporates the varying philosophies of their respective Surgeon Generals and top administrators. Because the mission of each service is different, the program content varies somewhat although the main emphasis is on primary care. Each program is highly structured with extensive documentation of the curriculum, this provides the required continuity of training in an environment where instructors are frequently moved in and out of the military educational system.

A notable feature of all three military programs is their affiliation with major civilian academic institutions. Such affiliation creates a mechanism for the awarding of college credit for work undertaken in military operated PA program. Having the oversight provided by representatives of academic health centers undoubtedly helps the military program administrators and enhances the image of the graduates as they later seek civilian employment.

A major issue for each military service is the proper placement of the graduate physician assistant in the rank or grade hierarchy. This is an extremely significant issue because it affects not only the monetary awards which accrue to the PA but also the status of those in the profession. The Air Force decided that the PA should be a commissioned officer whereas the Army and Navy took the position the PA should serve as a warrant officer, a rank between the commissioned officer and the non-commissioned officer ranks. After a long period of intraservice negotiations, and finally congressional intervention, the issue was resolved to the satisfaction of all three services. It was agreed the Air Force could commission its physician assistants, and the Army and Navy could grant warrant officer status to its PAs. The compromise on the status of the PA did include a provision that a PA may not advance above the rank of Major. This limitation on rank was intended to preclude the physician assistant from holding more rank than their supervising physicians.

A major policy question facing the military has been whether to procure physician assistants from the civilian sector or to train their own. On the surface, it appears to many that it would be less expensive to staff the military with civilian educated PAs similar to the staffing of nurse and other health professional positions. Experience, however, has caused the services to opt to train their own personnel selected from the ranks of an experienced enlisted medical corps. Such a policy accomplishes two important things. It assures that the physician assistant is well oriented to the military medical care system and the unique characteristics of that system. Secondly, the policy allows for the professional growth and development of many career minded individuals who clearly possess the intellectual ability to function in more responsible positions.

A common concern among the military services is in the area of quality of care and patient acceptance of the physician assistant. A well publicized research effort for the Air Force by the Rand Corporation, addresses the question of quality of care. The findings and conclusions, released in January 1980, provided encouragement and support to the proponents of physician assistant use in the military. In summary, the evidence was clear that the Air Force can deliver the same quality of care when PAs treat a sizeable percentage of patients formerly treated by physicians; PAs ordered diagnostic procedures at rates similar to physicians; supervision occurred with reasonable frequency;

and consultation took up only a modest amount of the physician's time. Another study by the Rand Corporation indicated substantial patient acceptance; patients exposed to PA services rated the quality of care as uniformly high.

Physician Assistants now are well integrated into the military services, enjoying a place of status, and the respect of their comrades while making significant contributions to the health care system.

II. THE ORTHOPEDIC PHYSICIAN ASSISTANT

A. Role

The Orthopedic Physician Assistant (OPA) is a specialized member of the health care team. The OPA serves as an adjunct to the orthopedic surgeon in four basic areas. These areas include: 1) applying of immobilizing devices, bandages, plaster and fiberglass casts and splints; 2) serving as a primary assistant in orthopedic surgery where the OPA retracts, positions, ties suture and assists the surgeon in other ways as directed; 3) aiding in the initial and follow-up assessment of the orthopedic patient; and 4) functioning in the office setting as an interface for the surgeon. The individual who serves as an assistant to the orthopedic physician allows the surgeon more time to pursue tasks that require his expertise.

Since our program's conception in 1968, the curriculum has been altered to meet the needs of the orthopedic surgeons using the services of the orthopedic assistant, but the original philosophy still holds true.

B. Curriculum

The curriculum followed by Kirkwood Community College is six quarters in length. Approximately 50% of the course of study is didactic, the remaining is clinical instruction.

A collection of core courses heavily weighted in the "hard sciences" provides a framework upon which the specialty courses are built. Human anatomy and physiology, microbiology and pathology provide the necessary background for courses such as orthopedic conditions, operating room techniques and immobilization techniques. The latter three courses are designed to inform the student about selected injury or disease processes and the treatment modalities available. The use of plaster and fiberglass casting materials, braces, and traction therapy are explored and practical experience is provided in the laboratory setting. Basic operating room techniques are developed with an emphasis on orthopedic surgery.

The rudiments of orthopedic assessment are presented. This includes obtaining an orthopedic history as well as the use of various diagnostic tests. Elementary evaluation of radiographs is presented throughout the course of study. Documentation of findings is stressed during all facets of the program.

Communication between the OPA and patients, and other health team members is improved by the incorporation of speech, composition studies and educational techniques. Both Faculty and Advisory Board Members feel such subject material is necessary to fully prepare the OPA as a patient-physician intermediary.

Kirkwood Community College offers clinical sites in several locations. This variety allows students to observe the basic thought behind this, which is that various treatments for similar dysfunctions exist. In an attempt to provide a well-rounded example of treatment diversification and practical experience in working with these situations, students are placed for varying lengths of time at the University of Iowa Orthopedic Outpatient Clinics; the Veterans Administration Medical Center located in Iowa City, Iowa; Ramsey County Hospital in St. Paul, Minnesota; and various private practices and hospitals throughout the Midwest. A final three-month preceptorship exposes the student to the daily workings of an office and surgical practice.

The prospective student should be aware that a high level of skills in reading, writing, and the sciences is necessary for completion of the program. Past experience in the health field is a major benefit in grasping the data presented. Inquiry may be made by contacting the Office of Admissions, Kirkwood Community College, 6301 Kirkwood Boulevard, SW, Cedar Rapids, Iowa 52406.

C. Graduates and Certification

Consistently high placement for graduates has been seen and is projected to continue. Graduates from Kirkwood Community College are practicing in many areas of the United States. The major region of placement exists in the central states; however, placement is also brisk in the southern states.

Three large employers of OPA's are identified: 1) the specialty physician's practice—In a majority of cases a group practice of between three and five physicians employ two or more OPAs. The assistants usually rotate between surgery and general office duties as well as sharing on-call responsibilities; 2) hospital affiliated assistants—These individuals usually function as an extension of nursing service. Their duties center around the in-patient care of orthopedic patients and may involve assisting in surgery. They may also occupy administrative positions within the orthopedic area; 3) sales—An area somewhat distant from the direct patient care arena is the sales/education field associated with major instrument and appliance firms. The OPA represents a person who is very knowledgeable about the supplies and equipment necessary to practice orthopedics and therefore represents a major asset to these companies.

A national certifying examination exists for the credentialing of Orthopedic Physician's Assistants. This examination is administered several times per year by the National Board for Certification of Orthopedic Physician's Assistants.

Information concerning this process may be obtained from the National Board, Mr. Tavo Guthrie, 393 SE Centurion, Apt 21; Gresham, Oregon 97030.

III. PATHOLOGIST ASSISTANTS

A. Historical Perspective

Dr. Thomas D. Kinney, past Chairman of the Department of Pathology and Dean of the Duke University Medical School, like Dr. Eugene Stead, recognized the need for Physician Assistants and their potential value and impact on the nation's health care delivery system. Dr. Kinney was perplexed by the fact that pathologists had for several decades utilized skilled allied health personnel to assist in the many responsibilities associated with the clinical laboratories and cytopathology, yet did not train or employ similar individuals to assist in the duties of anatomic pathology. In response to this need, Duke University Medical Center's department of Pathology, in conjunction with the Veterans Administration Hospital, established the first Pathologist Assistant Training Program in the United States in 1968. Since then, eight other programs ranging from on-the-job training to those offering formal training and a collegiate degree have begun. Presently, only five programs remain. Each is affiliated with a major medical center and a college or university which confers either a Bachelor or Master of Science degree.

B. Education

The training is two calendar years in length, consisting of four semesters of didactic and laboratory courses, and two summers of hospital-based practical experience. The average curriculum consists of pre-clinical basic science courses in human anatomy, physiology, histology, microbiology, and pathology, and practical training in autopsy and surgical pathology prosection, as well as medical photography and histopathologic technique. Students also have the opportunity of participating in elective rotations in such subspecialty fields as forensic pathology, pediatric pathology and neuropathology.

C. Role

Pathologist Assistants are trained to work under physician supervision, performing many of the rigorous tasks associated with anatomic pathology. They usually function under the direct supervision of one M.D. pathologist, even though their services may be available to several pathologists within a group or a hospital. They assist the pathologist in postmortem anatomic dissection and in the evaluation of disease by the compilation and correlation of patient data as it relates to postmorten findings. Pathologist Assistants also assume an important role in the surgical pathologist's dissection and examination of surgical specimens. In addition, they render valuable assistance in medical photography, in the organization of autopsy and surgical materials for conferences, in the procurement of organs and tissues for transplantations, and in medical center research projects. Many Pathologist Assistants are placed in managerial and supervisory positions, in addition to their service work.

D. Organization

The American Association of Pathologist Assistants recognizes approximately 175 Pathologist Assistants practicing in 38 states including Alaska and Hawaii. They are employed in a wide variety of anatomic pathology settings which include: private pathology laboratories and community hospitals; large academic medical centers, and state university hospitals; corporate and governmental research facilities; and state and county medical examiner systems.

The Association is presently working through the American Medical Association and the Committee on Allied Health Education and Accreditation in an effort to gain certification for the practicing Pathologist Assistant.

Chapter 7

MEDEX PROGRAMS:
HISTORY AND PROGRESS

WILLIAM M. WILSON, Ph.D.
RICHARD A. SMITH, M.D., M.P.H.

BACKGROUND

The MEDEX model for the training and deployment of primary care physician assistants was formally implemented at the University of Washington in 1968 by Richard A. Smith. M.D., after four years of planning and experimentation. The word MEDEX in capital letters refers to one of the programs using essentially the same model to train and deploy primary care physician assistants. The word in lower case letters "Medex" is the professional title of those individuals who have successfully completed MEDEX training. Initially, the MEDEX model was designed to utilize, in rural or inner city communities, the extensive medical training and otherwise wasted experience of former U.S. military corpsmen. Most of these corpsmen had served in Southeast Asia during the Vietnamese conflict. However, after the model was systematically replicated and, consequently, regionally refined across the United States by nine geographically disparate colleges of medicine, an organized consortium of MEDEX training programs was established by 1972 and a select group of graduate physician assistants (including non-corpsmen, nurses, and others with extensive medical backgrounds) had been trained and deployed to communities in need of additional primary health care manpower and services.

The sponsoring institutions included: Charles Drew Postgraduate Medical School, Los Angeles, California; Howard University College of Medicine, Washington, D.C.; Dartmouth Medical School, Hanover, New Hampshire; University of North Dakota School of Medicine, Grand Forks, North Dakota; University of Washington School of Medicine, Seattle, Washington; University of Hawaii School of Medicine, Honolulu, Hawaii; Pennsylvania State University College of Medicine, Hershey, Pennsylvania; Medical University of South Carolina, Charleston, South Carolina; University of Utah College of Medicine, Salt Lake City, Utah. A tenth program, at the University of Alabama, trained only one class of Medex and then disbanded. Today, only six of the original training programs continue to train physician assistants for the United States: Drew, Howard, Washington, Hershey, South Carolina, and Utah.

CONCEPTUAL FRAMEWORK

The MEDEX educational model was designed, at once, to address both the training and deployment of physician assistants in an integrated system. The basic factor which distinguishes MEDEX from other physician assistant training programs is that historically MEDEX has directly and systematically addressed the issues of both training and deployment. The vast majority of other programs have focused primarily upon training and curriculum development. Thus, the operational philosophies which undergird MEDEX activity concern the manner in which Medex trainees and graduates will be supervised, utilized, and distributed within the primary care delivery system. To insure that distribution reflects both the needs of the health care system and the demands of that system, and to insure that supervision and utilization of each graduate is carried out in such a way as to maximize his or her impact upon health care delivery, the MEDEX Programs have developed step by step procedures and systems which are distinct from more traditional approaches to health manpower education.

A. Identification of Job Placements Prior to Selection and Training of Students

This is the first and, perhaps, most critical tenet in the MEDEX training and deployment philosophy. MEDEX programs, working in collaboration with practicing physicians, organized medicine, health planning agencies, and in some instances consumer groups, identify communities and physicians who have a documented need for assistance. Once the identification of potential areas of demand and need has taken place, site visits are conducted by program staff to individual communities in order to discuss with physicians and others the implications and responsibilities of Medex utilization. The purpose of the site visit is three-fold: first, to explain in detail the operation of the program; second, to assess the physician's interest and need for a Medex; and third, to determine the adequacy of physical facilities such as the number of examining rooms for training and ultimately employing the Medex. Special attention is devoted also to review of record keeping systems, interest in and capabilities for teaching, type and scope of practice, attitudes regarding task delegation to assistants, and standards of care adhered to within the practice.

In order to become a preceptor, the physician must agree to: (1) accept the Medex as a professional with whom he can work in providing high quality patient care; (2) enter actively into a sustained teaching effort with his Medex; and (3) participate in both the ongoing and final evaluation during the Medex's traineeship.

In addition, to the extent possible, potential preceptors must be engaged in delivering primary care, well-accepted and secure in their communities, highly regarded by their peers, and willing to employ a Medex at the completion of training. Preference is given to those physicians who have the greatest need for assistance, who are under 60 years of age, and who practice in communities where additional health services are needed.

B. Identification of Candidates for MEDEX Training

The identification of suitable candidates to be trained as Medex is a complex and arduous process. Although individual programs establish specific screening criteria appropriate to regional needs, common criteria are that applicants have at least three years of combined medical training and experience (including substantial experience in primary care under physician supervision), be highly recommended by physicians familiar with their capabilities, and possess a strong motivation to pursue MEDEX as a career. After initial screening of the 300 to 500 applications received for each class, 20 to 40 outstanding candidates are invited to attend an intensive 2½-day selection conference. At the conference, the final selection of from 15 to 30 students is made based upon objective tests, personality measures, individual interviews with potential preceptors, psychiatrists, graduate Medex, and MEDEX staff. The interviews provide the opportunity to evaluate the candidates' personal qualifications, clinical knowledge, maturity, communication skills and, most importantly, their awareness of and willingness to work within their own skill limitations. Again, the number of trainees selected depends almost entirely upon the number of physician-preceptors available for each class, thus insuring for each Medex a place to work and learn from the outset of training.

C. Matching Students and Preceptors

Matching the Medex with their preceptors begins with the trainee selection conference where the potential Medex and preceptors meet for the first time. The stability of the Medex-preceptor match depends not only upon their mutual compatibility, but also upon the Medex and his or her family's successful adaptation to life in the preceptor's community. Accordingly, early in the didactic phase of training, the Medex and their wives or husbands make a series of personal visits to three or four practices and communities attractive to them. These visits give Medex and their families a chance to become better acquainted with the preceptor, his practice, and his community.

After all of the visits are completed, both preceptors and Medex prepare ranking lists indicating their top three choices in order of preference. The staff then matches the preceptor and Medex according to the preferences indicated. Thus, both individuals painstakingly select each other and, in so doing, greatly increase the probability that they will form a compatible and productive relationship.

D. Training

Again, there are variations among programs on the basic training model, but essentially training is divided into a didactic university phase, clinical rotations, and extensive preceptorship. The university phase of training takes place in the parent academic institution where student learning is focused upon data collection skills, identification of patient problems, and the planning and implementation of treatment procedures. The length of time spent in this setting varies, with most programs using an intensive university phase of training as the basic component for imparting supplemental knowledge and the acquisition of previously unacquired skills.

During the university phase, instruction is balanced between classroom and clinical sessions. Classroom teaching incorporates each of the many instructional techniques presently available within the medical center. Methods of instruction range from textbooks to standardized treatment protocols, pamphlets, programmed texts, audio-visual aids, and simulated and actual patients. The clinical sessions are largely conducted in local primary care settings and are designed to provide greater relevance to the classroom experience.

The preceptorship phase of training is designed to develop and refine these skills and involves placing the student with his or her matched preceptor in the day-to-day delivery of primary care. This "controlled apprenticeship" is carefully monitored by the program staff through on-site evaluation visits, periodic return of trainees to the university, mailback evaluation protocols and learning packages, and continual communication with preceptors. Upon the successful completion of all MEDEX educational objectives, the trainee is certified by the university and is graduated.

THE MEDEX MODEL OVER TIME

Geographical, institutional, and demographic forces have caused several of the MEDEX programs to substantially alter the original MEDEX model and others to close their doors. Some of the existing MEDEX programs have converted to the two-year model of physician assistant training, replacing the preceptorship phase with a series of clinical rotations. One of the remaining "true MEDEX" programs, Utah MEDEX, through advantageous geographical location, institutional support, and physician acceptance has managed to continue the original MEDEX model with only minor adaptations.

After nearly two years of coordinated local effort, Utah MEDEX was initiated at the University of Utah Medical Center in June, 1971. The first class consisted of twelve former military corpsmen, most of whom were recently returned Vietnam Veterans. Since that time, the program has trained and deployed 180 graduates—in twelve classes, and 98% of all graduates have passed the National Board of Medical Examiners Certifying Examination.

The advantages of a deployment system can be seen in the distribution of graduates over the program's target region. Eighty-six percent of the program graduates have remained in the eight-state region, and 68% have stayed with their original preceptors. Seventy-two percent are in communities of less than 10,000 people and over half of the program's students have been deployed to designated Health Manpower Shortage Areas.

MEDEX TRAINING AROUND THE WORLD

After working together successfully to develop a systems approach to domestic primary health care problems, it was natural for the MEDEX programs to share their experiences beyond America's borders. Thus, an invitation in the early seventies to help the government of Micronesia (in the Southwest Pacific) to strengthen its coverage of health services led to the establishment of the international MEDEX group, with its base at the John A. Burns School of Medicine at the University of Hawaii in Honolulu.

Since 1974, the MEDEX group at the University of Hawaii has been developing an approach to strengthen and rapidly expand basic health services to the majority of a developing country's population. The MEDEX technology is aimed at two critical intervention points: manpower development and systems development. The manpower development promoted by MEDEX emphasizes (but is not limited to) training of village health workers and mid level health workers. But the development of manpower, by itself, is futile. In order for health workers to function, they need medical and other supplies, e.g., kerosene to run the refrigerator that keeps vaccines from spoiling. They need supervision, reliable communications, and transportation to reach isolated communities with preventive services. In sum, the workers need to be supported by a rationalized and functioning management support infrastructure.

The MEDEX technical assistance approach includes:

1. Strategy and methods to facilitate improvements in the Primary Health Care (PHC) system on a national comprehensive basis (rather than on a basis of isolated, unrelated projects).
2. Field tested prototype competency-based training modules for PHC workers covering preventive, promotive, curative and managerial knowledge and skills.
3. Field tested prototype systems development materials for improving planning, evaluation and management operations.
4. Appropriate technology transfer methods for country-specific adaptation of prototype materials (that is, what to do and how to do it, in a way that works for each country.).

These aspects of the MEDEX technology have been undergoing development and field trials over the past eight years, beginning in Micronesia and Thailand (1974-1977). In the early programs, training was used an an entree to health systems development, thus the present official name of the group (Health Manpower Development Staff).

As MEDEX evolved to the larger job of developing a receptive framework for new manpower as well as to PHC delivery system strengthening and development, emphasis was placed upon improving management competence. It is apparent that poor management is the single most important cause of failure in development projects, especially when dealing with the most peripheral rural populations. By viewing development in its larger context rather than from the perspective of isolated projects, the MEDEX group, collaborating with host governments, helped to design and implement *national* programs in Pakistan, Guyana and Lesotho.

The MEDEX approach emphasizes appropriate technology and cost containment by maximizing effective use of limited resources in less industrialized countries. This provides a realistic perspective and thrust for health sector development at a time of dwindling global resources. MEDEX has pioneered promoting what have now become worldwide accepted concepts of PHC. In recognition of this, the World Health Organization has asked the MEDEX group to be a Collaborating Center with that U.N. agency since MEDEX is the only group anywhere in the world that has committed 100 percent of its resources and efforts to primary health care technology development and application, including the adaptation, field testing and evaluation of the technology with emphasis on results that can be applied on a large scale.

The MEDEX group has been collaborating with countries seriously committed to developing substantive primary health care programs. Medex has demonstrated its capacity to help adapt technology and methods to suit the individual and special needs of most developing nations. Guidelines and proto-type materials for adaptation in developing country settings that have resulted from those experiences will be published by mid-1983.

MEDEX facilitates involvement of both public and private sector profes-sionals to target their expertise and mobilize their resources in more effective directions. Further, using the MEDEX approach to design and implement a nationwide PHC strategy, small projects and vertical programs (e.g., Safe Water, Maternal and Child Health, Nutrition, Immunization), which are par-tial solutions to PHC, can be converted into strong components of a compre-hensive national primary health care program.

CONCLUSION

The MEDEX model provides a well-designed strategy for meeting acute needs for additional primary health care manpower, especially in rural areas. In recent years, the applicability of the model has been demonstrated in rural areas of the developing world, where health manpower shortages far exceed any of those encountered in the United States. This MEDEX experience sug-gests that the potential role for midlevel non-physician health care providers including physician assistants, nurse -midwives, and nurse practitioners is only beginning to be explored within the framework of the severe health manpower shortages of the developing world.

BIBLIOGRAPHY

Danforth, N.: The Current Status of the MEDEX Programs and their Relationship to the Physi-cian's Assistants Concept. *Physician's Associate, 2(4):*128-132, October 1972.

Jacobs, A., Johnson, K., Breer, P., and Nelson, E.: Comparison of Tasks and Activities in Physi-cian-Medex Practices. *Public Health Reports, 89(4):*339-344, July-August 1974.

Kane, R., Olsen, D., and Castle, C.: Effects of Adding a Medex on Practice Costs and Produc-tivity. *Journal of Community Health, 3(3):*216-226, Spring 1978.

Kane, R., Olsen, D., Wilson, W., Reynolds, L., Jr., Hogben, M., and Castle, C.: Adding a Medex to the Medical Mix: An Evaluation. *Journal of Medical Care, 14(12):*996-1003, December 1976.

Kane, R., Olsen, D., and Castle, C.: Medex and Their Physician Preceptors. *Journal of the American Medical Association, 236(22):*2509-2512, November 29, 1976.

Lawrence, D.: MEDEX — The Education-Deployment Interface. *Journal of Medical Education, 50(12):*85-92, December 1975, pt. 2.

Lawrence, D., Wilson, W., and Castle, C.: Employment of MEDEX Graduates and Trainees: Five-Year Progress Report for the United States. *Journal of the American Medical Associa-tion, 234(2):*174-177, October 13, 1975.

Nelson, E., Jacobs, A., and Johnson, K.: Patients' Acceptance of Physician's Assistants. *Journal of the American Medical Association, 228(1):*63-67, April 1, 1974.

Olsen, D., Kane, R., Manson, J., and Newman, J.: Measuring Impact of Medex Using Third-Party Payer Claims. *Inquiry, 15:*160-165, June 1978.

Pulsipher, V., and Kane, R.: A Model to Predict the Stability of Medex-Preceptor Matches. *The PA Journal, 6(4):*197-201, Winter 1976.

Riess, J., and Lawrence, D.: *Utilization of New Health Practitioners in Remote Practice Settings.* Final Report. Prepared under contract No. 1-MB-44168 between DHEW and Department of Health Services, School of Public Health and Community Medicine, University of Washington, Seattle, Washington, February 9, 1976.

Segal, R., Wilson, W., Hogben, M., Asahina, B., Murdock, R., and Gerity, P.: Deployment — A Six Year Perspective. *The PA Journal, 7(4):*198-204, Winter 1977.

Smith, R.: Health and Rehabilitation Manpower Strategy: New Careers and The Role of the Indigenous Paraprofessional. *Social Science and Medicine, 7(4):*281-290, April 1973.

Smith, R.: MEDEX — An Operational and Replicated Manpower Program: Increasing the Delivery of Health Services (editorial). *American Journal of Public Health, 62(12):*1563-1565, December 1972.

Smith, R., Anderson, Jr., and Okimoto, J.: Increasing Physician Productivity and the Hospitalization Characteristics of Practices Using MEDEX — A Progress Report. *Northwest Medicine, 70:*701-706 passim, October 1971.

Smith, R., Bassett, G., Markarian, C., Vath, R., Freeman, W., and Dunn, G.: A Strategy for Health Manpower — Reflections on an Experience called MEDEX. *Journal of the American Medical Association, 217(10):*1362-1367, September 6, 1971.

Stone, L., and Brosseau, J.: Cross Validation of a System for Predicting Training Success of Medex Trainees. *Psychological Reports, 33:*917-918, 1973.

Wilson, W., and Castle, C.: The Utah MEDEX Demonstration Project: One Approach to the Intermountain Region's Health Manpower Problems. *Rocky Mountain Medical Journal, 69:*53-56, January 1972.

Chapter 8

THE CHILD HEALTH ASSOCIATE

BONNIE SCHMIDT, M.S., CHA

Americans have the highest standard of living, but not the highest standard of life when measured by infant mortality and average life expectancy. A number of homogenous European countries surpass the Unites States in this regard. Americans deserve and can afford better health care services.

The need for improved pediatric medical services in the United States is indicated by the following statistics: each year 3.5 million children under five years of age have no contact with a physician. The Center for Disease Control reported an average of 37% of children are inadequately immunized for polio, diphtheria, pertusis, tetanus, measles, mumps and rubella: in 1979, the infant mortality rate was 13 per 1,000 live births; and the post-neonatal mortality rate is greater for blacks than whites. Almost half of all infant deaths are associated with low birth weight. The risk of delivering a low birth weight infant is increased when mothers have no prenatal care. The complication of low birth weight is the highest among infants whose mothers are under 15 years of age. The birth rate among teenage mothers is the only birth rate that is rising substantially in the United States. In 1979, there were over 1.1 million pregnancies to teenage girls in America and many of their infants suffered from low birth weight complications (1).

There is an average of one general pediatrician per 9,200 children in poorer areas of America compared to one per 3,125 children in the affluent areas. In a 1978 American Academy of Pediatrics survey, pediatricians are primarily in urban and suburban areas (2), while the census indicates 20% of all children live in rural areas. The National Council for Children and Youth reported in 1976 that 10.2 million children under the age of eighteen are from low income families, or one child in six now lives in poverty. The pediatric population of the United States, numbering 62 million children and youths under 18 (3), is underserved presently and in the face of "Reagonomics" and a growing recession, childrens' needs for basic health care services will probably continue to be unmet.

The Carnegie Commission of Higher Education identified in 1970 only one serious manpower shortage, and that was in the area of health care personnel. The Commission projected even more acute shortages in health care personnel as health insurance expands in the future (4). The expansion of third party reimbursement of health care services would create more demand and lead to more unmet needs. Out of this perceived need the physician assistant concept grew, with the goals of providing health care services of better quality and greater quantity to more Americans. Improved accessibility to higher quality health care is still a goal of physician assistant training programs.

The majority of physician assistants work in the primary care specialties. In a 1978 profile on the physician assistant profession, 52 percent were in family practice, 12 percent in general internal medicine, 1.9 percent in obstetrics and gynecology and 3.3 percent in pediatrics. The remaining physician assistants work in sub-specialties such as surgery and emergency medicine. Of the 3.3 percent of physician assistants practicing in a pediatric setting, a large number are child health associates. Nurse practitioners and physician assistants provide primary health care to ambulatory pediatric patients, but predominantly in family practice settings. The recent report of the Graduate Medical Education National Advisory Committee (GMENAC) pointed out that by 1990, the care given to children in about 15% of all visits in physicians' offices or public health facilities should be delegated to nonphysician health care providers. GMENAC recommended that there be no decrease in the number of nonphysician health care providers trained. Fifty of the fifty-five accredited programs of the Association of Physician Assistant Programs are presently training people for primary care, and the Child Health Associate Program is the only pediatric primary training program.

The potential value of nonphysician health care providers can be seen by a closer look at child health associates. Child health associates are graduates of an American Medical Association physician assistant program which prepares them to be providers of comprehensive and high quality primary health care to children of all ages. During the first two years of this three-year program at the University of Colorado Health Sciences Center, students have basic science and didactic courses similar to medical students. All courses for child health associates concentrate on practical application to ambulatory pediatrics. Students are exposed to a wide variety of clinical experiences on the wards, in the nursery, in pediatric outpatient departments, in pediatric specialty clinics (otolaryngology, dermatology, allergy, orthopedics), as well as in community settings such as private pediatric offices and neighborhood health centers.

The following year is a mandatory year of internship in child care in urban and rural settings which allows the interns to participate in the assessment and care of more than 2,000 children. As interns, child health associates apply and practice previously learned skills under the supervision of physician preceptors and they assume increased responsibility and greater autonomy in making independent value judgements regarding the health care of children.

On completion of the course of study and successful passage of a certifying examination given by the Colorado State Board of Medical Examiners, child health associates may, by law, engage in the "practice of pediatrics." The regulating statutes allow child health associates to counsel, diagnose, manage and treat children, as well as prescribe approved drugs.

Child health associates are trained in ambulatory pediatrics. They ultimately work in private and public outpatient settings. The assessment and evaluation studies of child health associates indicate they can care for at least 90-95% of children seen in a variety of practice settings and reduce by 95% the time physicians require to care for those pediatric patients seen by the child health associate without a decrease in the quality of care (5,6,7,8,9).

In a prospective study, financial and functional aspects of nine private practices were analyzed both prior to and one year after child health associates joined those practices (9). Significant findings of this study include:

1) The addition of a child health associate to each practice resulted in an average increase of 28% (range 10-62%) in the total number of patients seen in each practice, allowing overworked physicians the ability to decrease their own patient load.

2) The percentage of patients seen with each of the 25 most commonly encountered pediatric conditions was the same for physicians and for child health associates. The physicians studied felt comfortable delegating both well and sick child care to the child health associates.

3) There was no increase in return visits to see the physician when the patients were seen by the child health associates. This reflects patient acceptance of the care given by the child health associate.

4) Some form of consultation by the physician was indicated for less than 10% of patients. Most of the consultations were to confirm the clinical findings or to sign prescriptions. A detailed assessment was necessary in less than one percent of the patient contacts.

5) The average consultation required 2.8 minutes of the physician's time.

6) There was no difference between the dispositions made by the physician and child health associates of patients with any of the acute conditions studied. There was also no difference in the average number of tests and x-ray procedures ordered, indicating comparable care given by both physicians and child health associates.

7) Child health associates were used to screen medical complaints on the telephone and to see appropriate patients after hours when indicated.

8) Five of the nine physicians participating in the study reported a decrease in the number of "after-hours" telephone calls despite a significant increase in the total number of patients seen. The decrease in calls might be a result of increased patient education.

9) Several practices used the child health associates to develop new patient education and community service activities and new systems for
improving health care delivery.

10) Income generated by the child health associates in the first year of employment (between 1974 and 1976) averaged $37,807. With current
inflation the figure would be appreciably higher (5,10).

The productivity of a child health associate employed in an inner-city
neighborhood health center was compared with that of pediatricians working
in the same setting. The average number of patients seen by the child health
associates was approximately the same as seen by the clinic pediatricians. The
average cost of the visit was half of physician cost (5).

Children are dependent on their caretakers to determine their wants and
needs for medical services. Adolescents are now a growing force in creating demands on medical services. The Ambulatory Pediatric Association study of
pediatric care cites the unmet needs and wants of adolescents as a major area
for redirection in medical education. The Child Health Association Program
training for the past decade has directed a major thrust of the educational
program toward adolescent medicine. Child health associates are able to deliver health care services and education concerning: knowledge about
adolescents' physical, mental and emotional processes; sexual function and sex
education, including information on venereal diseases, birth control and pregnancy; parenting skills; screening for adult diseases, i.e. hypertension, counseling on diet and food fadism; and information and guidance on how to use
health services appropriately and effectively.

Much of pediatric practice is preventive medicine and patient education.
Patient education has been an important thrust in physician assistants education. Routine well child care encompasses approximately one third of child
health associate's patient contact time (11). The demand for preventive medical services has been traditionally low for all income levels. The number of
underimmunized children reflects the low demand for preventive medicine or
a gap between the "wants" and "needs" because of consumer ignorance. The
general population is unaware of what the medical profession sets as standards
for "good health" and need for more patient education and involvement in
their own medical care (12).

Another important factor that curtails families from seeking pediatric health
care services is the limited third party reimbursement for this type of medical
care. Close to thirteen percent of America's population have no public or
private health insurance and many millions more have inadequate coverage.
The present system for reimbursement is procedure oriented and directed and
does not adequately reimburse ambulatory care services. One could project an
increased utilization of health maintenance, guidance, counseling and health
education if ambulatory services were adequately reimbursed.

Utilization of pediatric health care personnel, such as child health associates, physician assistants, and pediatric nurse practitioners, has been shown to be medically and economically sound as a mechanism for delivery of quality health care. Public access to these services provided by nonphysician pediatric health care personnel has increased without a decrease in quality of care. The concept of physician assistants is little more than a decade and a half old. From this concept of health professionals were created who have the problem solving and decision making skills in the area of primary care far exceeding any thoughts conceived at their inception. Child health associates, and other nonphysician primary care practitioners for children, have brought America one step closer to eliminating the gap between pediatric health care needs and other silent demands of America's children.

REFERENCES

1. Advisory Committee on Child Development, Assembly of Behavioral and Social Sciences, National Research Council: *Toward a National Policy for Children and Families.* Washington, D.C., National Academy of Sciences, 1978.
2. Task Force on Pediatric Education, Ambulatory Pediatric Association: *The Future of pediatric education.* Tucson, Arizona, 1978.
3. National Council of Organizations for Children and Youth: *America's Children 1976: a bicentennial assessment.* Washington, D.C., 1976.
4. Carnegie Commission on Higher Education: Higher Education and the Nation's Health: Policies for Medical and Dental Education. McGraw-Hill Co., New York, 1970.
5. Silver, H.K., and Ott, J.E.: Assessment and evaluation of child health associates. *Pediatrics, 67:*1, 1981.
6. Fine, L.L., and Scriven, S.: The CHA: A non-physician primary care practitioner for children. *PAJ, 7:*137, 1977.
7. Fine, L.L., and Moore, V.M.: A successful new primary health care provider in the newborn nursery. *Clin. Pediat., 14:*845, 1975.
8. Silver, H.K., and Ott, J.E.: The child health associate; A new health professional to provide comprehensive health care to children. *Pediatrics, 51:*1, 1973.
9. Fine, L.L., and Silver, H.K.: Comparative diagnostic abilities of child health associate interns and practicing pediatricians. *J. Pediat., 83:*332, 1973.
10. Ott, J.E.: Financial feasibility of child health associates in private practice settings, abstracted. Ambulatory Pediatric Association, San Francisco, April, 1977.
11. Fine, L.L.: The pediatric practice of a child health associate. *Am. J. Dis. Child., 131:*634, 1977.
12. Sheffler, R.: A manpower policy for primary health care. *NEJM, 298:*106, 1978.

Chapter 9

THE MILITARY PHYSICIAN ASSISTANT

HENRY B. PERRY, M.D., Ph.D.

With the escalation of manpower costs and the termination of the physician draft, the concept of appropriately trained non-physicians as providers in primary care in the military is gaining increasing interest and acceptance as a practical policy for medical staffing. Physician assistants constitute one important occupational group currently active in the military, as well as in civilian life, in providing primary medical care with physician supervision. In a previous report (1), the status in 1974 of 99 physician assistants who had graduated from the USAF/USN Physician Assistant Program at Shepard Air Force Base was compared with the status of 840 civilian graduates. Military physician assistants constituted 13% of the physician assistant profession at that time. Military physician assistants were older, had less extensive education but more medical experience prior to beginning physician assistant training. Military physician assistants were more likely to be working in primary care disciplines than were civilians, and they also perceived themselves to have greater patient care responsibility, less physician supervision, lower incomes, and fewer career opportunities than civilian physician assistants. Multivariate analyses of the impact of type of program attended indicated that the USAF/USN Physician Assistant Program produced graduates who performed better, as judged by supervising physician performance evaluations, than did civilian training programs when background characteristics were controlled (2).

The information regarding military physician assistants presented in this chapter arise from an analysis of data from the 1974 and 1978 national surveys of physician assistants (3, 4).

DESCRIPTION OF MILITARY PHYSICIAN ASSISTANTS

The total number of physician assistants working in the military identified by the national surveys in 1974 and 1978 increased from 99 to 670. The overall

percentage of currently active physician assistants who were working in the
military increased from 13.3% in 1974 to 18.2% in 1978.

Table 9.1 compares a number of the background characteristics between
military and civilian physician assistants. As noted in the 1974 survey, military
physician assistants continue to be somewhat older, have more prior medical
experience but less prior formal education, and to be almost exclusively men.
Since 1974, the percentage of military physician assistants who are women has
increased from 0% to 5%. The types of programs attended by physician
assistants are shown in Table 9.2. Eighteen percent of military physician
assistants attended civilian physician assistant programs, while only 2% of
civilian physician assistants attended military programs. The USAF/USN
Physician Assistant Program at Shepard Air Force Base had 353 graduates
participating in this study and the Army Physician Assistant Program, in coordination with Baylor University, 240.

TABLE 9.1

COMPARISON OF BACKGROUND CHARACTERISTICS
OF MILITARY AND CIVILIAN PHYSICIAN ASSISTANTS, 1978

	Military (n = 670)	Civilian (n = 3849)
Average age	37.5	34.3
Percentage who obtained a college degree prior to beginning physician assistant training	22.7%	51.3%
Average number of years of medical experience prior to beginning physician assistant training	12.2	7.3
Percentage who are male	95.0%	65.3%

TABLE 9.2

TYPE OF TRAINING PROGRAM ATTENDED BY MILITARY
AND CIVILIAN PHYSICIAN ASSISTANTS, 1978

Type of Physician Assistant Program Attended	Current Military Status	
	Active Duty (n = 620)	Civilian (n = 3849)
Military (n = 593)	82.1%	2.2%
Civilian (n = 3876)	17.9%	97.8%
	100.0%	100.0%

74 *Alternatives in Health Care Delivery*

The specialties of military and civilian physician assistants are shown in Table 9.3. As in 1974, military physician assistants continue to work almost exclusively in primary care fields, with almost no employment in surgical specialties. Although civilian physician assistants are also concentrated in primary care fields, this is less so than for military physician assistants. The specialty distribution of military physician assistants remains virtually unchanged from than noted in 1974.

The incomes of military and civilian assistants are compared in Table 9.4. Although in 1974 civilian physician assistants earned an average of almost $2,000 more per year than did military physician assistants, by 1978 this difference had been narrowed to just over $1,000. If the dollar value of the fringe benefits were added to "take home pay," the average income for military physician assistants would probably exceed that for civilian physician assistants.

For those 724 physician assistants for whom cohort data are available in 1974 and 1978, their movement in and out of the military can be traced. As Table 9.5 indicates, there has been a net loss of 19 of the original 98 military physician assistants in the cohort between 1974 and 1978. Almost one-third of the original 98 military physician assistants in the cohort left the military to obtain civilian jobs.

TABLE 9.3
COMPARISON OF SPECIALTIES OF MILITARY AND
CIVILIAN PHYSICIAN ASSISTANTS, 1978

Specialty	Military (n = 620)	Civilian (n = 3849)
Primary Care	91.3%	70.3%
Surgical Specialty	0.8	13.8
Medical Subspecialty	4.6	6.4
Other Specialty	3.3	9.5
	100.0%	100.0%

TABLE 9.4
A COMPARISON OF INCOMES FOR MILITARY AND
CIVILIAN PHYSICIAN ASSISTANTS IN 1974 AND 1978

	Average Income 1974	Average Income 1978	Absolute Increase	Percentage Increase
Civilian PAs	$14,543 (n = 791)	$17,611 (n = 3153)	$3,068	20.4%
Military PAs	$12,598 (n = 121)	$16,412 (n = 532)	$3,823	30.4%
Absolute Difference:	$1,954	$1,199		
Percentage Difference:	13.5%	6.8%		

TABLE 9.5
CHANGES IN MILITARY STATUS FOR A COHORT OF 724
PHYSICIAN ASSISTANTS BETWEEN 1974 AND 1978

Military Status in 1974	Civilian	Military	Total
Civilian	616	10	626
Military	29	60	98
	645	79	724

IMPLICATIONS

These findings suggest that the role of the physician assistant in the military, particularly in primary care, is growing in importance. The rationale for developing the physician assistant concept in the military seems quite clear. Military physician assistants are able to provide primary care under supervision without any deterioration in quality (5, 6). The cost savings associated with the substitution of physician assistants for physicians in providing primary care services are substantial, particularly in institutional settings such as the military (7). The policy implications of these observations are quite consequential, especially in view of the fact that the military has difficulty in attracting a sufficient supply of physicians, particularly in primary care. Whether or not the military chooses to establish a pay scale for physician assistants sufficiently attractive to recruit civilian physician assistants remains to be seen (8). Between 1974 and 1978, however, it appears that, if anything, the reverse was true. More physician assistants were leaving the military to take civilian employment than vice versa. The issue of warrant officer status versus commissioned officer status for physician assistants has been under active consideration by all branches of the military. Currently, Air Force physician assistants are fully commissioned officers while those in other services are of the warrant officer type. According to one recent analysis of pay scales for physician assistant in the Air Force:

> The evidence strongly supports the contention that the Air Force can recruit significant numbers of civilian trained PAs (without weakening quality standards) only with commissioning . . . However, the failure of officer pay to even truly achieve comparability with civilian earnings may mean civilian recruiting alone cannot supply enough PAs for Air Force needs (8).

The military cannot afford *not* to invest heavily in the development of the physician assistant concept. The potential cost savings are too great.

The rationale for limiting the involvement of physician assistants in the military almost exclusively to primary care should be questioned. It is becoming increasingly clear that the broadly trained physician assistant can perform a very important role in the care of hospitalized patients. In a growing number of civilian medical institutions in the United States, civilian physician assistants are functioning as junior surgical residents and performing quite effectively (9-11). The utilization of physician assistants in roles of this type could also reduce the numbers of non-primary care physician specialists required in the military.

SUMMARY

The military's commitment to the utilization of physician assistants appears to be increasing. The cost-effectiveness of this new group of health professionals is becoming quite obvious to those with responsibilities for program policies in health care in both the military and the civilian sector. The development of effective pay policies which will ensure career retention among military physician assistants is still being negotiated. Although military physician assistants are now almost exclusively working in primary care fields, the development of roles for these persons in surgical specialties and in medical subspecialties would provide additional financial savings because of the fewer number of specialist physicians that would be required. The enhanced productivity of the supervising physicians and their capacity to devote more time and energy to those complex or challenging patients confronting them could conceivably enhance the professional satisfactions of the surgeons, medical subspecialists and primary care physicians in the military, thereby promoting career retention among them.

REFERENCES

1. Perry, H.B.: A Comparison of Military and Civilian Physician Assistants. *Military Med.*, *143*:763-767, 1978.
2. Perry, H.B.: An Analysis of the Professional Performance of Physician Assistants. *J. Med. Ed.*, *52*:639-647, 1977.
3. Perry, H.B.: Physician Assistants: An Overview of An Emerging Health Profession. *Med. Care*, *15*:982-990, 1977.
4. Perry, H.B., and Fisher, D.W.: The Physician's Assistant Profession: Results of a 1978 Survey of Graduates. *J. Med. Ed.*, *56*:839-845, 1981.
5. Goldberg, G.A., and Jolly, D.G.: *Quality of Care Provided by Physician's Extenders in Air Force Primary Medicine Clinics.* Santa Monica, California, The Rand Corporation, 1980.
6. Goldberg, G.A., Siegal, A.F., Chu, D.S., and Jolly, D.G.: *The Quality of Air Force Outpatient Care: How Well Do Physician Assistants Perform?* Santa Monica, California, The Rand Corporation, 1979.
7. Record, J.C. (ed.): *Staffing Primary Care in 1990: Physician Replacement and Cost Savings.* New York, Springer Publishing Co., 1981.
8. Hosek, S.: *Potential Civilian Earnings of Military Civilian Physician's Assistants.* Santa Monica, California, The Rand Corporation, 1980.

9. Miller, J.I., and Hatcher, C.R.: Physician's Assistants on a University Cardiothoracic Surgical Service: A Five-Year Update. *J. Thorac. Cardiovasc. Surg., 76:*639-642, 1978.
10. Heinrich, J.J., Fichlander, B.C., Benfield, M., *et al.*: The Physician's Assistant as Resident on Surgical Services. *Arch-Surg., 115:*310-314, 1980.
11. Perry, H.B., Detmer, D.E., and Redmond, E.L.: The Current and Future Role of Surgical Physician Assistants. *Ann. Surg., 193:*132-137, 1981.

Chapter 10

CERTIFICATION, REGISTRATION AND LICENSURE OF PHYSICIAN ASSISTANTS

CARL E. FASSER, PA-C
PETER ANDRUS, M.D.
QUENTIN SMITH, M.S.

The 1960's heralded the onset of turbulent times for American society and its health care delivery system. Limited availability of medical care for minorities and other disadvantaged groups accompanied a growing social consciousness with respect to those elements of society that were deprived of basic health care services. The effect of these forces contributed to a greater demand for health services, to complaints about the continued rise in health care costs, and to concern over the supply and geographic distribution of physicians and the trend toward increased specialization in the medical profession.

Criticism of the health care industry, the inability of physicians already in practice to keep pace with the demand for professional services, and the need for more equitable distribution of health care services among socioeconomic groups provided strong support for the argument that there was a "health care crisis" at hand (1). The perceived shortage of physicians prompted the federal government to place greater emphasis on incentives intended to increase the supply (2). Concurrently, closer examination of the potential use of medical auxiliaries was undertaken to determine if such approaches could be applied in the United States with the same positive results that had been attained in other countries.

While addressing a conference on medical education in 1961, Dr. Charles Hudson of the American Medical Association first postulated the notion of creating a category of patient care providers to serve as physician extenders. Dr. Hudson was of the opinion that one could expand the availability of medical services by using trained personnel functioning under the responsibility of the physician (3). While the proposal received somewhat positive support by physicians, it was not until 1965 that the formal training of physician assistants became a reality.

IMPEDIMENTS TO UTILIZATION

The first educational program for physician assistants began at Duke University Medical Center in 1965 with the goal of providing these future nonphysician care providers with an education which would make them competent to assist either a family physician or general internist after graduation (4–6).

The implementation of the physician assistant program raised a number of concerns. Some of these concerns have received considerable attention in the literature over the past decade and a half. Among the major concerns were the importance of defining the physician assistant's future role in the practice setting; assuring the assistant's ability to accept a work role dependent on the physician; assessing the physician's willingness to delegate traditional medical functions to a non-physician, and measuring the ultimate acceptance of the physician assistant by the consumer. The most pressing concern, however, centered around the capacity of the existing health care system with its array of licensure and certification regulations to accommodate the provision of medical services by a nonphysician. The uncertainty accompanying this concern was underscored by at least one case in a western state where the court allowed an inference of negligence to be drawn from the mere fact that a task was delegated to a person not licensed to perform it (7).

AUTHORIZING TASK DELEGATION

In 1965, existing legislation made the provision of health care services by anyone not licensed to provide that service a criminal act. The implications of such legislation for the physician's assistant were obvious. Indeed, in the opinion of Forgotson, Romer and Newman, the problem of delegation of function was "without question, . . . highly significant, if not the most significant problem requiring resolution" (8) among the many problems presented by the medical licensure law. Leff contended that the greatest danger in the use of paramedicals rested in "their unlicensed status" or lack of legal recognition in some way other than licensure (9).

Recognizing that without resolution of the issue of delegation, no overall implementation strategy for the training and use of physician assistants could be implemented, the faculty of the Duke physician assistant program sought a ruling from the Office of the Attorney General's Office of North Carolina as to whether the projected physician-supervised activities of the physician assistant would contravene the licensure laws of the state (10). The ruling, delivered in April 1966, stated that:

> nothing in this article should be construed in any way to prohibit or limit
> performance by any person of such duties as specified mechanical acts in

the personal care of a patient when such care or activities are performed under the orders or direction of a licensed physician, licensed dentist, or registered nurse (11).

While the program operated under the sanction of opinion delivered by the North Carolina Attorney General's Office, it was understood that the opinion was merely advisory and that the legal implications of using physician assistants to provide health care services would require further exploration. At about the same point in time, several states enacted general delegatory statutes to support physicians who became involved in litigation in which the delegation of tasks was at issue (12-14). Oklahoma's exemption statute is typical of these statutes and provided that:

> . . . (N)othing in this article shall be so construed as to prohibit . . . services rendered by a physician's trained assistant, a registered nurse, or a licensed practical nurse if such services be rendered under the direct supervision and control of a licensed physician (15).

These statutes recognized the physician's authority to delegate tasks. It had previously been assumed that such authority was available to the physician, although no legal sanctions were explicit prior to passage of these statutes. Passage of these statutes early in the evolution of the physician assistant concept also facilitated the establishment of physician assistant training programs in Colorado, Kansas and Oklahoma.

THE MODEL LEGISLATION PROJECT

As the Duke physician assistant program began sending graduates out into the world, physicians and lawyers expressed concern that utilization of the unlicensed physician assistant would result in increased risk of civil and criminal liability on the physician's part. Under the doctrine of *respondeat superior,* the physician is liable for the negligent actions of anyone in his employ or, in some cases, for the actions of a person who, though employed by another, is acting at his direction (16). By itself, this doctrine did not seem to unduly inhibit the use of physician assistants and served the useful function of giving the employer a personal stake in the quality of care delivered by his assistant (17).

Of more concern was the application of the doctrine of negligence *per se,* which holds that liability inheres where an injury results from an act committed in violation of a statute, regardless of whether *actual* negligence is involved (18). Additionally, it was felt that even if the physician assistant was not negligent, the delegation itself could be found improper (19).

A series of conferences were held in October 1969 and March 1970 at Duke University to discuss the merits of various proposals for the legal recognition of physician assistants. The conferences were made possible through funding provided by DHEW (now DHHS) for a "Legal Study on Health Manpower Innovations" under the directions of Martha Ballenger, J.D. and E. Harvey Estes, Jr., M.D. The final recommendations resulting from these conferences incorporated the features of three proposals. Major points of these proposals called for: licensure of users of physician assistants (20); promulgation by the state board of medical examiners or by a committee on manpower innovations of standards and regulations to govern the use of physician assistants; and enactment of a general exception statute (21) which, when part of the medical practice act of a state, would exempt:

> Any act, task or function performed by an assistant to a physician licensed by the Board of Medical Examiners, provided that
> (a) Such assistant is approved by the Board as one qualified by training or experience to function as an assistant to a physician, and
> (b) Such act, task or function is performed at the direction and under the supervision of such physician, in accordance with rules and regulations promulgated by the Board (22).

Adoption of the recommendations left the regulation of the category physician assistant to the medical profession, with control being exerted by both organized medicine, through the Board of Medical Examiners, and by the individual physician employer.

A MORATORIUM ON THE LICENSURE OF NEW HEALTH PROFESSIONALS

As first envisioned, the sphere of activities for the physician assistant encompassed all those areas in which physicians provided care: office, clinic, hospital, patient's home, operating room or nursing home. This degree of practice latitude was felt essential to facilitate, through proper delegation and responsible supervision, the effective use of the physician assistant's exceptionally broad range of skills. Because this level of involvement in the delivery of health care was unique (no other nonphysician provider functioned in such a broad fashion), the discussions concerning how best to accommodate the physician assistant became the subject of national interest.

As if these concerns were not enough, the physician assistant arrived on the scene at a time when licensure practices for all health professionals were being questioned. Enacted in the twentieth century to protect the public from quacks and incompetent practitioners, licensure laws were increasingly viewed as barriers to educational advancement, effective task delegation, and innovation in the use of health manpower. Further, they had failed to solve the problems of the incompetent or unethical practitioner (23–24). Consistent with the views of most knowledgeable observers of the scene, these conclusions appeared in position statements on the licensure of health professionals prepared in 1970 by the American Medical Association (25) and the American Hospital Association (26).

A moratorium on the licensure of additional health occupations was urged following a June 1971 Report on Licensure and Related Health Personnel Credentialing (27) issued by the Department of Health Education and Welfare, which had reached similar conclusions. The proposed moratorium further emphasized the need for a "proper umbrella for the delegation of medical tasks for physician assistants" (28), a view shared by the National Advisory Commission on Health Manpower (29).

STATE CODIFICATION OF DELEGATORY AUTHORITY

With the AMA, AHA, and DHEW recommendations urging individual states to enact amendments to their medical practice acts to codify the *Physician's* right to delegate tasks to nonphysician care providers, the stage was set for action. The initial statutory enactments affecting the physician's use of a physician assistant were met with mixed reviews. While Silver (30) thought the Child Health Associate Law (CHA) enacted in Colorado in 1969 was innovative, it was described by Curran (31) as "what should not be done with any licensed group of professionals." In 1970, California became the second state to enact legislation specific to physician assistants through the use of a registration act rather than a licensing law. To implement the enabling statute, the state required the Board of Medical Examiners to approve educational programs for assistants, the qualification of assistants, and the physicians expecting to use physician assistants (32).

To date, some 45 states have incorporated amendments to their medical practice acts to facilitate the use of physician assistants. The only states which have not yet enacted either regulatory or delegatory legislation are Kentucky, Minnesota, Mississippi, Missouri and New Jersey. Legislation is currently pending in three of these states, excluding Minnesota and New Jersey (33, 34). As reflected in Figure 10.1, the early trend of legislatively defining the physician's authority to delegate has largely been overtaken and replaced by legislative enactments which regulate physician assistants.

States which have enacted the general delegatory exception to the medical practice act include, Colorado, Connecticut, Delaware, the District of Columbia, Hawaii, Maryland, New Hampshire, North Carolina, North Dakota, South Carolina, Tennessee, Texas, Utah and Virginia. In a number of instances, a particular state agency, usually the board of medical examiners, is charged with devising administrative rules and regulations to guide the physician's employment and use of a physician assistant.

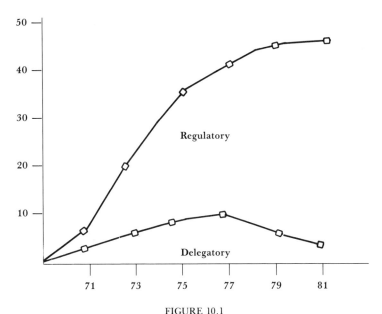

FIGURE 10.1
ENACTED LEGISLATION GOVERNING PA UTILIZATION

Source: Miller and Byrne 1978 and
American Academy of Physician Assistants 1981.

The laws enacted in most other states provides more regulatory framework permitting the performance of medical services by physician assistants within the state. These more comprehensive statutes typically provide for a mechanism for registering/certifying individuals as physician assistants, specifying the degree of supervision necessary, delineating the scope of clinical privileges and approving educational programs (see Table 10.1) (35).

As can be seen in Table 10.1, the majority of the 45 states require graduation from an approved physician assistant program. The process of programmatic accreditation, as formulated by the Committee on Allied Health Education and Accreditation (CAHEA) and specified in the "Essentials of an Approved Educational Program for the Assistant to the Primary Care Physician" and adopted by the organizations sponsoring the accreditation process, is recognized both in statute and the administrative rules associated with delegatory legislation. In such states as California and Michigan, however, a separate process of program approval has been established (36).

TABLE 10.1
OVERVIEW OF ENABLING PHYSICIAN ASSISTANT LEGISLATION

Characteristics	Number of States Requiring
State registration	38
Approval of physician supervisor	37
Graduation from approved program	35
National credentialing of proficiency	33
Specific delineation of privileges	28
Limited prescriptive privileges	14
Continuing medical education	10
Specific MD/PA ratio	37

STATE REGISTRATION

Most states require physician assistants to meet several criteria in order to be covered by the statute(s) governing physician assistants' involvement in the provision of health care. The process typically involves the completion of an application to be submitted to the examining board that includes proof of graduation from an approved program, possession of or evidence of eligibility for professional certification, submission of a recent photograph and registration fee, information on the prospective physician employer, a description of the proposed job description, and the nature of the responsible supervision to be applied to the physician assistant's activities. Where an alternate supervisor is to be used in the absence of the primary physician, the alternate physician must also be identified.

The delineation of clinical privileges approved for physician assistants as reflected in the various state statutes suggests involvement in a broad range of activities. The most frequently approved privileges include: obtaining a complete and accurate history; conducting a physical examination; performing routine procedures, such as urinary catherizations, injections and immunizations, venipuncture, and electrocardiography; and performing minor surgical procedures, such as removal of foreign bodies from the skin and suturing minor lacerations. In 14 states, the physician assistant has been extended limited prescriptive privileges, excluding prescription of controlled substances and parenteral preparations except insulin.

Along with granting of certain privileges, most boards also hold the right to terminate state registration for charges such as impersonating a physician, providing services without supervision, attempting tasks beyond the scope of the physician assistant's role, habitual use of intoxicants or drugs, felony convictions, mental incompetence or failure to comply with guiding regulations in the state. There are also limitations in the range of delegable tasks to include certain vision care functions (37), acupuncture, engaging in chiropractic, and billing patients for services provided.

Finally, in those states granting circumscribed health care delivery privileges to physician assistants, there exists a secondary form of registration. This process is internal and consists of maintaining lists of all certified physician assistants, those physician assistants approved to function in the state and physicians approved to employ and supervise a physician assistant.

THE CONFUSION IN TERMINOLOGY

Even as states were enacting delegatory and/or regulatory legislation, there continued to be confusion in the minds of many concerning the term "physician assistant." The label had come to represent a wide variety of support personnel from physicians' office and clerical aides to persons receiving postgraduate education as highly trained professionals. Not until publication of the National Academy of Sciences (NAS) report, *New Members of the Physician's Health Team: Physician's Assistants* (38) was any serious, wide scale attempt made to categorize the various levels of physician assistants.

The NAS identified three levels of physician assistants which they referred to as Types A, B, and C, according to their degree of specialization and the level of judgement involved. The Type A assistant is defined by the report as:

> capable of approaching the patient, collecting historical and physical data, and presenting them in such a way that the physician can visualize the medical problem and determine appropriate diagnostic or therapeutic steps (39).

Several months after the National Academy of Sciences published its definitive report, the American Medical Association officially, though vaguely, defined a physician assistant as:

> a skilled person qualified by academic and practical on-the-job training to provide services under the supervision and direction of a licensed physician who is responsible for the performance of that assistant (40).

While these definitions were somewhat generic, when taken together, they specified accountability by the physician and distinguished the Type A physician assistant from other trained assistants to physicians by an ability to integrate and interpret findings on the basis of general medical knowledge.

The "Description of the Occupation," included within the educational essentials adopted in 1971 for use in the review and accreditation of physician assistant training programs, did much to clarify the physician assistant's practice role while simultaneously approaching some degree of standardization in the nomenclature used by programs and their graduates. The role of the physician assistant was to include, but not limited to:

The initial approach to a patient of any age group in any setting to elicit a detailed and accurate history, perform an appropriate physical examination, and record and present pertinent data in a manner meaningful to the physician;

Performance and/or assistance in performance of routine laboratory and related studies as appropriate for a specific practice setting, such as the drawing of blood samples, performance of urinalyses, and the taking of electrocardiographic tracings;

Performance of such routine therapeutic procedures as injections, immunizations, and the suturing and care of wounds;

Instruction and counseling of patients regarding physical and mental health on matters such as diets, disease, therapy, and normal growth and development;

Assisting the physician in the hospital setting by making patient rounds, recording patient progress notes accurately and appropriately, transcribing and/or executing standing orders and other specific orders at the direction of the supervising physician, and compiling and recording detailed narrative case summaries;

Providing assistance in the delivery of services to patients requiring continuing care (home, nursing home, extended care facilities, etc.) including the review and monitoring of treatment and therapy plans;

Independent performance of evaluative and treatment procedures essential to provide an appropriate response to life-threatening emergency situations, and;

Facilitation of the physician's referral of appropriate patients by maintenance of an awareness of the community's various health facilities, agencies, and resources (41).

Concerned more with liability than with nomenclature and role responsibilities, hospitals, boards of medical examiners, physicians and other agencies, began to look for appropriate credentialing procedures by which to identify the incompetent or fraudulent physician assistant.

EARLY ATTEMPTS TO IDENTIFY COMPETENCE

In recognition of the need to deal with the diversity of educational experiences provided students and the subsequent range of skills they would bring to the physician's practice, the AMA was approached in 1969 and asked to adopt at least tentative educational guidelines that could lead to the responsible development of the emerging physician assistant profession. With the AMA remaining unresponsive, the leaders of three university-based physician assistant programs founded the American Registry of Physicians' Associates (42). Its purposes were to provide a mechanism for accrediting Type A physician assistant programs and registering those who had either graduated from such programs or those who, through education and experience, were able to function in the capacity of a Type A physician assistant.

With the need for a nationally accepted physician assistant credentialing process finally recognized, in 1971 the AMA directed its Council on Health Manpower to promote the development of a national program of certification for the assistant to the primary care physician (43). The use of national certification was felt to facilitate greater geographic mobility, provide the physician employer with some evidence of competency, and permit greater flexibility than state licensure. The National Board of Medical Examiners (NBME) agreed to collaborate with the AMA on development of the needed examination (44). The NMBE appeared to be the best available resource to develop the examination, since it not only had considerable experience in medical and psychological testing, but was also independent of the educational system, employers of medical personnel, and the medical profession. Additionally, it was felt that, because of the relationship between the physician and the physician assistant, a parallel credentialing process would be beneficial.

Initial efforts were aimed at defining skills physician assistants would be expected to possess, based upon the frequency with which these skills would be used and "criticalness" of the skill to the delivery of optimum health care. Some 900 tasks were screened and organized into areas representing various components of the clinical problem solving process. The identified core skills served as the basis for determining the content and methodology for the certifying examination. The first such national certifying examination, developed under a federal contract with the DHEW Division of Allied Health Manpower (45) was administered to some 880 persons on December 12, 1973.

NATIONAL CERTIFICATION COMMISSION

It was the consensus of opinion among parties involved that any ongoing mechanism to certify physician assistants should be responsive to and have input from not only the profession itself but from other groups such as the educational institutions, potential employers, closely allied nonphysician professionals and regulatory agencies. It was determined that the most appropriate vehicle to facilitate this process would involve the creation of a new, free-standing agency incorporating policy representation from appropriately concerned groups, but dominated by no one organization.

On September 8, 1973, the AMA's Council on Health Manpower transmitted, in a letter to the AMA's Board of Trustees, a proposal for the establishment of a "National Commission on Certification of Physician Assistants." With the concurrence of the Board of Trustees, an invitational meeting sponsored by the AMA was held in Chicago on November 28, 1973, to discuss the formation of the Commission (46). The purpose of the proposed national certifying body was to:

> safeguard patients and potential employers by maintaining high professional and ethical standards in the profession of physician assistants through recognition of those achieving and maintaining appropriate knowledge and skill in the field, and to safeguard properly qualified workers by providing them nationally validated evidence of their competency thus facilitating geographic and career mobility.

In 1974, the National Commission on Certification of Physicians' Assistants (NCCPA) was organized and, shortly thereafter, assumed responsibility for the administration of the 1975 and subsequent Certifying Examinations. The NCCPA is comprised of individuals from the following organizations:

American Academy of Family Physicians
American Academy of Pediatrics
American Academy of Physician's Assistants
American College of Physicians
American College of Surgeons
American Hospital Association
American Medical Association
American Nurses Association
American Society of Internal Medicine
Association of American Medical Colleges
Association of Physician's Assistants Programs
Federation of State Medical Boards of United States
National Board of Medical Examiners
United States Department of Defense

In addition, three Directors-at-Large, one physician knowledgeable about health manpower, and two public representatives, are chosen by the other membership.

The NCCPA's major responsibilities associated with the national credentialing process involve: determination of criteria for eligibility; review of applications and registration of candidates; development of the exam through subcontract to NBME; determination of pass/fail standards; issuance and verification of certificates; recertification of persons demonstrating continued competence; publication of lists of physician assistants certified each year for each state.

Functioning as outlined since its formation, the NCCPA has examined more than 13,000 persons (see Table 10.2). The number of people taking the written and psychomotor components of the credentialing examination had increased dramatically until about 1976, but have since leveled off. This stabilization in the numbers closely mirrors the overall number of students graduating annually from the physician assistant training programs.

TABLE 10.2
PROFILE OF CANDIDATE PERFORMANCE ON CERTIFYING EXAMINATION*

Years Taken	Number of Candidates	Number Passing	Percentage Failing
1973	880	770	12.5
1974	1303	1089	16.4
1975	1411	1129	20.0
1976	1615	1286	20.4
1977	1639	1289	20.9
1978	1649	1255	22.6
1979	1665	1276	21.9
1980	1781	1371	23.0
1981	1770	1363	23.0

*National Commission on Certification of Physician Assistants.

CONTINUING MEDICAL EDUCATION

Recognition that changes both inside and outside the profession gave rise to doubts about the permanence of qualifying standards for professional certification, coupled with an awareness of the need to be accountable to the public, the American Academy of Physician Assistants (AAPA), the professional organization of physician assistants, adopted a policy of mandatory continuing education for its members. The requirement called for each physician assistant to amass 100 hours of continued learning over two years. The nature of the continued learning experience was subject to approval by the AAPA before credit would be granted.

Discussions within the NCCPA regarding the reexamination intervals and criteria for the reregistration of certificates held by practicing physician assistants led to a collaborative agreement with the AAPA concerning the acquisition of continuing medical education as a means of demonstrating eligibility for reregistration of one's certificates every two years. Eligibility to do so is based on reporting to NCCPA of at least 100 hours of approved CME credits. At the end of three periods of reregistration, the physician assistant is expected to participate in a process of recertification by written examination as a means of demonstrating continued competence.

SUMMARY AND IMPLICATIONS

The concept of a formally trained assistant to the physician reached fruition in 1965 with the opening of the first training program to prepare physician assistants. The concept was borne out of an identified shortage and geographic maldistribution of primary health care providers.

The issue of the credentialing of physician assistants was of great concern to physician assistants, physicians, hospitals, and other employers. The 1971 moratorium on licensure of new health occupations, urged by the Department of Health, Education and Welfare, as well as the American Hospital Association and American Medical Association, effectively eliminated licensure as a potential credentialing mechanism for the physician assistant. State legislatures, however, initiated amendments to state medical practice acts to reduce barriers to further task delegation to nonphysicians. While these amendments paved the way for physician assistants to deliver health care services, pressure for some universal means for determining minimum competency continued to mount. In response to the pressure, the National Board of Medical Examiners, in collaboration with the AMA, set about to develop an examination process which might be of value in recognizing the competent assistant. The first of these examinations was administered in 1973 and was designed to measure competency in gathering information, synthesizing that information, interpreting patient data, and performing other tasks essential to the delivery of optimal health care services. Since 1973, more than 13,000 physician assistants have taken the national certifying examination.

Pressure for credentialing of physician assistants also influenced the nomenclature used to describe this new health practitioner and the system(s) used to train them. The push to standardize the physician assistants' educational process resulted in the 1971 adoption of minimum education standards for use in a process of programmatic accreditation by the AMA in collaboration with other physician groups. In a number of states, both the certification and accreditation mechanisms have been incorporated into statutes governing the activities of physician assistants. While some flexibility with respect to qualifications remains, most states have adopted policies which specify minimum requirements for entry into the profession. The requirements include graduation from an approved physician assistant training program and evidence of competency as demonstrated by successful performance on a national certifying examination. This trend toward more stringent entry requirements suggests that, in the future, only those physician assistants who come from formal educational programs and successfully complete the certifying examination will be allowed to deliver health care services as an assistant to the physician.

Another trend that has been observed, with respect to the use of physician assistants, has been the trend toward specialization. Just as the medical profession has become increasingly specialized, the physician assistant has found opportunities to more narrowly focus his or her skills and abilities. Currently, specialty training opportunities exist for the surgeon's assistant, and programs to train orthopedic and urologic physician's assistants have been operational, though the AMA withdrew accreditation from these last two programs in 1974 and 1977 respectively. Many would argue that specialization for the physician assistant would run directly counter to what this health care provider was originally intended to do—increase access to primary health care. These people would argue that the physician assistant should be assuming greater responsibility in health education, preventive health care, and health promotion, and leave specialized care to the physician specialist. Compelling arguments can be developed both for and against specialization for physician assistants.

The final outcome of the "specialization" issue could have significant impact on the certification process. The current certification process is intended to measure proficiency in certain core skills essential to the primary care provider. Should the trend toward specialization continue, specialized certification components would need to be added to the basic certification examination to document competence in the more narrowly focused practice area that the physician assistant had chosen. This development would parallel the process extant in the medical profession, in which the practitioner first must become licensed as a physician and then complete requirements for specialty certification.

The physician assistant profession is in its adolescence. Great strides have been taken with respect to credentialing, both in terms of enabling legislation at the state level, and the certification process at the national level. What the future will bring with regard to state licensure, specialty certification, and the ensuing changes that might occur in the certification process, one can only speculate. It is certain, however, that in a profession born in the midst of great controversy and debate, the credentialing issues which will be faced in the future will be carefully examined and most likely resolved through compromise.

REFERENCES

1. Hogness, J.R.: Why the Crisis: An Overview. In: *The Crisis in Health Profession's Strategy.* National Health Council, New York, November 1981, p. 9.
2. *Ibid.*, p. 10.
3. Hudson, C.: Expansion of medical professional services with non-professional personnel. *JAMA, 176:*95–97, 1961.
4. Stead, E.: The Duke plan for physician's assistants. *Med. Times, 95:*40–48, 1967.
5. Estes, E.H., and Howard, D.R.: Potential for new classes of personnel: Experiences of the Duke Physician's Assistant Program. *J. Med. Educ., 95:*149–155, 1970.

6. Carter, R.D., and Gifford, J.F.: The emergence of the physician assistants profession. In: *Physician Assistants: Their Contributions to Health Care.*, Perry, H.B. and Breitner, B. (eds.). New York, Human Sciences Press, Inc., 1982, pp. 25-26.

7. *Barber v. Reinking,* 68 Wash. 2d 122, 411 P.2d. 861 (1966).

8. Forgotson, E.H., Roemer, R., and Newman, R.W.: Legal regulation of health personnel in the United States. In: *Report of the National Advisory Committee on Health Manpower.* Washington, D.C., Government Printing Office, 1967, p. 332.

9. Leff, A.A.: Medical devices and paramedical personnel: a preliminary contact for emerging problems. *Washington U.L.Q., 332:*332-399, 1967, p. 395.

10. Ballenger, M.D., and Estes, E.H.: Model legislation project for physician's assistants. Durham, Department of Community Health Sciences, 1969.

11. Carter, R.D., and Gifford, J.F.: supra, note 6 at p. 26.

12. *Arizona Rev. Stat.* Section 32-1421, September 1969.

13. *Colorado Rev. Stat.* Section 91-1-6(3) (M) 1963.

14. *Kansas Rev. Stat.* Section 65-2872 (g) 1964.

15. *Oklahoma Stat.:* Title 59 Section 492. Supplement 1968-69.

16. Rabon v. Rowan Memorial Hospital, Inc. 269 N.C. 1,152 S.E. 2d 499 (1967).

17. Collins, C.M., and Bonnyman, G.G.: *Physician's Assistants and Nurse Associates: A review.* Washington, D.C., Institute for the Study of Health and Society, January 1971, p. 24.

18. Leff: supra, note 9 at p. 363.

19. Leff: supra, note 9 at p. 366.

20. Hershey, N.: An alternative to mandatory licensure of health professionals. *Hospital Progress, 50:*71-74, 1969.

21. Ballenger, M.D., and Estes, E.H.: supra, note 10 at pp. 18-21.

22. Ballenger, M.D., and Estes, E.H.: supra, note 10 at p. 38.

23. Forgotson, E., Bradley, C., and Ballenger, M.: Health services for the poor—the manpower problem: Innovations and the law. *Wisconsin Law Review, 3:*756-789, 1970.

24. Leff: supra, note 9 at pp. 332-413.

25. American Medical Association, Council on Health Manpower, House of Delegates: *Licensure of Health Occupations,* adopted November 8, 1970.

26. American Hospital Association, Special Committee on Licensure of Health Personnel: *Statement on Licensure of Health Personnel,* adopted December 1970.

27. Department of Health, Education and Welfare: *Report on Licensure and Related Health Personnel,* June 1971.

28. Sadler, A.M., Sadler, B.L., and Bliss, A.A.: *The Physician's Assistant: Today and Tomorrow.* Yale University Press, New Haven, 1972, p. 95.

29. *Report of the National Advisory Commission on Health Manpower,* Volume II (1967), p. 332.

30. Silver, H.: New allied health professionals: Implications of the Colorado Child Health Associate Law. *N. Engl. J. Med., 284:*304-307, 1971.

31. Curran, W.: New paramedical personnel—to license or not to license? *N. Engl. J. Med., 228:*1085-1086, 1970.

32. *California Business and Professions Code.* Division 2. Healing Arts, Chapter 13.7, Article 1, General Provisions, Section 1399:504-506, 1977.

33. Fasser, C.E.: Credentialing in the PA Profession. *Physician Assistant/Health Practitioner, 5:*64, 68, 1980.

34. American Medical Association, Legislative Department: *State Health Legislation Report: Allied Health Practitioners,* Volume 6, No. 3, Chicago, September 1978.

35. Fasser, C., and Anderson, S.: *Legislative Handbook: Summary of State Legislation.* American Academy of Physician Assistants, Arlington, May 1981.
36. Fasser, C., and Anderson, S.: *Ibid.,* see note 35 at p. 2.
37. American Medical Association: supra, see note 34 at p. 4.
38. National Academy of Sciences, Board of Medicine: *New Members of the Physician's Health Team: Physician's Assistants:* Washington, D.C., May 1970.
39. National Academy of Sciences: *Ibid.,* May 1970, p. 3.
40. American Medical Association, Council on Medical Education: *Essentials of an Accredited Educational Program for the Assistant to the Primary Care Physician.* Chicago, 1971.
41. American Medical Association: *Ibid.,* 1971, pp. 1-2.
42. Howard, D.R.: The History, Utility and Greater Advantages of the Term "Physician's Associate." *Physician's Associate, 2.1*:4-5, January 1972.
43. Todd, M.C.: *Proposed National Certification of Physician's Assistants by Uniform Examinations.* Paper presented at Federation of State Medical Boards of the United States, February 4, 1972, p. 8.
44. National Board of Medical Examiners: A National Program for Certifying Physician's Assistants. *The National Board Examiner, 20*:1-4, 1972.
45. Confrey, E.A.: Physician Extenders: A Review of the Field in Relationship to DHEW Roles. U.S. Department of Health, Education and Welfare, Health Resources Administration, March 1974.
46. Minutes, Special Organizational Meeting on Proposal for National Commission on Certification of Physician's Assistants, American Medical Association, Chicago, November 29, 1973, p.1.

Chapter 11

PHYSICIAN ASSISTANTS WORKING IN SURGERY: AN OVERVIEW

HENRY B. PERRY, M.D.
REGINALD D. CARTER, Ph.D

The concept of physician assistants working in surgery has evolved *considerably* from that of a technician trained in a narrow scope to that of a mature professional functioning with the responsibility and judgement of a junior level general surgical resident. This rather remarkable evolution over the past several years has occurred because of the outstanding abilities demonstrated by physician assistants in tasks considered initially to be far beyond their capability. In spite of this marked role expansion within surgery, it must nevertheless be emphasized that no practice settings allow the functioning of surgical physician assistants without the close supervision and legal authorization of a practicing surgeon.

BACKGROUND

In the late 1960's, a number of training programs were developed for physician assistants in specific surgical subspecialties such as orthopedics, urology, and ophthalmology. The programs were narrow in scope because they were organized, administered, and taught exclusively by personnel within the surgical subspecialty of a medical center or medical school. Emphasis was placed on technical skills and not on general knowledge and judgement. Because federal funding became limited to programs training primary care physician assistants and because of the limited skills these surgical physician assistants were perceived to possess, these programs fell into disfavor and most were discontinued. An exception was the Surgeon's Assistant Program at the University of Alabama at Birmingham where a rigorous two-year training program provided surgeon's assistants with a broad set of patient care and technical surgical skills which made them highly attractive to surgeon employers. The Surgeon's Assistant concept has been highly regarded and quite successful. The overwhelming majority of physician assistants who work in surgical specialties today, however, are graduates of primary care physician assistant programs. For instance, the 1981 survey of physician assistants identified 589 physician assistants working in surgery. Ninety-nine of these (17%) were graduates of the three Surgeon's Assistant Programs currently in existence. The view is commonly held that training in primary care is highly appropriate for the physician assistant who obtains employment in a surgical field (see Chapter 13). The broad exposure to general patient management provides a strong basis for considerable responsibility in patient care. The particular technical skills required can be acquired quickly within this general framework of broader medical knowledge.

In a 1979 survey of 552 Chairmen in departments of surgery in hospitals of more than 400 beds throughout the United States, surgical physician assistants were found to be working in a third of these institutions (1). In those hospitals where surgical physician assistants were working, two-thirds of the department chairmen felt that patient care had been improved, and only 2% felt that patient care had been adversely affected following the introduction of surgical physician assistants. Among the 120 hospitals with both surgical housestaff and surgical physician assistants, almost half (45%) of the surgical department chairmen felt that the quality of surgical housestaff training had improved, while only 3% felt that housestaff training had been adversely affected. The beneficial effect on housestaff training can be attributed to the capacity of surgical physician assistants to handle routine, time-consuming tasks which have lost their educational value for surgical housestaff.

CURRENT STATUS

The 1981 Association of Physician Assistant Programs' survey of the physician assistant profession identified 589 persons working primarily in a surgical specialty. We estimate that currently approximately 1,500–1,600 physician assistants are working in surgical specialties. This estimate is derived by assuming that there are 12,000 to 12,750 active physician assistants in the United States. Ninety-five percent of these work primarily in patient care, and 13% of those working in patient care are working in surgery.

PROFESSIONAL PRACTICE CHARACTERISTICS

Eighty percent of surgical physician assistants are working in one of three surgical specialties: general surgery, orthopedic surgery, or cardiothoracic surgery (see Table 11.1). Of these 589 surgical physician assistants, 68% work primarily in hospital settings. The remainder work primarily in office (28%) or other (4%) settings. For the 480 surgical physician assistants working at least part-time in hospital settings, almost half (45%) work primarily in the operating room, and 43% work primarily with inpatients on the wards. A small percentage work primarily in ambulatory or emergency room care (see Table 11.2).

Surgical physician assistants earn approximately $1,000 more than physician assistants working in other fields ($22,942 vs $21,781). Thirteen percent of surgical physician assistants had worked as an operating room technician prior to entering physician assistant training.

TABLE 11.1

SUBSPECIALTIES OF SURGICAL PHYSICIAN ASSISTANTS, 1981

Surgical Subspecialty	Percentage (n = 589)
General Surgery	37.3
Orthopedic Surgery	23.6
Cardiothoracic Surgery	19.2
Neurosurgery	6.6
Urology	5.8
Plastic Surgery	3.0
Otolaryngology	2.9
Ophthalmology	1.6
	100.0

TABLE 11.2

MAJOR SITE OF HOSPITAL WORK FOR SURGICAL PHYSICIAN ASSISTANTS
WHO SPEND AT LEAST PART OF THEIR TIME IN HOSPITAL SETTINGS

In-Hospital Site	Percent (n = 480)
Operating Room	45.0
Inpatient Wards	43.3
Ambulatory Care	7.9
Emergency Room	1.9
Other	1.9
	100.0

As one might expect, surgical physician assistants are more likely to locate in urban areas than non-surgical physician assistants (see Table 11.3). There are some notable differences in regional distribution between surgical and non-surgical physician assistants. Surgical physician assistants possess a greater relative concentration in the Northeast and a smaller relative concentration in

the West than non-surgical physician assistants (see Table 11.4). This is probably related to the fact that eastern medical centers such as Yale, Johns Hopkins, Tufts-New England Medical Center, Montefiore, and Duke have been
leaders in developing roles for surgical physician assistants, while the concept
still remains relatively new in the West.

TABLE 11.3
COMMUNITY SIZE IN WHICH SURGICAL AND
NON-SURGICAL PHYSICIAN ASSISTANTS WORK

Community Size	Percentage of Surgical Physician Assistant (n = 582)	Percentage of Non-Surgical Physician Assistant (n = 4173)
Greater than 250,000	48.8	32.6
50–250,000	24.8	17.8
10–50,000	20.7	20.8
Less than 10,000	5.7	28.8
	100.0	100.0

TABLE 11.4
REGIONAL LOCATION OF SURGICAL AND NON-SURGICAL PHYSICIAN ASSISTANTS

Region	Percentage of Surgical Physician Assistants (n = 579)	Percentage of Non-surgical Physical Assistants (n = 4161)
West	6.6	19.4
North Central	18.3	19.7
South Central	11.2	14.9
South East	29.5	22.3
North East	34.4	21.2
Overseas/Shipboard	0.0	2.5
	100.0	100.0

THE DEMAND FOR SURGICAL PHYSICIAN ASSISTANTS

Although the percentage of physician assistants working in surgical specialties has not increased since 1974, the number of physician assistants working in surgical fields continues to grow yearly. In a 1979 national survey of
surgical department chairmen in hospitals with more than 400 beds, the utilization of surgical physician assistants was expected to almost double by 1984
(1). It is anticipated that surgical and labor-intensive high technology
specialties such as cardiothoracic and orthopedic surgery constitute fruitful

areas for increased physician assistant utilization. As technological advances make new operations feasible and increase the demand for time-consuming patient care activities, a need arises particularly for the supportive services of surgical housestaff. The time-consuming activities are not so much the actual operation as the preoperative and postoperative care of the surgical patient.

With the growth of coronary artery bypass surgery, surgical housestaff have been insufficient in number in many institutions to meet the need for assistance in the operating room and, more importantly, in the care of the patient during the early critical postoperative period. Furthermore, increasing numbers of hospitals without surgical housestaff have established open-heart surgical programs which rely upon surgical physician assistants for this important physician-support activity.

The percentage of foreign medical graduates (FMGS) among surgical housestaff in New York City has been as high as 40%, and FMGs constitute a majority of the housestaff in half of New York City teaching hospitals (4). In New York City, the demand for physician assistants to function as surgical house officers (and to function as house officers in other specialties) has risen sharply with the growing inability of medical institutions there to fill housestaff positions with physicians, foreign or otherwise.

The favorable experience of physician assistants working in surgical specialties has led to proposals to consider reducing the numbers of physicians training in overpopulated surgical specialties and medical subspecialties, and utilize physician assistants for the provision of many of the patient care responsibilities previously provided by physician housestaff in these specialties (5, 6). Surgical physician assistants have also made it possible for busy surgical practitioners to expand their patient volume without diminishing the quality of services. By serving as a liaison between the surgeon, the nursing staff, and the patient, communication is facilitated. Improved satisfaction of all health team members *and* of the patient is frequently observed.

The long-term career viability of surgery as a specialty for physician assistants remains to be established. In a cohort study of 516 physician assistants between 1974 and 1978, 21 of the 91 physician assistants working in surgery in 1974 were no longer working in surgery four years later (7). The work hours tend to be quite long for surgical physician assistants, and evening, night, or weekend on-call responsibilities frequently are required.

CONCLUSION

The implication of the very favorable experience of physician assistants working in surgical specialties is only now beginning to be understood. It can be anticipated that both practicing surgeons and hospitals will increasingly come to see advantages in incorporating surgical physician assistants into the web and fabric of surgical patient care.

REFERENCES

1. Perry, H.B., D.E. Detmer, and E.L. Redmond: The Current and Future Role of Surgical Physician Assistants: Report of a National Survey of Surgical Chairmen in Large U.S. Hospitals. *Annals of Surgery, 193:*132-137, 1981.

2. Goodman, L.J., and L.E. Wunderman: Foreign Medical Graduate and Graduate Medical Education. *Journal of the American Medical Association, 246:*854-858.

3. Perry, H.B., and D.E. Detmer: Factors Affecting the Demand for Surgical Physician Assistants. *Public Health Reports* (in press).

4. Way, P.O., L.E. Jenson, and L.J. Goodman: Foreign Medical Graduates and the Issue of Substantial Description of Medical Services. *New England Journal of Medicine, 299:*745-751, 1978.

5. Perry, H.B., and B. Breitner: The Physician Assistant's Future Role in Non-Primary Care Fields. In: *Physician Assistants: Their Contributions To Health Care.* New York, Human Sciences Press, 1981, pp. 235-256.

6. Detmer, D.E., and H.B. Perry: The Utilization of Surgical Physician Assistants: Policy Implications for the Future. *Surgical Clinics of North America, 62:*669-675, 1982.

7. Perry, H.B., and E.L. Redmond: Career Trends Among Physician Assistants: *Physician Assistant* (in press).

Chapter 12

THE SURGEON'S ASSISTANT CONCEPT

J. GARBER GALBRAITH, M.D., F.A.C.S.
MARGARET K. KIRKLIN, M.D.
ARNOLD B. DIETHELM, M.D., F.A.C.S.
M.I. CULPEPPER, JR., LL.B.
JACQUELINE HALL, S.A.
JOHN W. KIRKLIN, M.D., F.A.C.S.

HISTORY

When the first physician assistant program was initiated by Dr. Eugene Stead at Duke University in 1965, Dr. John W. Kirklin, former Chairman of the Department of Surgery at the Mayo Clinic, had just accepted the position of Chairman of the Department of Surgery at the University of Alabama School of Medicine in Birmingham. The idea of the surgeon's assistant was conceived by Dr. Kirklin. The experiences which stimulated him to initiate this program in the University of Alabama Department of Surgery in 1967, and to continue it, are threefold.

The seed was first planted in 1955 when open heart surgery was begun at the Mayo Clinic and with it the use of the pump oxygenator. Most surgeons doing open heart surgery depended on the use of a resident to run the pump oxygenator. Of course, surgical residents do not remain in that category for prolonged periods. Running the complicated pump oxygenator required a person who could devote all his energies and attention to it and who could be depended upon to remain in that job for months and years. It was proven at that time that intelligent and highly motivated individuals, even though not having an extended scientific and medical education, could be taught to run efficiently and responsibly this complicated apparatus under the direction of the surgeon. Today, the pump technician is a recognized and important member of the group of individuals providing care to the person in need of open heart surgery.

Second, an experience leading to the concept of the surgeon's assistant was the changing role over the years of the resident in surgery at the Mayo Clinic. In the early years, a surgeon at that institution would have been a resident for a full year. This was really a beautiful arrangement for the surgeon, because he would have the same assistant in the operating room over this long period of time and the same man taking care of the patients. The resident became thoroughly familiar with the way the surgeon wanted things done. But this arrangement disappeared as residents were assigned to surgeons for shorter periods of time. At the present time, some surgeons in practice have a resident working with them for short periods of time if they are fortunate to be associated with a residency training institution. But, of course, many surgeons have no resident at all. So the question arose: Wouldn't the surgeon with a busy clinical practice working outside a medical center find it very helpful to have a trained professional assistant who, although not a physician, would have learned several basic skills by which he could, working under the direction of the surgeon, help in providing the many details of surgical patient care?

Thirdly, it became apparent that medical centers may be training more surgical residents than are needed to provide surgical care to the population. On the other hand, a variety of types of surgery are carried on in a medical center which require many people to carry through the various aspects of patient care. It seems unwise and wasteful to determine the number of surgery residents to be trained merely on the basis of the number of hands needed to get the work done. So it seems reasonable that the surgeon's assistant would also play an important role in the medical center setting.

This was the history and thinking that caused Dr. John W. Kirklin to initiate the surgeon's assistant program at the University of Alabama in Birmingham in 1967.

PRECEDENT AND LEGAL RECOGNITION: LEGISLATION

Nationally, in the late 1960's and early 1970's, emergence of these new categories of trained professional assistants presented a variety of potential legal problems. In most states, surgeon's assistants and physician assistants had no legal precedence. Moreover, medical malpractice claims and awards were, at this point in time, on the rise against physicians and hospitals. This factor complicated discussions with appropriate entities in Alabama to support enabling legislation.

In 1971, after almost two years of discussions, the University of Alabama in Birmingham, the Alabama Board of Medical Examiners, and the Alabama Hospital Association supported an "agreed on" bill for introduction in the 1971 Regular Session of the Alabama legislature. M.I. Culpepper, Jr., Administrative Assistant to Dr. Kirklin, authored the bill and lobbied its passage. Then, Governor George C. Wallace signed Act Number 1948 into law on September 20, 1971. The definition of an "assistant to physician" and provisions giving the Alabama Board of Medical Examiners the authority to approve programs and to promulgate rules and regulations for the training and use of new categories of paramedicals are perhaps the most important provisions in the Act. As structured, the Act does not have to be amended to legally recognize new categories of trained professional assistants. Since its passage in 1971, Act 1948 has remained unchanged. Presently, in Alabama, surgeon's assistants and physician assistants can legally function under the Act. However, surgeon's assistants and physician assistants function under separate rules and regulations promulgated by the Alabama Board of Medical Examiners.

THE EARLY PROGRAM

In 1967, the Surgeon's Assistant Program at the University of Alabama in Birmingham, under the direction of Dr. Alan Dimick, accepted its first class of six men and women, including two minority members. All but one member of the first class had either military or civilian allied health experience. All but one had completed at least two years of college. Mr. Jerry Wood, former Assistant to the Chairman of the Department of Surgery at the University of Alabama, arranged for the initial funding of the program and a student stipend from the Veterans Administration Hospital, which provided one of the clinical training sites for the students.

The first year's didactic instruction was obtained through the mechanism of having the surgeon's assistant students sit in on classes in biochemistry, physiology, gross anatomy, neuroanatomy, pathology and pharmacology in the School of Medicine without academic credit. The following year Dr. Margaret K. Kirklin assumed the directorship of the program and developed a distinct and separate curriculum taught by her and other physician members of the University of Alabama School of Medicine.

Beginning with the class of 1968, and without variance thereafter to the present, all students accepted into the program had completed at least two years of college work, including six hours of biology, six hours of chemistry, physics, precalculus math, and courses in the humanities and social sciences, all at the level of "C" or above.

Following completion of the first year's basic science courses, a second year was spent in various clinical rotations all within the Department of Surgery at the University of Alabama. These included cardiovascular surgery, oncology, gastrointestinal surgery, emergency trauma, general surgery, thoracic surgery, and so forth. There, the students learned the technical skills necessary to work with surgery patients, including the taking of patient histories and performing physical examinations, first- and second-assisting at surgery, performing central venous cutdown procedures, lumbar punctures, and para- and thoracentesis.

The graduates of the classes of 1969, 1970 and 1971 received certificates of proficiency upon completion of the two-year program. In 1972, in order to provide academic credit for the program and a Bachelor of Science degree, the Surgeon's Assistant Program reached an association agreement with the School of Community and Allied Health at the University of Alabama. Thereafter all students entering with the proper distribution of college credits received the B.S. degree upon successful completion of the program.

In 1974, Dr. Henry L. Laws became Director of the Program, with the addition of an Assistant Director, Jacqueline B. Hall, a Surgeon's Assistant who had graduated from the first class of the program in 1969. In 1982, Dr. J. Garber Galbraith, chairman emeritus of the Department of Neurosurgery at the University of Alabama at Birmingham became Director. Jacqueline Hall continued her role as Associate Director.

ACCREDITATION

Following publication by the American College of Surgeons of the *Essentials of an Approved Educational Program for the Surgeon's Assistant* in 1974, the Surgeon's Assistant Program at the University of Alabama applied for and received accreditation by the Joint Review Committee of the American Medical Association Council on Medical Education in collaboration with the American College of Surgeons. This unqualified accreditation has been continuous since that time.

EMPLOYMENT OPPORTUNITIES

Since 1967, surgeons over the United States and in Europe have been highly accepting of the Surgeon's Assistant from the University of Alabama in Birmingham. Of the 133 graduates, all but 7 are currently employed as Surgeon's Assistants. Four are in medical or dental school, two on maternity leave, and one has left the field for personal reasons (as of 1983). There has been very little lateral movement among graduates working in 26 states and Europe. These moves have been mostly for geographic preferences. The class of 1982 selected jobs from a list of 150 prospective surgeon employers. Many surgeons return to the school year after year to add to their surgical teams. Satisfaction has been high. Cardiovascular surgeons lead all other subspecialties in employment of the Alabama surgeon's assistant. Other graduates are distributed among 11 other surgical subspecialties.

Voluntary statements of employer surgeons regarding their approval of the level of technical expertise, medical knowledge, and professional comportment of the surgeon's assistants have been very positive. We shall attempt to examine some of the reasons for this strong and steady support of the Alabama surgeon's assistant.

The efficacy of the philosophy and insight of Dr. John W. Kirklin from the inception of the program has proven correct in experience: the selection of appropriate candidates for the rigorous training appears to be a crucial factor, both to the success of the graduate in meeting the surgeon's requirements for an assistant, and in providing job satisfaction for the surgeon's assistant. Graduate attrition has been very slight over the 15 years of the program despite typical long hours of work approaching 70–80 hours per week on the average. Surgeon's assistants do not receive hourly compensation for overtime, but function as professionals.

As the curriculum and training of the program was gradually widened and intensified in response to graduate experience and surgeon feedback, so, too, the educational level of the candidate increased. Since 1974, over 90 percent of accepted applicants held a bachelor's degree, and a few held a master's degree. Many of the students have extensive technical backgrounds and experience in other allied health fields such as nursing, medical technology, respiratory therapy, perfusion technology, and research. However, previous medical experience is not a deciding factor in evaluating candidates for admission. Rather, the admissions committee analyzes the strong academic background of the candidates in the basic sciences, the applicant's motivation for service, and his ability to deal with work that involves long hours and stress. The interview visit is utilized to assess these traits and also as an orientation period for the applicant. He is directed in informal interface with current students and with graduates working at the University of Alabama Medical Center. Realism and facts are emphasized in order to prepare the candidate for thoughtful consideration of the training and work as a surgeon's assistant.

CONCLUSION

In 1967, Dr. John W. Kirklin, Professor and Chairman of the Department of Surgery at the University of Alabama School of Medicine in Birmingham, originated the first program in the nation to train surgeon's assistants. The program was accredited by the Joint Review Committee of the American Medical Association, in collaboration with the American College of Surgeons, in 1974. The 133 graduates of the program have been well received by surgeons in the United States and Europe. They function in 11 surgical subspecialties. Approximately one-half work for cardiovascular surgeons. About one-half work in large teaching medical centers, and the remainder in private group practices. Although they are distributed in 26 states, most are located in the Northeast and Midwest. Starting salaries are good, but working hours are long. Surgeon approval is high. Jobs are abundant for these graduates. Given the continuation of careful selection of candidates, we predict continuing demand for the surgeon's assistant from the University of Alabama in Birmingham.

Chapter 13

PRIMARY CARE PHYSICIAN ASSISTANT TRAINING PROGRAMS AND PHYSICIAN ASSISTANTS IN SURGERY

SUZANNE B. GREENBERG, M.S.
HAROLD F. RHEINLANDER, M.D.

When the American College of Surgeons implemented a policy to limit the output of surgeons, surgical training programs were required to reduce the number of their trainees. Consequently, a gap in the provision of service appeared imminent. It was necessary to find personnel to provide some of the services previously carried out by surgical house officers and to do it quickly. How the teaching hospitals solved this problem depended partly on where they were located and what resources were available to them.

One approach, particularly common in the Northeast, was to hire graduates of primary care physician assistant programs. This may have been accelerated because the hospital staffs were already involved in teaching part of the physician assistant curriculum and were familiar with their preparation. Of the nearly twelve percent of physician assistants working in surgical subspecialties, a large percentage are graduates of primary care programs.

It is interesting to note that at present, there are fifty-one active primary care programs and three surgeon's assistant programs. The two orthopedic and two urologic programs which were at one time approved by the national accrediting body, the American Medical Association's Council on Medical Education, have closed. This small number of programs training specialists in surgery may reflect the lack of funding available to support training for non-primary care physician assistants, and the interest of program developers.

The job to be performed varies from hospital to hospital. Typical responsibilities of the surgical physician assistant include admission history and physical examination (often checking on the medical student's work-up), ordering preoperative studies (some routine service orders and some written after discussion with the resident or staff), assisting at operations (in some hospitals, first assisting the surgeon becomes one of the physician assistant's primary duties), providing postoperative care (including procedures such as cut-downs, arterial puncture, insertion of tubes and drains, dressings and sutures, writing progress notes, writing orders for drugs—usually on verbal order of surgeon, arranging for procedures and consultations, family and patient counseling including nutrition and rehabilitation, and attendance in ambulatory clinics for new and postoperative patients). Liaison with nurses, dietitians, and various therapists must be maintained. Relationships with physicians on the surgical team must be developed and their respect and support earned.

In each of the subspecialties, there are also specific techniques to be performed. This means that it is necessary to identify and orient individuals with some basic medical knowledge and clinical skills who are interested in the more routine aspects of the patient's care.

The primary care physician assistant showed great potential for filling the job description and was the most available, particularly in the Northeast. In the Southeast and Southwest, primary care physician assistants are employed mainly in private practices; in the Northeast, graduates are employed in hospitals in larger numbers. Initially available and subsequently proving their worth, this pattern of hiring has continued and has proven to have many advantages.

The major objectives of every primary care physician assistant program are for its students to learn to collect data, organize it, present it effectively and follow through with appropriate management and treatment under the supervision of a physician. This coincides almost exactly with what surgeons are looking for to fill the developing gap in the provision of services in a surgical setting.

If one accepts the definition of a surgeon as a physician who masters the skills and theory of surgical practice and techniques, it follows that the surgical physician assistant should also have exposure to the broader aspects of the field of medicine. The primary evaluation of a surgical patient requires the same skills of eliciting a history, performing a physical examination, establishing a working diagnosis with appropriate tests as does every other branch of medicine. The appropriately employed surgical physician assistant must be well trained in these basic skills to be able to make his or her contribution to the surgical team. Once this basic general medical education has been mastered, specific skills, techniques or procedures can be readily taught since students already understand why certain things are being done.

Primary care programs teach interviewing and history taking skills, physical diagnosis, basic sciences, pathophysiology and medicine including emergency medicine, pharmacology and clinical pharmacy as well as electrocardiography, basic diagnostic radiology, nutrition, patient counseling and education, and rehabilitation medicine. These subjects are taught in such a manner as to apply to all ages and types of patients. This basic general education provides an excellent basis on which to add skills.

Primary care programs also introduce students to principles of surgical intervention and usually allow for some clinical experience in surgery in the course of the two-year program. The didactic material includes sessions on sterile technique, wound healing, principles of surgical intervention in gastroenterology, cardiac-thoracic, genito-urinary, oncology, vascular, and otolaryngology patients as well as principles of anesthesia. Some programs also include aspects of neuro-surgical intervention.

The clinical experience usually focuses on pre- and postoperative management of the patient. Students do spend some time in the operating room, both to understand better what happens when a patient has anesthesia and undergoes surgery, and to observe their patients so they will be able to follow them appropriately postoperatively. They often hold retractors and may help close incisions. The overall emphasis is on how to approach the surgical patient and collect relevant data.

Professionals become adept at their work as a result of practice. Each surgical subspecialty requires slightly different skills. Each practitioner uses a slightly different approach and cadre of therapeutics. Physician assistants must learn to adjust to a wide variety of styles. By being trained broadly they are well able to make the necessary adjustments.

For physician assistants who have had training in primary care, there seem to be two possible methods of introducing physician assistants to surgery and surgical care. One technique is to apprentice the physician assistant to a surgeon in private practice, the second is to attach the physician assistant to a surgical unit in a teaching hospital.

Apprenticeship is an appropriate technique the effectiveness of which is based almost entirely on the interests and talents of an individual surgeon. Many surgeons are knowledgeable, but not all of them have the patience, aptitude, interest, or time to indoctrinate the physician assistant student properly. Another problem resides in the necessarily narrow experience which the average surgical practice encompasses. The individual surgeon's practice in most hospitals is limited to a relatively well-defined area. This restricts the learning experience of the physician assistant to that area. Although this may be appropriate, it does not prepare the physician assistant for other fields of the surgical specialty. Another drawback is the lack of exposure to a number of different surgical opinions and practices. Much of surgical practice depends upon individual experience and training. Not all surgeons approach the same problems in the same way. Although different techniques may be equally effective, it may be valuable for an individual to be exposed to several points of view in order to be flexible and develop a better and deeper understanding of surgical practices.

For these reasons, it seems more appropriate to train primary care physician assistants on a teaching surgical service. In this setting, the physician assistant will be exposed to a number of surgeons who have demonstrated their aptitude and abilities to teach. More importantly, they become members of a surgical team with residents, interns, and students all participating in a learning experience revolving around patient care, both at the bedside and in the operating room. In such a setting, formal teaching sessions are built around medical student and resident needs and time is made available for the team not only to attend but to participate. The physician assistant with a primary care background fits very well into this pattern and in most instances has no problem with the content or complexity of these sessions. In addition, everyone on a teaching service is expected to contribute to those who are less knowledgeable. The physician assistant also must contribute in this manner and must read and study to keep abreast and even ahead of others.

Physician assistant instruction on teaching surgical services has taken several forms. The first is a formal "internship" usually lasting one year. In this role the physician assistant is regarded more as a student but is expected to provide a major service function and is suitably reimbursed for these services.

A successful technique used in some institutions over the past eight years is an "on-the-job" training program. This plan involves assigning the new physician assistant to a particular surgical team consisting of senior and junior surgical residents, experienced physician assistants, and medical students. The experienced physician assistant on the service sets up a training schedule based on a list of skills which the neophyte must master before he or she can assume a full role on the patient care team. This list involves technical skills as well as clinical skills and includes a plan of increasing responsibility for a variety of clinical responsibilities. The development of decision-making capacity and judgment is carefully weighed. Conferences with the supervision surgeon are held as frequently as is required by the performance of the physician assistant. When, in the opinion of the surgeon and senior physician assistant, the new member is ready to stand night call with the supervising resident in a different area of the medical complex, the new physician assistant is judged to have become a full-fledged member of the team. Three months appears to be a sufficient training period for the average candidate.

There are presently at least thirty physician assistants working on surgical services in six Boston teaching hospitals. These institutions represent three different medical schools. Nineteen of these are employed in two Tufts-affiliated hospitals, and the details of their duties, training, and performance are well known to the authors. Physician supervisors are, without exception, pleased with the performance of the physician assistants and are enthusiastic about their usefulness in improving patient care in both the ambulatory and in-patient settings.

During the past eight years, one of us (H.F.R.) has had personal experience with the training of twenty-six physician assistants for general or cardio-thoracic surgical services. Without exception, these individuals have come from primary care programs. Initially, a six month program was designed to orient the physician assistant to his or her role. As we have gained experience and confidence, the training period has been shortened. Our present requirement is for a three month gradual breaking-in period following which most physician assistants have been able to assume full responsibilities for their assigned duties. Training of new physician assistants is greatly facilitated by the presence of mature experienced physician assistants on the service, all of whom are interested in teaching and assume a major role in the orientation process.

The performance of physician assistants on the Tufts surgical services has been of high quality. In reviewing their performance, three factors have become apparent. The history and physical examination is very complete and accurate. The general quality of the patient's record is high as evidenced by well-written progress notes and summaries. Finally, medication orders tend to be more legibly and accurately written than those of surgical house officers, based on a six month study at Tufts New England Medical Center hospitals.

There is no question in our own minds that with an appropriate orientation period of approximately three months, graduates of primary care physician assistant programs can perform competently on surgical services.

Chapter 14

RESIDENCY TRAINING PROGRAMS FOR SURGICAL PHYSICIAN ASSISTANTS

J. JEFFREY HEINRICH, PA-C
BRUCE C. FICHANDLER, PA-C
MALCOLM BEINFIELD, M.D., F.A.C.S.

During the past decade, there have been three significant developments that pointed to a future shortage of surgical housestaff manpower. First of all, the Health Professions Educational Assistance Act of 1976 (Public Law A-484 and amendment PL-95-83) has reduced the number of foreign medical school graduates that may immigrate into the United States (1). Secondly, the Study on Surgical Services for the United States (SOSSUS), conducted by the American College of Surgeons and the American Surgical Association, showed that the number of physicians entering post-graduate surgical training programs should be decreased (2). Lastly, careful review of the educational components and other aspects of physician surgical residency programs, especially in community hospitals, has resulted in a phasing out of a number of these programs. These three developments have created in many hospitals a manpower shortage for the continuous inhouse coverage of the surgical patient. One solution offered has been the utilization of the surgical physician assistant.

Two formal surgical training programs have been developed to educate the physician assistant who has successfully completed a primary care physician assistant program. The existing programs are the Surgical Internship Program for Physician Assistants sponsored by the Montefiore Hospital and Medical Center/Albert Einstein College of Medicine (Montefiore) and the Norwalk Hospital/Yale University School of Medicine Physician Assistant Surgical Residency Program (Norwalk). Both programs are designed to teach the primary care physician assistant how to deal with common surgical problems seen daily in both the inpatient and outpatient setting. From the outset, it needs to be clearly understood that the surgical physician assistant works as a dependent practitioner under the direction and supervision of an attending surgeon.

The advent of postgraduate surgical training for physician assistants raised many questions in the minds of surgeons and administrators. The key questions were as follows:

1. Would this program be a valuable educational endeavor for physician assistants?
2. Could a physician assistant provide quality care of the surgical patient?
3. Would this endeavor be accepted by patients, surgeons, other physicians and nurses?
4. Would the hospital administration and board of trustees find this program acceptable and worthwhile?
5. What job opportunities would the physician assistant have upon completion of the program?

Montefiore and Norwalk both developed their programs with these and other questions in mind. Both programs were committed to evaluating this approach as a potential solution to the surgical manpower problem.

SURGICAL PHYSICIAN ASSISTANT PROGRAMS

The selection process for the two programs is highly competitive. An applicant must first be a graduate of a physician assistant program accredited by the Committee on Allied Health Education and Accreditation of the American Medical Association and/or have successfully passed a national board examination administered by the National Commission on Certification of Physician Assistants. Montefiore selects 15 physician assistants and Norwalk accepts 10 residents each year for their respective programs. Each program seeks applicants with a strong academic background, good interpersonal skills, and a strong commitment to a career as a surgical physician assistant. The programs receive numerous applications from all over the country each year.

While structurally different, both programs have similar goals. Unlike a physician surgical training program, however, the purpose of the programs is to develop the skills of a surgical assistant, not those of an independent operating surgeon. An overview of the two programs is provided to highlight their similarities and differences.

The Norwalk Program is divided into a 4 month didactic/clinical phase which takes place at Yale and an 8 month clinical phase at Norwalk. The Yale didactic/clinical component is offered to 5 of the physician assistant residents during the fall semester, and the remaining 5 physician assistant residents during the spring semester. During this phase of the program, both structured and unstructured instruction is provided. There are three courses offered in the structured curriculum; anatomy, animal surgery, and a general lecture series. The anatomy course emphasizes the clinical importance of anatomy rather than the abstract anatomy that most of the physician assistants were exposed to in their basic physician assistant training. This approach is reinforced by the use of surgeons in clinical practice as instructors. Although all of the physician assistant residents have had an opportunity to assist in a variety of surgical procedures, the animal surgery course is designed to enhance their technical proficiency in manual skills to make them more efficient and effective as surgical assistants. Each resident is required to participate in a minimum number of surgical procedures under the supervision of a surgeon. The last component in the structured curriculum is the lecture series which emphasizes topics related to the surgical specialties, as well as lectures in both cardiology and general medicine as they relate to surgery.

The unstructured curriculum consists of all of the conferences scheduled for the medical school and medical center and all of the classes being given to the first year physician assistant students in the Yale Physician Associate Program. In addition to the didactic curriculum, the resident's clinical responsibilities while at Yale include 5 rotations, 4 mandatory and 1 elective. The mandatory rotations are: anesthesiology, plastic surgery/burns, surgical emergency service, and surgical intensive care unit. Any other surgical or medical specialty is available as an elective.

The eight month rotation at Norwalk Hospital provides a broad clinical experience on the general surgical, genitourinary, and orthopedic services. The physician assistant residents actively participates in all aspects of peri-operative care. Their responsibilities include performing history and physical examinations, gathering and evaluating laboratory data, writing orders and progress notes, and making regular rounds with the attending surgeons. They suture wounds, perform thoracenteses, paracenteses, insert central venous lines, apply casts and perform cutdowns. Special emphasis is given to life threatening problems as they pertain to the surgical patient. In addition, each resident is assigned for one month to the surgical intensive care unit where he or she works closely with the staff surgical physician assistants and the full-time intensive care unit internist. The physician assistant residents under the direction of the surgical attendings have a decision making role in keeping with their level of competence.

The clinical aspect of the Norwalk Hospital rotation is supplemented by a daily structured lecture series which is designed to emphasize the pathophysiology of surgical disease. The physician assistant residents actively participate in the selection and presentation of cases at the weekly Surgical Grand Rounds and clinical surgical conference. A course in medical writing is offered to provide training in the utilization of library resources. The Norwalk Hospital Surgical Service offers rotations for undergraduate physician assistant students from several primary care programs. The surgical resident is involved in this educational experience. The fact that the entire surgical housestaff is physician assistants at varying levels of training provides an environment where the physician assistant residents do not compete with M.D. housestaff (3).

The Montefiore program is divided into two phases, a three month lecture series followed by a 12 to 24 month internship. The lecture series includes such topics as endocrine and metabolic response to injury, fluid and electrolytes, shock and wound healing. Also covered are anatomy, physiology and the diagnosis and treatment of surgical diseases of each organ system. There is a series of pharmacology lectures and the physician assistant interns attend the same radiology lectures as the medical students.

After successful completion of the didactic component, the next 12 months are devoted to a clinical internship. The majority of the physician assistant intern's time is spent on the General Surgical Services at the two private and two city hospitals of the combined Department of Surgery. The remaining time is spent on the surgical subspecialties, in the burn unit, and in the surgical emergency room. During this phase, they are required to attend the same conferences and lectures as the M.D. interns and residents.

Among the duties they perform on the surgical services are obtaining patient physical examination, gathering appropriate laboratory data, writing daily notes, and writing appropriate diagnostic and therapeutic orders. Although the physician assistant interns act as first and second assistants in the operating room, the emphasis in the training program is preoperative and postoperative care. All activities are performed under the supervision of the responsible attending surgeon.

The Montefiore program has been in existence for ten years and the Norwalk program, for five years. The programs have been shown to be a valuable experience by the enthusiastic reception they have received by the physician assistant population at large, by the surgeons and administrators at the participating hospitals, and by patients. To date, the experience at both institutions has primarily been positive, and all of the early questions have been answered in the affirmative.

Surgical physician assistants have demonstrated their ability to provide excellent pre-, intra-, and post-operative care to the surgical patients. They have shown this through their active participation on various inpatient surgical services, as well as through oral and written testing mechanisms.

The physician assistants in both programs have been well received by patients. They have the time to listen and easily communicate with their patients. The surgeons have also benefited from teaching these students of surgery and are supportive of this educational endeavor after having observed the physician assistant's willingness to learn and their capacity to contribute.

Physicians from other specialties have mixed feelings concerning the surgical physician assistant since he cannot provide independent consultation to their patients. The relationship to the nursing staff has been extremely favorable. The physician assistants are willing to learn from the experienced surgical nurse with ease and equanimity. Hospital administrators have also accepted and are in support of these worthwhile programs.

The job opportunities for the surgical physician assistant upon completion of training are excellent (4). For the most part, the graduates of these programs have been able to find employment in whatever part of the country where they wish to settle. Their positions and roles vary greatly with the practice setting, ranging from a general rural practice to a surgical subspecialty in a university based practice.

CONCLUSION

The Montefiore and Norwalk porgrams are making a positive contribution to the delivery of surgical care. The programs provide a new educational challenge for the institutions and produce a well trained surgical physician assistant for the medical community. The surgical physician assistant has demonstrated his willingness to learn and capability to contribute to the care of the surgical patient. Patients, surgeons, nurses and administrators have all enthusiastically accepted and supported this new health professional. The programs have clearly shown that manpower needs can be served by the addition of a surgical physician assistant to the team.

REFERENCES

1. Politzer RM, Morrow JS, Sudia RK, *et al.:* Foreign-Trained Physicians in American Medicine: A Case Study. *Med. Care, 16:*611-627, 1978.
2. Study on Surgical Services for the United States. Chicago, American College of Surgeons and American Surgical Association 1976.
3. Heinrich JJ, Fichandler BC, and Beinfield M, *et al.:* The Physician's Assistant as Resident on Surgical Service. *Arch. Surg., 115:*310-314, 1980.
4. Perry HB, Detmer DE, and Redmond EL: The Current and Future Role of Surgical Physician Assistants. *Ann. Surg., 193:*132-137, 1981.

PART TWO

**CLINICAL ROLES FOR
PHYSICIAN ASSISTANTS**

Chapter 15

THE PRIMARY CARE PHYSICIAN ASSISTANT IN A RURAL OFFICE-BASED SETTING

TIMOTHY N. FRARY, PA-C
LANNY B. REIMER, M.D.

INTRODUCTION

Even in these days of the projected physician surplus, millions of Americans are confronted with a very real shortage of health care services. A large percentage of these people live in rural areas where the glaring inequity of physician distribution between urban and rural locales is painfully obvious. For numerous reasons, some real and some imagined, it has become increasingly difficult to attract and retain young doctors in rural America.

The very concept of physician assistants is rooted to a great extent in the fertile soil of medically underserved rural areas. Initially, it was small towns and small town physicians who voiced the need for and saw the potential of this new profession. Today, more than ever, the opportunity and demand for the primary care physician assistant in rural areas is great. In many ways, the physician assistant is uniquely suited to this type of environment. In this chapter, we will explore the role of the physician assistant in an office-based rural primary care practice.

THE SETTING

In discussing the role of the physician assistant in any rural setting, it is important to realize that the geographic, demographic, and economic characteristics of a community will be major determinants of the type of health care services which are demanded and provided. No two communities will have the same mix of these characteristics. Therefore, it seems desirable to briefly describe this particular practice setting so that the reader may take these factors into consideration when extrapolating from this practice to other rural practices in other locales.

Newcastle, the county seat of Weston County, is located in the northeastern section of Wyoming. The population of Newcastle is approximately 3,600 persons. The only other community of significant size in Weston County is Upton, with a population of nearly 1,500. Much of the economy of Weston County, Wyoming, is directly related to oil, coal, and timber. Ranching and tourism play smaller but still significant roles. Newcastle is situated on the eastern fringe of the tremendous development which has taken place in northern Wyoming as a result of surface coal mining in nearby Campbell County. By virtue of its location on the perimeter of the coal basin, the community has managed to avoid most the "boom town" crisis while sustaining steady growth. However, being on the fringe also has its drawbacks, since nearly all of the tax revenue and state impact assistance goes to Campbell County and its principal city of Gillette.

The nearest city to Newcastle of any significant size is Rapid City, South Dakota, with a population of nearly 60,000. It lies on the eastern slope of the Black Hills about 75 miles distant. Because Rapid City is the largest city in a nearly 200-mile radius, it serves as a major medical referral center for western South Dakota, north-eastern Wyoming and northwestern Nebraska. It is well-equipped with modern medical facilities and has attracted a well-rounded complement of specialists and subspecialists.

THE PHYSICIAN'S VIEWPOINT

I returned to Newcastle, which, incidentally, is my hometown, following the completion of my family practice residency in California in 1978. Initially, I joined a group of three older physicians who had served the community for over 25 years. Several other doctors had come and gone over those years, but these three had remained as a stable group.

Shortly after joining the practice, I pushed to expand the delivery of the group's service to Upton, 30 miles to the northwest. I took this action for two reasons. First, the community of Upton was somewhat medically underserved, and, second, I had a National Health Service Corps scholarship obligation which I could repay by working in Upton, which was a designated manpower shortage area. Newcastle, at that time, was not so designated. Three of the four physicians in the Newcastle Clinic shared duties in Upton, rotating days in the smaller clinic.

Even though I was working in a well-established group, my long-term goal had always been to start my own clinic. The retirement of one of the older physicians in late 1980 and the lengthy illness of another made my decision to branch out a little more imperative. During late 1980 and early 1981, I began looking for another young family physician to join me. However, I met with no success, and, as the target date of July, 1981, loomed close, I began to get more and more discouraged. It was at about this time that I first considered employing a physician assistant.

I had worked with both physician assistants and nurse practitioners during my residency at the University of California-Davis, and, in general, had been favorably impressed. However, I confess that the idea of employing a physician assistant never really occurred to me until I visited with a young physician assistant who is on the teaching staff of one of the family practice residency programs of Wyoming. As I was telling him my sad tale of being unable to attract a colleague, he suggested that an experienced physician assistant might be a good, and perhaps in some ways better, alternative.

As we talked, I realized that a physician assistant might be just the person for my fledgling practice. Through the efforts of this physician assistant, I was soon contacted by a couple of well-qualified physician assistants who expressed an interest in working in Newcastle.

During these initial contacts, I asked as many questions as I answered. I still was uncertain that a physician assistant would fill a large enough gap to enable me to start my clinic. It was fortunate that one of the physician assistants with whom I talked had some fairly extensive experience in a rural community quite similar in many respects to Newcastle. He was able to answer many of my questions, such as: How are physician assistants accepted in the community? Will a physician assistant be able to pay his or her own way? How is call handled? With these answers and with a few phone calls to other doctors who employed physician assistants, I became convinced that the addition of a physician assistant would indeed enable me to open my new clinic in July as planned.

THE PREPARATIONS

Once the decision had been made that a physician assistant could fill this position, several other things needed to be done as soon as possible. First, even before I had made a definite commitment to hire a physician assistant, I contacted the State Board of Medical Examiners both by letter and telephone. I studied copies of the law and regulations pertaining to "physician support persons" as they are called in Wyoming. In areas which seemed vague, I asked the Director of the Board for clarification. He was able to give me the "official" interpretation. However, I felt it was also very important to learn how the law and regulations had been interpreted and enforced at the actual community practice level. I was able to get this information from a few practicing physician assistants and their employing physicians.

Secondly, at the same time I was researching the legal aspects, I was testing the waters of opinion within our own local medical community. I spoke with the other staff physicians, the hospital administrator, and the director of nursing in regard to their attitudes towards physician assistants. I also went to the Hospital Board with my plan and explained to them the role, functions, and legal aspects of hiring a physician assistant. I wanted to be as sure as I could that there would be no substantial resistance to my idea.

Third, and perhaps most important, was the actual selection of a physician assistant to help me in my practice. Because of conditions in our community, I had some criteria in mind which I hoped I would be able to fill. First, since this area was basically unfamiliar with physician assistants, I wanted to find someone who had been a physician assistant for some time and who was secure in his or her role. I felt that this would ease the "introduction period." Secondly, since there would only be two of us in the practice initially, I wanted to find someone who had experience in primary care. This would enable him or her to share more of the workload responsibility and, it was hoped, require less direct supervision. Thirdly, since Newcastle is a small and relatively isolated town, I wanted to find someone who had small town living experience and who knew what to expect. I did not want to hire someone and move him to town only to have him discover that he disliked the rural lifestyle. Once again, I turned to the administrators of the Family Practice Residency Program. Since they often get employment inquiries from physician assistants in other states, I was given the names of several likely candidates, and, fortunately, one of them met my criteria to a very large extent. After several phone conversations to get acquainted, we arranged a personal interview and eventually were able to reach a mutually satisfying agreement. This physician assistant joined the practice on August 1, one month after I had opened the Black Hills Medical Clinic.

I had learned from other physician–PA teams that the first few weeks would be a very critical time. Since Newcastle was basically unfamiliar with physician assistants, it was doubly important to get off on the right foot.

In a very real sense, our professional association started well before the physician assistant moved to town. I was busy helping to draft a proposal for an amendment to the medical staff by-laws allowing limited hospital privileges to non-physicians. I was also busy channelling the necessary papers and completing forms for the staff application as well as the materials required by the State Board of Medical Examiners.

I knew that it would be very important to gain the initial support (or at least to avoid the active resistance) of the hospital staff. Therefore, I circulated several copies of the curriculum vitae of my new associate. I wanted the staff to feel they knew him before he arrived. I also posted a short article about my physician assistant, with his picture on the bulletin board in the nurses' lounge. I think this helped to personalize the "mysterious stranger" who was neither physician nor nurse.

I also took a number of small but, I feel, very important steps to get our practice started right. I made sure that the physician assistant's name was displayed prominently on our office "shingle." This not only helped the physician assistant to feel immediately like a part of the practice, but it also helped to present a positive image to the public: "Here is a new provider whose name appears right beside the doctor's." For the same reason, I had both our names printed on clinic business cards. It was clear from the outset that this person was to be a big part of my practice. It displayed my confidence in our association, and I think this confidence was conveyed to the public. We also placed a brochure on physician assistants in our office waiting room. Last, but not least, as an introductory step, I had the newspaper come by for a story and photo. We appeared side by side in the photo and here again we helped to convey the "team concept" of health care to our community.

Our first week of working together was really a "get-acquainted" period. We spent the week together seeing patients and discussing management and diagnosis strategies. It is critically important in an MD–PA association that each learn how the other thinks and acts in common situations. I know that if the physician assistant I employed had been less experienced, I would have wanted more than a week's orientation. However, I knew from our conversations and interviews that we shared many ideas about medical, behavioral, and ethical issues. Therefore, I felt comfortable with this relatively short introduction. This week enabled the nurses and other doctors to see that a supervisory relationship did truly exist. I think it was time well spent.

THE OUTCOME

Following our introductory week, we settled into a routine which has been very successful and only occasionally modified. Our practice consists basically of four components: hospital, nursing home, the clinic in Newcastle, and the Upton satellite clinic which I took over when I established my own practice.

In the hospital, we usually make morning rounds together. I am responsible for the management of all hospitalized patients, but I feel it is very important for the physician assistant to know the status of each one. When I am in Upton or not immediately available, the physician assistant may be asked to clarify an order or to perhaps write new orders as the case may dictate. Also, the physician assistant does the history and physical on each patient he has seen prior to admission.

I have not asked the physician assistant to play a major role in the nursing home segment of my practice. First, it represents only a small percentage of my patients, and, second, because of current Medicare regulations, his services would not be reimbursable anyway. However, he does occasionally see patients who have acute problems when I am not available.

Following hospital and/or nursing home duties, we both generally see patients in the Newcastle office. Then, every afternoon, one of us travels the 30 miles to Upton to see patients in the satellite clinic. Unless there are extenuating circumstances, we generally alternate days of traveling. Such extenuating circumstances might include a seriously ill hospitalized patient or an impending delivery. In these situations, I stay in Newcastle to be near the hospital, while the physician assistant sees our Upton patients.

The two of us alternate the night calls, taking every other night and every other weekend. Of course, I am always available for back-up when the physician assistant is on call, unless I have another physician immediately available to cover for me.

ISSUES AND IMPRESSIONS THUS FAR

My association with a physician assistant has not been without a few problems, but I must truly say that the benefits have far outweighed the difficulties. I am not sure I could have survived the first months of practice without the help of the physician assistant.

What have some of the problems been? First of all, the laws and regulations vary from state to state. A physician cannot depend on *any* degree of standardization between states. Therefore, one cannot assume to know what is legal or illegal. Legality must be verified. Physician assistants are closely regulated in most states. Conforming to these regulations, many of which do not make any sense from a patient protection point of view, can be a real headache.

Secondly, one can count on the fact that some health professionals in your community are going to feel threatened by a physician assistant. There will be some resistance to the idea, both open and covert. Even the most careful preparatory work did not take care of all the misgivings and minor misunderstandings. However, we were fortunate that they were short lived in our community.

Thirdly, perhaps the biggest disadvantage to me, as a solo physician, is that I must always be available for backup call. I feel that this is important, but it makes it difficult to ever truly be "away" unless I hire a locum tenens or other form of backup physician. Our ideal situation, I believe, would be two physicians with one, and perhaps eventually two, physician assistants. This way the call and backup responsibilities could be shared.

As I mentioned, however, the advantages far outweigh the disadvantages. The first advantage has simply been one of survival. I am able to spend some quiet time with my family knowing that the minor problems are being well-handled. I am able to take one or two mornings to get office business chores done or to catch up on my hospital charts, knowing that the clinic is still running smoothly. I am, at times, almost able to be two places at once through the eyes, ears, and skills of my physician assistant.

The second advantage is one of focus. I am able to spend more time with my first love, which is obstetrics, because the physician assistant handles many of the acute illnesses and a lot of our pediatrics. He also does many of the school and employment physical examinations. This gives me a lot more "quality time" during my work day. The third advantage is one of patient convenience. We are able to maintain two clinics and to serve nearly twice as many people with less waiting time. If I am called away on an emergency, the patients which previously would have been cancelled can now usually see the physician assistant. Our patients have responded very positively to this arrangement.

The fourth advantage is educational. We continually prod one another with questions and suggestions. We learn from each other and I have frankly been surprised more than once by the breadth of clinical knowledge which many physician assistants have. Having the physician assistant around makes me a better physician, because I can learn by teaching and also by observing.

The fifth advantage is financial. There is no question that in this practice setting a physician assistant can more than pay his or her own way. If the physician assistant has been introduced to the community in a positive way and is willing to work hard, he can prove to be a real financial asset to the practice. I am not sure many physicians realize this.

There are other advantages to be sure, but I can sum it all up by saying that employing a physician assistant was perhaps the most important step I took in establishing my practice.

THE VIEWPOINT FROM THE PHYSICIAN ASSISTANT

The role of the physician assistant in a rural practice is usually rewarding, sometimes frustrating, and always challenging. The limited size of the community in general, and the medical community in particular, tends to place the physician assistant in quite a different position from that of his or her urban colleague. There are several factors which need to be considered in some depth by any physician assistant who thinks he or she might want to locate in a small town environment.

The first of these factors is the decision to live in a rural environment in the first place. Most people who choose a rural lifestyle have some fairly specific reasons for doing so. Often among these reasons are a slower, more leisurely pace of life, a friendlier community, a safer environment, and a better place to raise children. These are all valid reasons and most of them do apply to many small towns. However, on the minus side of the balance sheet we often find a lack of social and cultural opportunities, limited shopping, lack of privacy, and a shrunken housing market, as well as other "problems." How can one tell in advance whether the pluses will outweight the minuses? Probably the surest way is to be familiar with the small town lifestyle, and the best way to achieve this familiarity is to grow up in a small town.

Physician assistant programs have learned the same lesson that medical schools and businesses have learned. "If you want to place people in rural areas, then select applicants from rural areas." This does not rule out the possibility that our city cousins cannot find contentment in country living. However, those with no rural life experience are often in for some pretty rude surprises. If a person really thinks he would like to become a physician assistant in a rural primary care practice but does not have any rural life experience, then, at the very least, he should select a Physician Assistant Program which has a rural, primary care orientation. As a general rule, these tend to be the programs in the midwestern and southern states with large rural populations. Ideally, a fairly large portion of the clinical curriculum should actually take place in the community. A wise person once said that trying to learn about small town medicine at a medical center is like trying to learn about forestry at a lumber yard.

As a second observation about selecting the rural lifestyle, it is worth noting that many of the positive attributes of small towns are much more attractive to "family persons" than to young or single physician assistants. The lack of privacy and of social life often drives the young singles to larger communities with more variety in all aspects. Again, this is not a universal truth, but even some very committed young physician assistants have found that small town living was too sedate once the newness of the experience had worn off.

Another factor for consideration is the role of the physician assistant in the community. This, like the rural lifestyle, is a two-edged sword. In a general sense, the physician assistant in a small town tends to be a minor VIP. He is usually seen as an integral part of the small professional community. Also, as a health care provider, he is often cast in the role of helper, counselor, healer, and even savior. This usually accords him a position of esteem in the community and sometimes of civic responsibility as well. This can be pretty heady stuff and indeed can be quite enjoyable. It can also be a source of much trouble if the physician assistant is not prepared or not careful.

For example, important people in small towns are usually expected to do important things. This can include teaching a community education class, starting an EMT course, spearheading the Community Chest fund drive, leading a scout troop, or running for city office. These demands are for worthwhile causes, but may become unmanageable when they conflict with practice or family responsibilities. As another example, people who are perceived as "above the norm" in small towns are usually prime targets for gossip. This is a natural phenomenon, but, if a person is easily bothered by such things, then small town living may be a bad choice. This situation is in sharp contrast to physician assistants in urban areas who can often be lost in the health care shuffle among hundreds of doctors and thousands of nurses. If a physician assistant desires public recognition, public service, and responsibility, then small town life may be an avenue. However, if a physician assistant desires privacy, anonymity, and undisturbed free time, then an urban setting might prove more suitable.

A third (and perhaps most important) factor to be considered is the role of the physician assistant in the practice itself. Physician assistants who accept positions in "real" small towns (as opposed to suburbs) will usually find themselves in a community which is medically underserved. In these practices, the physicians are almost always busier than they want to be. This situation generally leads to three things as far as the physician assistant is concerned: (1) the physician assistant will usually be very busy too, (2) the physician assistant will tend to see a wider variety of problems because there is less opportunity for pre-visit triage, and (3) the physician assistant will likely be less closely supervised than in better staffed or slower paced practices. Let us look at each of these three areas in a little more depth.

First, it is true that physician assistants in most rural practices tend to be busy. A recent study of physician assistants in rural primary care showed that they saw an average of 110 to 120 patients per week in all settings. This is close to most averages which have been reported for physicians. The physician assistants reported working 50 to 60 hours per week on the average, and all of those surveyed were sharing emergency call duties with their supervising physicians (1). My personal experiences in small town practice support these figures very well. I generally see three to six inpatients, fifteen to twenty-five clinic patients, and one to four emergency room patients each day. On weekends when I am on call, I see fifteen to thirty outpatients and emergencies on Saturday and Sunday. I always work at least ten hours per day and often twelve to fourteen hours. This is a rigorous schedule.

Secondly, it is true that physician assistants in rural type practices see a wide variety of problems. This same study of rural primary care physician assistants also showed that the twenty to twenty-five most common problems seen by physician assistants paralleled very closely those reported by family physicians. Physician assistants, like family physicians, tend to see a high proportion of minor acute illnesses, minor trauma, and health care maintenance type problems. However, they also see more complex problems and illnesses, either by design or often by necessity. Again, my own experience verifies this. Some days, it seems that all I see are earaches, sore throats, and well baby checks. However, as I look back over the past six months at some of the cases I have seen, or diagnoses I have made, it is a little surprising. There have been lymphomas, systemic lupus erythematosus, thyroid carcinoma, Henoch-Schonlein purpura, idiopathic thrombocytopenia, carcinoma of the colon, pulmonary emboli, tubal pregnancy, encephalitis, rheumatic fever, and black widow spider bites, to name a few. This is a variety that many urban physician assistants would not encounter.

Finally, it seems true that many rural physician assistants are less closely supervised than their urban colleagues. The same study previously mentioned showed that those primary care physician assistants managed about 82% of problems seen at the "independent" level (1). I do not know what the percentage would be for urban physician assistants, but I suspect it might be somewhat lower. In fact, some rural physician assistants participating in this study reported "independent management" of 90-92% of problems seen. These figures and my own work experiences lead me to believe that very often in rural areas it is the physician assistant who determines when and which patients to refer, and when they have reached their limits as a physician assistant. This can be a very positive situation because who better knows the limits than the individual involved? It can also be a potentially disastrous situation if a physician assistant does not recognize his or her limitations, or, worse yet, chooses to ignore them. I have rarely known a physician assistant to consciously step over that fine line of ethics and skill. However, realistically, the pressure is sometimes there, especially in rural areas. To refer a patient may mean a rescheduled visit for a rancher who lives 30 miles from town. It may mean a log jam in the office schedule while the physician-supervisor checks the patient with the physician assistant just observing. It may mean a 100-mile trip to a specialist just to confirm a hunch. In these situations, it is easy to "temporize," easy to "try this and if you aren't better in a few days, give me a call." This is not always bad. Indeed, physicians often do the same thing. However, the judgements are often harder to make for the physician assistant; the line that we walk is often a little thinner. For this reason, rural practice tends to weed out two varieties of physician assistants: those who aren't sure of themselves and those who are too sure of themselves. Most rural physician assistants I know wish that they had a little closer access to their supervising physician. I know that as closely as I work with my "doc," I still wish I could call on him more often. However, I know that he often wishes he had an endocrinologist or an orthopedic surgeon around the corner to consult with. In the final analysis, all the laws and regulations ever written about supervision do not really cover most rural practices. Eventually, one comes to rely on three kinds of knowledge: knowledge of medicine, knowledge of supervisor, and knowledge of self limitations. Laws do not cover these areas.

Much advice can be given to physician assistants who think they want to work in rural areas. There are many factors to consider. However, the one I believe should be considered above all else is the supervising or employing physician.

Because of the closeness of one's relationship with his or her supervising physician, all those "little things" ignored when the job was accepted will come back to haunt just like in a marriage. Therefore, just like marriage, one should shop around a lot, get to know the intended as well as possible and *never* take anything for granted. Try to find out certain very important things before taking a job. Is his philosophy of medicine the same as yours? Is he intent on being wealthy? How hard does he like to work? He is likely to have the same standard for you. How long is he going to stay in this practice? Does he view you as an employee or as a colleague? Do you get along with his spouse? Does he get along with the other physicians in town? Does he go to Continuing Medical Education Conferences? The questions go on and on. You can live in the most attractive little community in your state, but if you do not get along with your supervisor, you will be miserable. Choose your boss before you choose your town. As a physician assistant, this is especially vital.

Having a good relationship with your physician does not mean that everything will be rosy, but it takes care of about 75% of the job. It is also important to cultivate a good working relationship with other health professionals, such as pharmacists, nurses, and hospital administration. These people can be invaluable allies or intolerable foes. It is much better to ease them towards your corner.

In moving into a small town and its medical community, it is really important to remember that change comes more slowly in the country. You will be all the "new" that they will want for awhile. Do not forget about your ideas for progressive parenting classes or stress management seminars, but do not rush to implement all of them in the first month either. Give people a little time to study you before jumping into the phone booth to change into "Super PA".

One final word of caution—never assume that the paperwork has been done! Write, call, and visit to insure that the state has given you the authority to go to work. Make sure that your malpractice insurance is in force. Be certain that the Hospital Board has approved your privileges before you see anyone in the ER. It only takes one little accident to make a routine case into a financial or legal nightmare.

I really enjoy the atmosphere and pace of small town living. As a physician assistant who loves family medicine or primary care, it is hard to imagine a setting which is more challenging, demanding, or rewarding than a small town practice. However, it should be obvious that it is not a setting for every physician assistant. It is a decision which must take many factors into account. It is our hope that this chapter has highlighted some of those factors and has helped shed some light on the role of the physician assistant in a rural, office-based primary care practice.

REFERENCE

1. Frary TN, Somers J, Edwards J, Gallagher TF: A descriptive analysis of physician assistant practice patterns in rural primary care. Association of Physician Assistant Programs 8th Annual Conference, New Orleans, 1980.

Chapter 16

THE PHYSICIAN ASSISTANT
IN A RURAL PRACTICE

JAMES LOVE, PA-C

When it comes to writing about the physician assistant in a rural office setting, I should be qualified, if in no other respect than to describe the "rural." I live in Wishek, North Dakota, a town of approximately 1,300, sitting out in the middle of the rolling Great Plains. Its existence and location were determined not by any great act of history or significant detail of geology, but rather by the location of a railroad, which allowed the farmers to market their grain and livestock.

Wishek shares the many strengths and weaknesses of other rural areas. From my point of view, the advantages of rural existence greatly outweigh the disadvantages, but that certainly is a personal bias. I readily acknowledge the problems inherent with the isolation and provincialism, the disadvantages of a homogeneous and predominantly elderly population, the weakness of a poorly diversified economy which forces the young to leave, the smallness and therefore the lack of programs at school, and the lack of cultural outlets. Nevertheless, I am impressed by the cleanliness of the town and the pride people take in what they have, the sense of security I have knowing my loved ones and possessions are quite safe, the honesty, industriousness, and independence of most of the people, and the opportunity I have to make a significant contribution. Our economy is dominated by the fate of the surrounding farms and ranches. Services, entertainment and shopping are limited, but all the essentials are available locally.

If a person needs more than is available locally, he can drive 96 miles to Bismarck, a very complete "small city" of about 50,000, 180 miles to Fargo which is North Dakota's largest city at approximately 80,000, or 8–9 hours to Minneapolis/St. Paul.

This part of North Dakota has not been affected by the coal and oil development occurring in other parts of the state and the West as a whole. Nonetheless, Wishek is somewhat unusual in that its population has grown very slowly over the last 10 years while most other towns have lost people. Much of that growth can be related to the existence of a fine nursing home and retirement apartment complex as well as a continuity of reliable medical services.

The medical establishment here consists of Dr. M. Wiest, Dr. D. Kosiak, his partner, and myself. We service an area of approximately 4,000 square miles including parts of three counties. The closest doctors are located 30 miles west, 30 miles south, 50 miles east and 60 miles north. We work out of a new clinic located across from the 30 bed community hospital. Both buildings are owned by the Hospital Association. We provide services to a community 30 miles north of here on a four day per week basis. To round out our practice, we are responsible for 143 nursing home patients in two homes.

The local hospital can hardly be called a modern wonder, but what it lacks in spaciousness and interior decoration it makes up for with warmth and caring by a staff of hard working nurses and aides. It is difficult for someone who has experienced only a large hospital to appreciate how supportive the staff of a "home town" hospital can be for both patients and medical staff. Most patients are known as friends or relatives by the staff, and the "extended family" atmosphere is beneficial. Although I cannot in any way support this statement with evidence from scientific research, I feel that friendliness is a definite factor in patient recovery.

Essential laboratory and x-ray services are available on a daily basis, and diagnostic x-rays, ultrasonography, and nuclear medicine are available weekly. We have arrangements with an internist to visit weekly, an orthopedic surgeon twice monthly, and a cardiologist monthly. Patients whose problems need referral are generally sent to the specialists in Bismarck; very infrequently referrals are made to the Mayo Clinic or the University Hospital in Minneapolis. Physical therapy, respiratory therapy, and outpatient nursing services — such as a Public Health Nurse — are not available at this time.

The fact that the hospital laboratory is somewhat limited and diagnostic x-rays and scans are available only weekly is a source of frustration and adds a definite challenge to the practice of medicine here. For example, cardiac isoenzymes are usually not on the chart until the patient has been treated for four or five days. If a patient with a suspected GI problem presents to the clinic on the wrong day, there is no choice but to treat empirically until the next week when x-rays can be obtained. If the case is more serious, the decision must be made either to treat the patient supportively until diagnostic procedures can be obtained or to transfer the patient to Bismarck. Since our size is too small to support a true ICU/CCU or intensive care nursery, really difficult cases must be transferred.

At first glance, the decision to transfer to Bismarck should be easily made, but it is not. Some patients do not want to go so far from home; they would rather be treated by their primary physician. From our point of view, it is frustrating to transfer challenging cases we are fully capable of managing simply because hospital support services are not available.

There are definite advantages in working at a small hospital. Since there are only two doctors on regular staff, this comes as close as is possible to being a privately-controlled hospital. The only admissions made are by our group, so the hospital administration has only one group of people to satisfy, and thus there is very little politicking and bickering. The hospital budget does not allow for all the latest equipment and gadgets, but what is purchased is our own choice.

Prior to moving to Wishek, I had lived in communities ranging in size from New York City to a small town in central Pennsylvania. I have lived all over the country and have been in various parts of the world as a member of a U.S. Air Force family.

I am a registered nurse and worked in a busy emergency department before going into the FNP/PA program at the University of North Dakota. The program is based on the Medex model with periods of intensive didactic experience followed by clinical rotations. I took my clinical rotations in Colorado in a busy family practice office.

By virtue of my personality I am a generalist, a trait which certainly carries over into my professional life. To me, the appeal of primary care is the variety. I enjoy having regular contact with many different types of problems. Obviously, as a "jack-of-all-trades" I cannot hope to possess the depth of knowledge or expertise of the specialist in his field, but my experience is broader, and to me that is satisfying.

The first time I saw Wishek, I was not impressed. In fact, I could think of no good reason to move there. Fortunately, my roommate at school was much more perceptive than I and was very impressed by the town and the practice opportunity. It was in large measure his assurance which persuaded me to give this small town a try.

The difference between working in a suburban office and a rural office was an adjustment to make. Dr. Wiest was practicing by himself when I arrived and was desperately overworked, so I immediately found myself working harder and being given more responsibility than I had ever had before. Concommitantly, I found myself contributing more and being more appreciated. At first, I was somewhat awed by the sense of responsibility inherent in being one of only two primary care providers in a large area, but that has worn off. Initially, I was on call quite frequently. This provided me with several occasions demanding a strong antiperspirant. Now, with another doctor around, I do not need to take first call as often.

The definition of "Family Practice" differs significantly from the rural area to the city/suburban area. In the rural setting, the family practitioner for the most part is limited only by the facilities available and his realization of his own limitations and sense of ethics.

It is not uncommon for the family practitioner in a rural setting to be performing a variety of surgeries and diagnostic procedures which simply would not be permitted in a larger institution with its restricted staff privileges and competition. In the same way that few restrictions exist for the doctors, there are also fewer restrictions for the physician assistant, and the atmosphere is much more supportive because of it.

My role in this practice has developed over time. Initially there was a period of adjustment as the two of us got to know one another and develop a workable relationship. By now, we have a fairly set routine. The day begins at approximately 8 A.M. with hospital rounds. If I am early, I will start seeing patients by myself or catch up on dictation. I am responsible for all discharge summaries and most of the history and physical examinations. I do most of the newborn physical examinations, so if there has been a delivery overnight, I will start there. Our inpatient census averages 12–15 patients per day, so rounds usually last until 9:30. If I finish rounds by myself, the patients are always seen later by Dr. Wiest, so that frequently the patients are seen at least twice daily.

After rounds, Dr. Wiest goes next door to the clinic, and if scheduling permits, I stay at the hospital to finish my duties and dictation. When a patient is admitted, I see the patient first, do the history and physical examinations, and write admitting orders for the appropriate work-up and therapy. Later in the morning, I will head over to the clinic. Unless there is a particular patient to be seen by Dr. Wiest, patients are seen by either of us, depending on which of us is free. I do not carry any presigned prescriptions, so we consult on almost every patient and most patients are seen briefly by both of us. As a result of this method of handling patients, I have not developed any "independent" caseload of my own. This is not necessarily the most efficient method, but the patients like it.

In our practice, we see the entire spectrum from the newborn to the elderly with all their problems, but the majority is definitely adult medicine and much of that approaches the realm of geriatrics. If there is such a thing, the profile of a "typical" patient would be a female in her late 60's or early 70's, coming to the clinic for evaluation and regulation of her chronic hypertension, arthritis, or diabetes. She will inevitably be moderately to severely obese, with little real desire to lose weight. She will be pleasant and cooperative, but will have only a very limited knowledge of her problems and the functioning of her body and will require quite a bit of ongoing teaching to ensure compliance.

During a typical day, we will do some minor office surgery such as wart removal or removal of a lesion for biopsy. Frequently, I do the entire procedure myself or will assist and do the suturing. If casting or splinting is required, I get to play in the "mud." All the routine physical examinations for school, athletics, insurance, and so forth, are my responsibility. The only category of patient care in which I generally am not involved is obstetrics. Dr. Wiest enjoys this specialty and chooses to follow his patient entirely by himself. I do very little office laboratory or x-ray work myself since we have an excellent nurse who is much more proficient than I.

Now that Medicare allows physician assistants to recertify nursing home patients, I am solely responsible for that aspect of our practice. In addition, I frequently make the routine nursing home rounds.

My role has changed somewhat with the arrival of another doctor. I find myself seeing fewer clinic patients and spending much more time in the hospital, primarily because our hospital census has increased considerably. I certainly am not interested in "competing" with the new doctor for patients. He needs to build his practice, so if there are excess patients to be seen, he usually sees them.

Patient acceptance has simply not been a problem here. It was perhaps advantageous in that no other physician assistant had been here previously, so I had no positive or negative expectations to fulfill or overcome. Frankly, even after a year many of the patients are not entirely certain what I am except they know I am not a doctor and not a student. Nonetheless, they are not overly concerned, because they know I work with the doctor and they have found out I know what I am doing and that I can do many things at both the office and the hospital. As would be expected, there are some few patients who prefer to be seen only by the doctor, but on the other hand, an equally insignificant percentage wish to see me everytime. As a rule, those who are well-aware of my role have no qualms about my participation in their care; on the other hand, those who will not see me are not sure who I am.

I hold very strongly to the opinion that the attitude of the supervising physician is the single most important aspect in determining patient acceptance. Almost without exception, in those instances where a patient steadfastly refuses to see me, it is at least partially because the doctor has tacitly reinforced this behavior by failing to support my role or has failed to educate the patient. When the doctor has been supportive of my functions, patients have been most cooperative and receptive.

The contributions that can be made by the physician assistant in a rural practice such as this are many and are a real source of gratification. Simply by working in a rural area you make a very important contribution and the townspeople are sincerely appreciative of your work. In a small town, you are not just another face but rather a known and appreciated person whose presence is felt by the entire community. The obvious corollary to this fact is that an unpopular physician assistant would have a strong negative impact on the community and could prove an insurmountable liability to a practice.

The physician assistant offers a very cost-effective and efficient contribution to a practice which is not equaled even by the addition of another staff doctor. I am comfortable with this statement because from a cost-production point of view, the physician assistant is very efficient. Furthermore, the physician assistant enables the physician to work more effectively and productively by handling many of the important but less remunerative tasks such as hospital paperwork. For the harried doctor in solo practice who has no prospect of obtaining a partner, this contribution can literally be lifesaving. Whatever liabilities there may be in having a physician assistant in the practice are very much overshadowed by the positive contributions.

For the physician assistant who is so inclined, it is possible to branch out widely in a small town and make much needed contributions in areas indirectly related to the office. For example, the area athletic teams usually do not have a trainer and need help. The scouts always need someone for first aid. The school can use help in health classes. The local paper would welcome a well-written weekly column on health issues. Your imagination, time and talent are your only limits. I even found myself becoming the co-founder and director of a community choir, a dream I have had before but could never fulfill in a larger community where imminently more qualified individuals rightfully fulfilled this function.

If I were to offer advice to a physician assistant contemplating a move to a rural setting, it would be to appraise your family and its ability and willingness to settle into a small town. If you have never lived in a small, isolated town, the transition could be traumatic. A primary reason for discontent among young professionals in rural practice is an unhappy spouse. No matter how exciting the practice or how remunerative, you are not likely to last long if your spouse and family are unhappy.

For myself, I am quite content and my family and I are more satisfied than we have ever been. I would strongly urge anyone to give careful consideration to a rural practice.

Chapter 17

THE PHYSICIAN ASSISTANT IN A SMALL TOWN PRIMARY CARE PRACTICE

THOMAS K. JOHNSTONE, PA-C

A physician assistant in a small town practices preventive medicine, manages acute illnesses, and assists with the long-term care of chronically ill patients. Like his physician supervisor, the physician assistant must remain current on new drugs and diagnostic procedures used for a broad range of medical problems. He should provide patients with sound advice and attempt to educate them about their medical problems and about medications. He must always remember that it is not the illness but the patient's understanding of the illness that is foremost. Proper nutrition and good health habits are also important matters to be discussed with patients.

While in training, I had the opportunity to work in several different practice settings. The most unique experience was working in a rural clinic in western North Carolina. The clinic was set up to do laboratory work, take x-rays, and dispense medications from a small pharmacy. It was here that I was exposed to a wide range of problems and saw first hand how a physician assistant could help extend a physician's practice. By using a citizen's band radio, I could make house calls while the physician remained at the office. I would relay my findings and he would indicate what he wanted me to do. It was a rewarding experience, but one thing was missing—the ability to follow-up on a patient who was sent to the hospital. The two nearest hospitals were located 30 miles from the clinic and it was not practical to make rounds when so many patients needed to be seen in the clinic. This led me to seek employment in a small town that had a hospital serving a predominantly rural community.

Reidsville is a pleasant town of about 18,000 people located in the northern piedmont region of North Carolina. The county in which it is located is mostly rural with tobacco, corn, and soy beans as major crops. It has a diverse industrial base, such as textiles, a major tobacco company, and a beer distillery. Reidsville is a good place to live, to rear a family, and to work.

The town has an excellent 160 bed hospital which happens to be located across the street from my supervising physician's office. This allows me to follow a patient's care from the time of diagnosis, through hospitalization, to recovery—depending on the problem. Medical and surgical consultations are available in the hospital allowing us to continue in the care of our patients.

I work for two general practitioners and divide my time equally between them. We make rounds on hospitalized patients twice a day. I round with one physician in the morning and with the other in the evening. This arrangement provides continuity of care. The physicians view this as a definite plus for having a physician assistant in their practice. It is during the morning that we see patients who were admitted by the emergency medical staff at night. While I order and collect laboratory data, the physician is freed to see newly admitted patients or to return to the office. Most of our hospitalized patient records are done in the evening when there is more time. There are times when I round on patients alone. For example, I make solo rounds on Saturday afternoons. I enjoy this experience for the most part. It enables me to review charts in more detail, and the added responsibility is welcomed. Visiting patients on a one-to-one basis is also a plus.

After rounds and a short coffee break, the office work begins at about 9:00 am and continues until about 12:30 or 1:00 pm when we break for lunch. Of course, we stay until the last patient is seen. We begin again at 2:00 pm and see patients in the office until about 5:00 to 6:00 in the evening. Then we are off to make evening rounds.

We see patients by appointment and on a first-come, first-see basis. There are no limitations placed on whom I see except for medicare patients. There is no reimbursement for services rendered by a physician assistant to a medicare patient so they must be seen by the physician unless there is an emergency and I am the only one available at the time. For the most part, I see about the same type of problems seen by the physician. When I am unsure or feel uncomfortable about a patient's problem, I immediately consult my supervising physician. Any practitioner who believes that he is above error and refuses to seek help is asking for trouble. It is important that you know your limitations and that you are honest about them.

In certain cases, I initiate therapy, order diagnostic laboratory work, and make referrals. In North Carolina, physician assistants can write prescriptions for commonly used medications for upper respiratory and urinary tract infections, gastrointestinal problems, and so forth. Physicians who do not employ physician assistants sometime have difficulty appreciating the time-saving benefits that this offers a practice and patients.

I believe that it is important for a physician assistant to adopt as closely as possible the practice style of his supervising physician. It is not necessary to become the mirror image of the physician or to lose your own professional identity, but it is important that you appreciate how your supervising physician approaches a particular medical problem and his manner of treatment. The physician assistant and the physician have their own personalities and philosophies, but each should know what the other is thinking. This develops by closely working together on problems and by keeping lines of communication open. Patients can sense this feeling of trust that develops between the physician and the assistant. Confidence and trust result in a good team effort and enhance the care rendered to patients.

I see a large number of patients who return to the office for routine cardiovascular checkups, suture or cast checks, and other types of medical problems. I assist with physical examinations to determine disability or time off from work. Counseling patients about how to care for themselves also takes time. It is easy to forget or become so busy as to place less emphasis on patient education. I must continue to remind myself that this is one of the reasons that I am here. Emergency situations do occur in the office, and it is important that any practitioner know how to handle these problems. A physician assistant should know basic life support techniques and be able to provide assistance until additional help arrives.

I am not laden with insurance physicals, forms for social service, and other paper shuffling details. The work comes as it may. The same is true in the hospital. I am not assigned all the write-ups and other dictation. If I admit a patient to the hospital through the emergency room or office, then I will do most of the paper work. There are occasions when my supervising physicians become swamped with paper work and I volunteer my service which is always welcomed. Admitting patients to our local hospital creates no problem. The hospital administrators view me as an extension of my supervising physicians. If I see one of our regular patients in the office or emergency room who needs hospitalization, I will admit without consulting the physician at that moment. I immediately inform the physician of any patient who is critically ill and needs their attention. In an emergency situation, it is standard procedure for me to notify other physicians who might be needed to assess the patient, such as a surgeon, cardiologist, or gastroenterologist. When in doubt, I always consult my supervising physician. Knowing one's limitations and abilities at this point are paramount for the patient, the physician, and the physician assistant.

There are barriers in my job. The greatest obstacle for me initially was a lack of understanding of my role by both patients and by medical personnel. No one knew what a physician assistant was before I came to town. I remember one physician felt extremely threatened by my presence at first, but he now seems to accept me as a member of our medical community. In general, I would say that I am well accepted by physicians in our community. The nursing staff accepted orders written by me, but also had difficulty deciding into what "slot" I fell. If I was not a doctor or a nurse, then what was I? It seemed that the younger and more informed nurses were easier to work with at first. To help them understand my role, I spoke to the local nursing association soon after my arrival. Also, I spoke at the high school on career day and at the local pharmacy club. These occasions to educate various groups about my role made the difference in my case. I would recommend this approach to any new physician assistant.

I find few people who refuse to accept my services, but there will always be people who want to be seen only by a physician. Initially, this was hard for me to accept, but I soon realized that one provider cannot please all people. This is no different from any other profession. My time and effort is better spent working with people who know and respect my role.

Another physician assistant in a similar practice setting may have a somewhat different routine, but I believe what I do is typical and representative of physician assistants working in a small town primary care practice. As you can see, I am proud of my role as a physician assistant. Without sounding too egotistical, I do feel that I have helped to improve the delivery of health care services in our community and that the town and surrounding area is now aware of the beneficial role of physician assistants. Eight years ago when I arrived on the scene, no one knew what a physician assistant was. Now that has all changed. Physician assistants can make a valuable contribution to primary care.

Chapter 18

THE ROLE OF THE PRIMARY CARE PHYSICIAN ASSISTANT IN AN OFFICE-BASED GENERAL INTERNAL MEDICINE SETTING

FRAN PIAZZA KAHLER, PA-C
WINTON BRIGGS, M.D.

THE PHYSICIAN ASSISTANT'S VIEW

Prior to entering the Physician Assistant Training Program at Bowman Gray School of Medicine in Winston-Salem, North Carolina, I had earned a Bachelor's degree in psychology, worked as a nurse's aide on a medical surgical unit, worked as a psychiatric aide, and as an abortion counselor in a women's abortion/gynecology clinic. I searched for a career that would challenge me as well as utilize my talents and interests in psychology. I was intrigued by the concept of the physician assistant with its emphasis on patient communication and teaching, improvement in quality and availability of health care, and potential for preventive medicine. I entered the physician assistant profession as an idealist with little appreciation of the possible barriers or prejudices I might encounter. Training in North Carolina, where the first Physician Assistant program began at Duke University in 1965, was advantageous. There are approximately 450 practicing physician assistants and two training programs in that state. Consequently, physician assistants have, to a large extent, been assimilated into the health care system there.

I soon realized that the fate of physician assistants depended on tolerant laws, a supportive view from the American Medical Association and the medical community, and an awareness and acceptance by the general population. Obviously this requires a strong national organization (the American Academy of Physician Assistants) and individual involvement beginning at the student level. Thus, I ran for and became the President of our Student Society, an involvement that continues to shape my thoughts about my profession.

After graduation, I worked with two psychiatrists in Winston-Salem. Their practice had utilized a physician assistant for many years, so my role was clear-cut. I helped with rounds, did hospital admission histories and physicals, and cared for many minor inpatient medical problems. I also helped with consults, often doing the initial interview. Afternoons were spent in the office doing initial histories and post-hospital visits. I followed a select number of patients and consulted the supervising physician as necessary. In addition, there was considerable phone work involving crisis intervention and routine problems. This experience in psychiatry served as a helpful foundation in my later job working in an internal medicine practice.

I chose internal medicine to practice primary care with a diverse patient population and a variety of medical problems. However, a large motivating factor was purely academic. Throughout my education I felt frustrated by the volume of material I wanted to learn and the limited amount of time in which to learn it. Internal medicine could provide me with the vehicle for the learning I desired. I was assured by many internists that my interest in psychiatry would be satiated.

Since September of 1980, I have worked in a busy internal medicine practice in Cape Elizabeth, Maine. I was hired when 1 of 3 doctors left to pursue a sub-specialty. In July of 1981, a third internist joined the practice. Cape Elizabeth is a relatively affluent "bedroom" community near Portland, Maine. Patients are mostly private paying or have insurance, are often well educated and thus medically sophisticated. Prior to my arrival, the physician assistant was virtually unheard of as there are only three of us working in the Portland area, and I am the only one in a private practice setting. Nevertheless, I have been remarkably well accepted in our practice.

Our office has two receptionists, one nurse, three full-time medical assistants, a billing person, and a part-time typist/insurance person. We have our own x-ray department and technician and a well-equipped lab for routine tests. We do our own EKG's, spirometries, sigmoidoscopies, and minor surgeries such as repair of lacerations and incisions and drainages.

The fee is the same for seeing either the doctor or me, and according to the billing office, few people have complained. The fee schedule is based on the assumption that I am providing the same quality care that would be delivered by the physicians. Our policy is that if I have any questions, I consult one of the doctors. Therefore, even if the doctor does not see a patient with me, the patient may be receiving the benefit of the doctor's expertise. For initial physicals and most periodic exams, I discuss the case in great detail with the doctor. I have a DEA number and can write prescriptions from a formulary which excludes class I and II narcotics as well as certain other medicines. This freedom has been a distinct advantage and has never posed a problem.

I have been introduced gradually to the patients, often seeing someone initially if the physician is behind schedule. If someone is tied up at the office or called away for an emergency, patients are asked if they would like to see me or reschedule. Usually patients prefer to see me.

The receptionists schedule me for an hour and a half per initial physical, one hour per periodic exam, and one half hour per office call. The staff tells me that patients frequently voice their appreciation of the extra time spent with them. Patients are given a choice of practitioners and oftentimes my availability is attractive. Thus they will often choose to see me earlier rather than wait for the doctor. It is this flexibility that is so helpful for school, camp, sports, company, and insurance physicals which often need to be scheduled on short notice. Understandably, patients consider this an asset. This also applies to walk-ins and minor problems such as sore throats, cystitis, vaginitis, and so forth. I occasionally make house calls as well. In addition, I see many patients who present acutely ill. This expedites the evaluation and possible hospital admission process, and benefits the patients while saving the physician valuable time.

Many patients were left without a physician when the third partner left the practice. Consequently, I saw many of his patients for problems and periodic exams. Many of these people have now been absorbed by the other doctors but I continue to see some primarily or assist in their interim care.

The longer I am here, the more referrals I receive from other patients. Many females, especially adolescents, are eager to see a woman practitioner. This works out well since I particularly enjoy gynecology. I spend considerable time doing PAP smears, first pelvic exams, birth control counselling, diaphragm fitting, and treating vaginal infections. There are patients who refuse to see me under any circumstances. However, it is not unusual that an initially skeptical person will later call and ask to see me or speak to me. Much of my time is spent explaining my role to the patients and despite this, many will ask if I will "go on" to be a doctor.

The feedback from the office staff has been positive. They appreciate the convenience of having someone who is available for questions, who can refill routine prescriptions, and who can take phone calls. In addition, they can satisfy the patients who need or want to be seen quickly.

Another convenience I afford is sharing call. Our system provides for me to be on call with each doctor every other time he is on. We share call with another group of internists so I work one weekend per month. Incidentally, the other group has commented that they are pleased with my services to their patients. I take all office-related calls and the doctor takes all hospital and nursing home calls referred by the answering service. On Saturday morning, I see patients in the office for acute problems allowing the doctor to devote his time to hospital rounds with limited interruptions. Of course, any complicated problems are discussed with the physician.

Overall, my position has added a new dimension to the practice. Patients benefit by getting first quality health care that is more available than ever before. I can provide more time for teaching, counselling, clarifying treatment plans, and answering questions both in the office or on the phone. The physicians have increased capabilities in terms of their emphasis on more complicated patients and the delivery of service to regularly scheduled patients. Interruptions and "work-ins" are reduced. Their days off and vacations are more easily executed with minimal disruption in the continuity of care provided to their patients. Clearly, I am cost-effective. I have generated almost three times my salary the first year alone in total charges including lab work.

Regretably, Medicaid will not reimburse for services rendered by a physician assistant in nursing homes not considered "rural health clinics". This option would be a tremendous asset to our practice and most certainly would improve the availability, thus quality, of care to the nursing home patients. I would enjoy the opportunity to get out of the office, particularly on slow days when I could be easily spared. Similarly, there are times when I would like the opportunity to be in the hospital. For example, I may see a patient for pancreatitis or an upper gastrointestinal bleeding episode whom I evaluate in the office and determine the need for hospital admission. Once I refer them to the doctor, I essentially lose track of them. Not only is this difficult in terms of my emotional investment in the patient (especially if I am the primary health care provider), but it is also frustrating not to learn the inpatient care of these conditions. In addition, my lack of familiarity with the hospital alienates me from the mainstream of the medical community. This bothers me personally but also professionally, because I feel the medical community needs to be exposed to physician assistants and the services they can provide.

The Maine Medical Center employs only two physician assistants and they work exclusively in the Emergency Room. Recently, the hospital's policies on physician assistants have been revised to allow these health professionals to provide patient care under the supervision of their employing physician. Hopefully with more exposure to physician assistants, the medical community will realize the physician assistant's value and will begin to utilize them in the hospital. In my case, our hospital practice is quite variable and my supervising physicians feel that I am more valuable to them in the office.

My limited personal experience with the physicians in this community has been basically favorable. It is disappointing, however, to write a letter of introduction in referring a patient and to enclose records that clearly indicate my role in the care of that patient, only to have all return correspondence directed solely to the physician. Occasionally, a doctor refuses to discuss a patient with me, despite my being the primary health care provider in that case. This can be frustrating and a blow to one's ego. Happily, this does not occur often.

Generally, though, I get enough positive feedback from my patients and the staff to provide me with the necessary job satisfaction and self-esteem.

However, the struggle that lies before the physician assistant profession cannot be overemphasized. There are many physicians who combine all middle-level health-care practitioners (physician assistants, nurse practitioners, nurse-midwives) and see physician assistants as desiring to become independent practitioners. Many see us as "frustrated doctors," thereby robbing us of the job prestige that should be credited to our unique, complimentary profession. Still others perceive us as a threat in view of the forecasted surplus of physicians. This perception ignores the fact that physician assistants contribute substantially to the solution of maldistribution of health care, a problem which will not be solved by the predicted excess of physicians alone.

My personal belief is that physician exposure to physician assistants and public awareness are the keys to the success of the profession. Once experienced, the physician assistants and their services speak for themselves.

THE SUPERVISING PHYSICIAN'S VIEW

Our group of three "workaholic" internists had been functioning smoothly for seven years when one of us had the opportunity to complete his nephrology training and enter a position as a full-time nephrologist locally. Within one and-a-half months, my associate and I had enlisted one of our local senior internal medical residents to join us in the following July. However, that left nine months with two-man coverage. Experience had previously demonstrated that two of us could handle the triple load only two to four weeks without undue stress.

We thus interviewed several nurse practitioners trained locally and three physician assistants trained elsewhere in search of a mature, competent "extender" to help us bridge the gap. We talked with other internists in our area and received cautious or hesitant comments. Two internists had experience with nurse practitioners. In the first case, the relationship terminated in less than a year because of less than ideal results. In the second case, a husband and wife team had worked successfully for several years. A physician assistant had not been used in a private practice of primary care in our area.

Our selection of Fran was based primarily on our interviews demonstrating an intelligent, mature person. Her previous experiences in counseling and in psychiatric practice could only be an asset, as a significant portion of our primary internal medical practice involves recognizing and treating psychiatric problems. We also had some concern, possibly unfounded, that a nurse practitioner might present a problem of being more independent than we supervising physicians would be comfortable with.

We presented our patients with a letter making the triple announcement of the one physician leaving, the arrival of one physician assistant, and the anticipated arrival of the third internist months away. We reviewed these changes with our office staff, basically feeling that a personal contact with Fran's assets would prove more to the staff and the patients than words of explanation from us. Indeed, I believe that an attempt to "hard-sell" the concept of a physician assistant, or Fran in particular, would have been harmful. In any event, Fran's introduction was gradual and quiet. No deleterious gossip occurred within the community. Indeed, at least one physician's wife expressed her preference for Fran's competent care.

Fran brought to us not just the manpower to handle the anticipated patient load, but also a very thorough style of histories and physicals, a superb understanding and handling of the multiple personalities within our community, and a continuing and avid learning attitude in interpretive and therapeutic skills.

As was hoped, the addition of a physician assistant in the office was accepted by my associate and myself, by the office staff, and by the overwhelming majority of our practice. The unusual stresses anticipated from the increased patient load failed to materialize with Fran's help. Vacations were still possible and our continued work on the teaching service in internal medicine at our local hospital was still possible.

With the arrival of our third internist, there was some question as to whether we would still need a physician assistant. Given the assets that Fran brings, we have continued now with a four person office practice. We anticipate gradually broadening our patient base to support the four professionals more adequately.

We have encouraged our physician assistant to maintain her interests in participating in professional associations for physician assistants, to continue with continuing educational conferences at least in part at our expense, and to utilize local hospital conferences. We have not expanded her field to inpatient care based on our philosophy that any individual ill enough to require hospitalization requires significant interpretative and therapeutic capabilities that our physician assistant has not learned. We feel that she lacks the direct experience necessary to expand her inpatient capabilities. The additional involvement in the nursing home environment continues to be a possibility, somewhat depending upon financial support from third party payers.

Since the arrival and successful use of a physician assistant in this office, we have had several other primary care physicians discuss this with us, although none have yet hired such a professional. I would like to believe that our positive experience will enhance the utilization of physician assistants in this community.

However, this medical community is structured around a tertiary medical facility (the Maine Medical Center of Portland, Maine) which is in an environmentally comfortable location. Thus, the area has more than an ample supply of physicians. It is likely that other groups will hire another physician rather than risk the utilization of a physician assistant.

Chapter 19

EMERGENCY DEPARTMENT
AND THE PHYSICIAN ASSISTANT

ROBERT J. MEYER, M.D.
GEOFFERY A. BECKETT, PA-C
JOSEPH P. CONRAD, PA-C

Emergency room utilization has nearly doubled since 1960, and the basic nature of emergency room care has been changing radically. Increasingly, traditional rotating call and "moonlighting" coverage by physicians has proven inadequate for the needs of individual emergency departments. In many emergency rooms, the employment of fulltime physician specialists has been a superior alternative, but economic considerations limit this possibility to the busier facilities. Since the early 1970's, the use of emergency room physicians assistants has been carefully studied as a possible part of a solution to the staffing crisis. The consensus of investigators detailed in numerous articles that have appeared in the medical literature is that physician assistants represent a particularly valuable resource for emergency medicine and can be utilized in a wide variety of settings. In both rural and metropolitan emergency departments, they have been perceived favorably by the public and the medical community and are seen as contributing to increased cost effectiveness and an improved quality of care. It seems probable that their role will continue to expand in helping to meet the demands facing the emergency medical system.

The reasons for the phenomenal growth in emergency medicine are complex, reflecting social developments as well as problems intrinsic to the health care delivery system. Through an unplanned evolutionary process, the "accident room" of the 1950's developed into the "emergency department" of the late 1970's, a concept bearing little resemblance to its predecessor. By 1979, emergency medicine became a recognized medical specialty. Technological advances demanded both more complex and expensive equipment and a staff with the expertise to manage critical care problems and supervise sophisticated pre-hospital life support by emergency medical technicians and paramedics.

Emergency room physicians are now expected to demonstrate competence in both traumatology and cardiopulmonary emergencies, though true emergencies constitute less than ten percent of most hospital emergency room visits. The bulk of the emergency room case load is non-critical. In fact, many emergency rooms now function as outpatient clinics in addition to handling the severely ill. It is routine medical care that accounts for most of the increase in utilization.

There are several explanations for this. The decrease in availability of general practitioners in the 1960's coupled with the postwar increase in mobility served to interrupt long-term doctor-patient relationships so that fewer and fewer Americans had a "family doctor." This was particularly true in low-income areas of the inner city where the absence of primary care physicians forced many people to seek out emergency rooms for all their health needs. In the general population, as expectations were rising about most aspects of life, so too did the demand for rapid, expeditious health care.

The emergency room is frequently perceived as offering increased convenience. A significant group of young and basically healthy people seem to see no advantage in a private physician when they require health care only once or twice annually. Still others come to the emergency room for acute care despite the availability of their family physicians. Another source of patients is a small but a growing population of people alienated from the mainstream who rely on the ER for a variety of medical and emotional needs and occasionally as a source of food and shelter. Derelicts, psychiatric outpatients, and others who are marginally functional have come to regard the emergency room as their "family doctor," while some patients are referred by local police and various social agencies.

In response to public demand and improved technology, medical staffs have enlarged and facilities have been expanded and upgraded with the generation of more "career oriented" physicians and specialized allied health workers. Expansion of services in turn has resulted in a greater utilization. While the increasing availability of primary care physicians will probably alter this trend, it is unlikely to effect radical change in the next two decades. The emergency care structure, therefore, needs to remain malleable and to adapt to changing social and economic conditions while continuing to provide high quality care.

STAFFING PATTERNS

The traditional approach to emergency room staffing in community hospitals has been the rotating call system. In this model, each private practicing physician takes an equal responsibility to cover the emergency room on a rotating basis. Such physicians may take call weekly, biweekly, or with whatever frequency might be necessary to effect full coverage. In some hospitals, a common call schedule for all physicians is maintained while in others, separate surgical and medical call schedules are kept. Call is taken from home and from the office. Many hospitals have abandoned this system due to both the frustration of overextended staffs and community unhappiness over quality of care. This system has been shown to have produced many deficiencies in the quality of care provided because the on-call physician may not be available to attend to an unstable patient or a true emergency or the on-call physician is required to attend to a patient with a problem outside of his area of competence.

Many emergency rooms have been staffed in the past by physicians trained in other specialties, often semi-retired or awaiting more permanent positions. More recently, groups tend to be composed of physicians who have developed an interest in emergency medicine as moonlighters or residents and have chosen to make it their career. This latter group evolved into an important force in the 1970's which created the new specialty of emergency medicine. Postgraduate training in emergency medicine was introduced. Scientific and clinical research flourished and a new sense of professionalism raised standards of care nationally. Protocols for advanced cardiac life support developed by the American Heart Association gained wide acceptance. Good prehospital care began to grow with a network of competent EMT's and paramedics. The experience of military medicine in Viet Nam and Korea, which demonstrated the value of triage, rapid transport, and definitive care of trauma in centralized facilities, fostered the development of regional trauma centers.

As in any other rapidly growing field, there has been considerable difficulty in assimilating new technologies and organizational ideas into well-established structures. While recognition of the needs of area wide planning and rational use of facilities is slowly overcoming traditional practices, jurisdictional disputes between hospitals, communities, and governments have often hindered attempts to reorganize. This lack of coordination has frequently resulted in the duplication of services and a waste of resources. Every department should be capable of meeting fairly diverse needs and stabilizing the critically ill, yet it is sensible for each to understand its primary functions and its limitations. Rescue services should triage and transport their patients to the most appropriate facilities. Staffing should be tailored to the nature and volume of patients the department projects. Clearly, larger and busier facilities demand skills of the full-time emergency room specialist, while smaller emergency departments find it difficult to bear the expense and may question the need for a physician with such an advanced level of training. Skill loss and boredom contribute to the poor professional longevity of career physicians in low volume departments. Staffing must be individualized and adapted to each setting. The balancing of cost efficiency, physician satisfaction, and a high quality of care is often a difficult proposition.

PHYSICIAN ASSISTANTS

The use of mid-level practitioners to provide emergency care first intrigued investigators in the early 1970s. They were concerned with the dual issues of economy and availability of services, particularly in rural hospitals. Golomb, in 1974, concluded that physician assistants could adequately treat over half of the patients who presented to the emergency room of a 200 bed hospital. He suggested a model of one physician and one physician assistant jointly covering a busy facility (1). In New Hampshire, Maxfield studied the role of physician assistants in a rural 90 bed hospital as an alternative to rotating emergency staff call. After a gradual development over a three year period, Maxfield showed in 1974 that physician assistants could adequately manage 93% of the patients they saw with telephone consultations with supervising physicians or by requesting later physician followup. Physicians, nurses and patients, perceived significant improvements in efficiency without loss of quality (2). In 1980, Newkirk compared the use of physician assistants to rotating night time physician staff coverage in rural Maine emergency departments. His findings demonstrated a marked increase in patient utilization in departments with full-time physician assistants, financial benefits to both hospital and medical staff, and an increase in the consistency and predictability of good quality medical care (3). In two large urban teaching hospitals with tertiary care responsibilities, Goldfrank reported the successful use of physician assistants to replace moonlighters and interns in the emergency department. In a setting replete with surgical and medical specialists, physician assistants provided a liaison role between these two groups and were observed to "broaden the interest and skills" of the specialist physicians. The physician assistants were able to stabilize a previously erratic service, limit the variability of care, and gain overwhelmingly positive patient acceptance (4).

In the early 1980s, physician assistants utilization in the emergency department is widely practiced and accepted. In the State of Maine, 38% of hospital emergency rooms use physician assistant coverage (5). A 1978 national survey revealed emergency medicine as the third most practiced physician assistant specialty (6). A 1980 editorial in the *Annals of Emergency Medicine* stated "proper utilization of well trained and motivated physician assistants in the emergency department is an ideal use of physician extenders." A general consensus exists that physician assistants can handle the initial management of 80 to 90% of the emergency room cases and can stabilize life-threatening situations until physician consultation is available. Adequate physician backup is necessary, obviously. Patterns of use vary widely and have been adapted to meet individual department needs. Several models can be cited.

1. The small rural hospital which has been unhappy with rotating staff call can improve its services by hiring two physicians and three or four physician assistants to effect 24 hour coverage. One physician is always present during 12 hours of every day, with night time duty taken by a physician assistant who has specialty backup from the staff. Each physician assistant also works 25 to 50% of his or her hours during the day with one of the physicians. This provides quality control, continuing medical education for the physician assistant, and of course, additional manpower during busy hours.

2. In another model, two emergency rooms are covered by a single group consisting of four physicians and three physician assistants. The larger of the two hospitals has 24 hour physician coverage while a smaller satellite facility remains open 12 hours per day with physician assistant staffing. A direct phone hookup enables the physician assistant to rapidly communicate with the physician preceptor in the event of a critical problem. Chart reviews take place daily. The three physician assistants spend 25% of their clinical time with the preceptors at the larger facility. At the smaller facility during night-time hours, private patients are seen by their family physicians, and drop-in traffic is referred to the "parent" facility.

3. In a 600 bed teaching hospital, two physician assistants complement a staff of five attending emergency physicians and house officers serving their rotations. The attending physicians are allowed more time for teaching and critical care while the physician assistants handle most of the noncritical care and assist in teaching and with critical care. As in the previous models, physician assistants actively work with prehospital personnel by acting as intermediaries and as a learning resource for EMTs.

Physician assistants are frequently able to spend more time with each patient than the physician might be able to. By being physically present when a patient walks in the door, physician assistants can cut waiting time considerably. Variability in care is decreased, and close monitoring of their practice is not difficult. Because their interests and activities are focused on emergency medicine, physician assistants can develop and maintain a high degree of proficiency in acute medical care. Teaching interactions with physicians stimulate intellectual exchange and frequently increases the physician's job interest. Several postgraduate training programs have developed that allow physician assistants to strengthen their emergency room skills. Procedures such as endotracheal intubation, central line placement, and insertion of chest tubes are taught along with advanced cardiac life support.

As emergency medical systems are streamlined, it seems likely that physician assistant utilization in emergency rooms will expand. The categorization of facilities will cause many departments to narrow their scope and concentrate on ambulatory care, enhancing the desirability of physician assistant obligation. By virtue of their cost effectiveness, community acceptance, and proven competence, physician assistants are clearly part of the solution to the dilemma of emergency care.

REFERENCES

1. Golomb, M.H., *et al.:* Alternative Staffing Proposals for Emergency Rooms. *J.A.M.A.*, Vol 228, No. 3, April 15, 1974.
2. Maxfield, R.G., *et al.:* Utilization of Supervised Physician's Assistants in Emergency Room Coverage in a Small Rural Community Hospital. *The Journal of Trauma*, Vol 15, No. 9, 1975.
3. Newkirk, W.: Rural Emergency Department Coverage. *The Journal of Maine Medical Association*, Vol 71, December 1980.
4. Goldfrank, L.: The Emergency Services Physician Assistant: Results of Two Years Experience. *Annals of Emergency Medicine, 9:*2, February, 1980.
5. *Special Study of the Use of Physician Assistants in Emergency Rooms.* Medical Care Development Inc., Augusta, Maine, 1980.
6. National Data on Physician Assistants. *American Academy of Physician Assistants,* Appendix 4, 1979.

Chapter 20

THE PRIMARY CARE PHYSICIAN ASSISTANT IN A FAMILY PRACTICE TRAINING PROGRAM

PAULA MONTGOMERY-KOWALSKI, PA-C
KAREN G. HOLMAN, M.D.

One of the newest recognized specialties in medicine is family practice. It is unique because not only does it encompass the role of primary care providers, diagnosing and treating illnesses, but assumes longitudinal responsibilities for the whole family regardless of the presence or absence of disease, thereby being responsible for the family's total health care. Since this is a new specialty, the authors believe that to better understand the utilization of physician assistants in the residency it is first important to have some knowledge of the training of family practice residents. Only a brief explanation of the University of Oklahoma Health Sciences Center Family Practice Residency Program will be given since no two residencies are exactly alike.

The University of Oklahoma Health Sciences Center Family Practice Residency is three years in length. The first year consists of specialty rotations (general surgery, 2 months; internal medicine, 3 months; pediatrics, 3 months; obstetrics and gynecology, 3 months; and emergency medicine, 1 month). During these rotations during the first year, the resident is required to return to the family medicine clinic one-half day per week to see patients. These clinics are designed for the residents to begin assuming the responsibility of patient care and to begin providing health care for the entire family. The residents continue to follow these families until completing the residency.

Residents in the second year are on a split schedule. Four months of the year are spent full-time in family practice. During this time, the residents care for their own patients and cover the practice for residents on elective. The majority of their time is spent in the family practice clinic, but also includes hospital coverage of family practice patients. During the other eight months of the year, the residents divide their time between the family practice clinic and rotations in other specialty areas, except one or two months of the year when the residents are not available to care for their patients. The residents are also assigned approximately ten patients from one of several nursing homes used in the residency. They are required to make monthly visits on their patients and provide acute care as necessary. Home visits are made on patients as the residents and attending physicians believe are necessary.

In the third year of the residency, residents average seven months working full-time in the family practice clinic. The remaining five months are spent divided between the clinic and specialty rotations. Nursing home and home visit responsibilities continue as in the previous year. During the residency, residents develop a small private practice and provide patient continuity of care for up to three years. The residents learn to provide care in settings other than the hospital, primarily in the clinic setting, but also in the home and nursing home. There is also sufficient time to gain experience in the other specialties which contribute to family practice.

One of the important secondary goals of the residency is a direct personal experience with the role of physician assistants in family practice. Before physician assistants can be effectively utilized, residents and faculty must accept the philosophy of health care teams and the resultant sharing of patient care responsibilities. The Department of Family Medicine at the University of Oklahoma supports the concept that health extenders are an important asset to family physicians, especially for those practicing in rural areas. In order to understand the various possibilities of how physician assistants can be utilized, the residents have the opportunity to work with physician assistants during their training. The following is a general, perhaps idealistic, approach to utilizing physician assistants in a family medicine residency training program which has arisen out of our experience at the University of Oklahoma.

Most residencies begin each day with a check-in. The residents, attending physicians, and physician assistants exchange information about recent admissions and the current status of hospitalized patients. After check-in, each health care team (consisting of residents, an attending physician, and a physician assistant) make hospital rounds. The team approach to health care is more personalized for everyone including the patient, and gives residents a better concept of a small practice. After the physician assistants complete rounds with their team, they usually have clinics with their supervising physician and a team resident or they are assigned to see emergency patients. The clinics are structured to allow residents to work directly with the physician assistant. This helps the resident obtain a better understanding of how health care teams provide medical care. For the physician assistant, the time with the resident is beneficial because the physician assistant will have the opportunity to meet the resident's patients and also learn the resident's protocols. Continuity of care is enhanced by this policy because the residents are on rotations much of the time during their training. If acute care is needed while the resident is on elective, the patient has a choice of being seen by another physician and/or by the physician assistant. It is not unusual for the patient to choose the physician assistant because he usually has provided health care to the patient in the past and the patient recognizes this health professional as part of the health care team of their regular physician. The physician assistant will see the patient, make a diagnosis, and then institute a treatment plan according to the physician's protocol. If any questions should arise concerning the patient's case there is always an attending physician in the clinic available for consultation. If the problem is minor, a notation is made to inform each physician that their patient was seen, the diagnosis, treatment and follow-up (if arranged). When follow-up is needed, the physician assistant tries to schedule the patient to return when his regular physician is in the clinic. If this is not possible, the patient returns to see the physician assistant for follow-up care. If the problem is serious enough for hospitalization, the attending is consulted. If the attending agrees with the need for hospitalization, the resident is immediately notified. The resident then follows his patient during the hospitalization. Physician assistants also assist residents in minor outpatient procedures such as circumcisions, casting, and biopsies. Physician assistants should have expertise in these areas so they can help the residents perfect their techniques in these procedure-oriented areas.

Another aspect of the physician assistant's role in a residency program concerns nursing home visits. The health care team is assigned to a specific nursing home and makes rounds once a month. The physician assistant provides direct care to the patient and helps resolve any psychosocial problems which might arise. The physician assistant is the key to providing continuity of care when acute care is needed and the physician is unavailable. The physician assistant will make the nursing home visits by himself, manage the patient's problem if possible following the physician's protocol, but consult an attending if necessary.

Home visits still play an important though limited role in providing health care to selected patients. Home care is most frequently provided to the aged or to the chronically ill whose mobility is restricted. In most instances, only routine care is provided, but occasionally acute care is rendered. Usually, only one member of the health care team makes the home visit. If the resident is not available, then the physician assistant will make the visit. Home visits are also useful to assess the home environment and family interactions. For instance, if a family has an infant with poor weight gain, a home visit might reveal some of the contributing factors to this medical problem. The information obtained by one member of the health care team would be shared with the others.

During regularly scheduled clinics, physician assistants work with their supervising physicians. This allows the attending, with a limited amount of time, to see personal patients and to see more patients more efficiently. Again, the physician assistant provides continuity of care when the supervising physician is not available to see acutely ill patients, using other attendings for consultation if necessary. This form of team collaboration serves as a role model to the residents, accentuating the positive aspects of the team approach to health care delivery.

Most family practice departments are involved in student education. During the time the medical students and physician assistant students are rotating in family practice, lectures are given explaining the concept of family practice and the team approach to patient care. Some of the round table discussions are about physician assistants, their utilization, how they fit into the health care team, and the benefits to the patient and the physician. While the students are in the clinic, they can observe the physician and the physician assistant working as a team. For instance, if the physician is busy with one student, other students can present their findings of a patient encounter to a physician assistant and the necessary tests can be ordered. Since the student must present the patient prior to ordering tests, this procedure of presenting to the physician assistant decreases patient waiting time and more effectively utilizes the physician's time. By working within a health care team context, the students observe practicing physician assistants as role models. Medical students, even if they do not intend to specialize in family medicine, acquire knowledge regarding physician assistants and the health care team approach.

Research is another important activity in many family practice residency programs. Most of the research is conducted by physician and non-physician faculty, although residents are also encouraged to participate in research during their training.

Most of the research conducted within family practice residencies is family or patient care oriented. Topics such as compliance, effective utilization of health care teams, surveys of diagnoses encountered in an ambulatory care setting, the effectiveness of a particular treatment plan, and the correlation of stress and illness are examples of areas in which research is being done.

Residents participating in research projects can be assisted by the attending physician and the physician assistant on their team. The attending physician and the physician assistant can offer expertise to the resident because of their past experiences in other research projects. This would include selecting and organizing an appropriate and feasible project, obtaining the results, and summarize the findings. The paper describing these findings is presented at a family medicine conference and may be submitted for publication.

Physician assistants can also generate income for the department and patients for the residents by being involved in employee health services of companies and institutions in the area. These services usually consist of new or annual physical examinations for large businesses and industries, hospitals, city employees, or companies with only a small number of employees. Before the employees are seen they sign a consent form releasing all medical information found during the exam to the employer and, if needed, to their private physician. The cost of performing the physical examinations is minimal to the department since very little of the supervising physician's time is needed, yet the examinations bring in a large income. The physician assistant informs the patient of any abnormalities found during the examination and of any necessary follow-up care using the supervising physician's protocols. The employee health service becomes a source for new patients, some who have abnormalities that need to be followed up or others who need an ongoing personal family physician.

Family practice residency training programs have many responsibilities involving resident education, student education, patient care, research, and community services. In all these areas, physician assistants can play a vital role. The approach and resources used by each training program to achieve these various goals will differ. Thus, the role of physician assistants in each program will vary. Some of the ways that physician assistants can be utilized has been discussed in this chapter. It is anticipated that as family practice residency programs continue to evolve the role of the physician assistants within these residencies will also change.

REFERENCES

1. Rakel, Robert E.: *Principles of Family Medicine.* Philadelphia, W.B. Saunders Company, 1977.
2. Medalie, Jack H.: *Family Medicine Principles and Applications.* Baltimore, The Williams & Wilkins Company, 1978.
3. Mendenhall, Robert C., Repicky, Paul A., and Neville, Richard E.: Assessing the Utilization and Productivity of Nurse Practitioners and Physician Assistants: Methodology and Findings on Productivity. *Medical Care,* 1980, June 17(6) 609-623.
4. Kapp, David F.: A Plea for Physician Assistants. *Journal of Iowa Medical Society,* 1971 December 61:730-733.

Chapter 21

PHYSICIAN ASSISTANTS IN HEALTH MAINTENANCE ORGANIZATIONS

GARY R. SCOFIELD, M.S., PA-C
REUBEN GULL, M.D.

THE PHYSICIAN ASSISTANT'S VIEW

Health Maintenance Organizations (HMOs) are prepaid health plans providing complete medical, surgical, and hospital benefits to members paying a monthly fee. The plan is usually offered through employers and the companies usually pay a portion or all of the monthly fee. This plan differs from indemnity plans in that the patient must see the doctors who are either employed by or contracted to the HMO. In non-emergent situations, the patient is admitted to contract hospitals or hospitals owned by the HMO. Other ancillary medical services, such as dental care, optometric care and so forth, are usually offered to members for an increased monthly payment.

When the recent graduate of a physician assistant program or the physician assistant contemplating a job change considers a practice setting, there are several factors that require careful thought. Is there adequate supervision and consulting services if and when needed? Since most HMO's use a physician/PA team in their practice settings, this allows for interaction between practitioners. For the recent physician assistant graduate, the availability of the supervising physician for consultations is a necessity and HMO's generally allow easy access to physician supervisors. Physicians who are hired by HMO's are told of the need for them to supervise the physician assistant. The lack of desire to supervise physician assistants has never been a problem in our HMO. In addition, specialists who are employed by the HMO are readily available for physician assistant referral and consultation. Contracting specialists who do not actually work for the HMO have no obligation to accept physician assistant referrals or consultations. In my early days of practice, there was some difficulty in referring patients to contract specialists. This problem faded over the years as the contract specialist became more familiar with the physician assistant concept and with individual physician assistants. Since the HMO has hired its own specialists who understand when they are hired that referrals and consultations will be coming from physician assistants, there appears to be no further conflict.

Another question any physician assistant should ask when considering his practice setting should be: Is the patient population diverse and/or suited to my interests and training? The HMO provides primary care services to all age groups, including gynecological problems, trauma, and health education. Obstetrical cases in most HMO practices are referred to obstetrical specialists for prenatal care and delivery. However, the physician assistant in an HMO will see all types of patients with a wide variety of medical and psychological complaints, including prenatal patients in selected situations.

The question of acceptance by patients is an interesting one. It should first be noted that any patient in an HMO is never required to see a physician assistant. The patient may select the primary care practitioner of his choice. All physician assistants in California where we work and in the HMO are required to wear identification badges. All patients are told that they will be seeing the physician assistant when their appointment is made. Once the patient understands the physician assistant's qualifications, scope of practice, and most importantly, once the patient is examined and treated by the physician assistant, acceptance has not been a problem. An occasional patient wants to see a physician assistant specifically. In five years of patient care in our HMO, there have been only a handful of patients who have rejected seeing a physician assistant.

A typical day in the primary care office of an HMO practice would be very similar to a private family practitioner's day. Generally, the physician assistant has an assigned number of exam rooms with scheduled morning and afternoon patients. The physician assistant maintains his own appointment schedule. Screening patients for assignment is generally not done. In California, written protocols are required and, therefore, certain cases seen by the physician assistant require immediate consultation with a physician. Included among these are chest pain of suspected cardiac origin, lacerations involving deep structures, and displaced fractures. The majority of cases seen in a primary care office can be handled by an experienced physician assistant with little or no consultation.

Patients are placed in rooms by the nurse who takes and records the vital signs. The nurse may also inquire as to the complaint. The physician assistant examines the patient, makes a provisional or definitive diagnosis, and initiates treatment. In California, physician assistants are not allowed to write prescriptions. Therefore, if a prescription is needed, the physician assistant discusses the appropriate drug for the condition with the physician. The physician then writes and signs the prescription.

Other patients seen in a typical day may require routine complete histories and physical examinations, well-baby checks, repair of lacerations, casting of non-displaced fractures, or minor surgical procedures.

All patients admitted to the hospital in our HMO are followed by the appropriate staff specialist. Neither family practice physicians nor physician assistants admit patients to hospitals. Not all HMO's function in this manner, and if a physician assistant desires hospital-based work he should check with the individual HMO to determine policy.

Another point that may be the most important consideration of all when choosing a practice setting is security. By nature, a dependent practitioner such as the physician assistant must rely upon the stability of his employer/ physician for his livelihood. Many of my physician assistant colleagues who have established a job in private practices find themselves out of work when the physician retires, dies, moves, or decides to hire a second physician in lieu of a physician assistant. In an HMO, the physician assistant is employed by the health plan and the plan provides a physician supervisor. The physician assistant's position is secure even though that particular supervisor may leave. This factor is crucial to any physician assistant who cannot afford unexpected job changes. As a rule, HMO's provide excellent job security to dependent medical practitioners.

Physician assistants in an HMO environment do not earn the salary of a physician assistant in fee-for-service practice. However, in my opinion, this is compensated for by excellent benefits and job security. An HMO also provides greater opportunities for career advancement because a physician assistant works for a company with different job categories.

In conclusion, practice for the physician assistant in an HMO setting provides for adequate supervision, diverse patient care experience, professional interaction, job security, and career advancement.

THE PHYSICIAN'S VIEW

In most cases, the HMO is a relatively new concept. Many of the medical directors *and* the primary care physicians in an HMO setting have had prior practice experience in a conventional fee-for-service solo or group practice. In my case, which may be regarded as typical, I was first introduced to the idea of an adjunctive physician assistant in a medical office while still engaged in combined private and pre-paid medical practice. I had been promoted to part time Medical Director's duties while still engaged in full-time primary care as a family practitioner and a well-qualified physician assistant was hired to practice full-time in my office previously staffed by myself plus one other full-time physician. As a result, instead of cutting down on numbers of patients seen we were able to *increase* our services to the community in that we now had two full-time practitioners (one physician assistant and one physician) supplemented by my part-time activities in the office. Our HMO had already placed 4–5 other primary care physician assistants in other offices always with one or two supervising family practitioners also working full-time. Without reservation, I can state that the transition from M.D. exclusively in an office to M.D.–P.A. offices was made with a minimum of disturbance. This transition, in my own case, became complete when, in 1979, I assumed the position of Medical Director full-time and switched from medical practice to administration exclusively.

There are several reasons for hiring a primary care physician assistant in an HMO setting:

1. We are a pre-paid health plan offering a complete service to the membership including medical, surgical, maternity and hospital care and including many ancillary and supporting fields such as optometry, podiatry, health education, psychologic counseling, and chiropractic. In inflationary times such as we have at present, the HMO is strapped by ever increasing medical costs, but confined to a single pre-paid monthly or quarterly fee which cannot be changed except at an annual renewal date. The primary care physician assistant commands a salary which is approximately 50% of that required to hire a new physician, yet the physician assistant, if properly chosen and adequately supervised, can perform the work of a physician.

2. In many areas, although the supply of physicians is increasing, the practice settings may often be in low-income neighborhoods catering to a high percentage of Medicaid patients. It has been most difficult to staff such offices at least for the present, with physicians exclusively. On the other hand, the primary care physician assistant has no such illusions about "desirable or undesirable" settings. He has entered the medical field with a definite dedication to helping the sick and the disabled and is not interested so much in the "ideal location" as he is in fulfilling his vows to help.

3. In a primary care setting, particularly in a small to medium-sized HMO, many primary clinics would normally be staffed by a single physician with no alternative offered to the member dissatisfied with his physician–patient relationship except to disenroll from the plan. Adding a physician assistant to an office permits a member an "alternative" choice. In addition, some physician assistants prefer to do episodic care exclusively, thereby making available a more flexible appointment schedule to the member so that more minor illnesses and complaints need not be put off until the infirmity is major.

4. The physician assistant, although intensively trained in several aspects
   of primary care, has no illusions about being unavailable for the simpler
   complaints such as "runny nose," a cold, or an ingrown toenail, whereas
   a physician in an HMO setting is often more oblivious to such complaints particularly in many places where primary care is delivered exclusively by internists rather than family practitioners.

The primary issues in introduction of the physician assistant into an HMO
practice setting are similar to those encountered in Fee for Service (FFS)
practice:

1. Careful screening of candidates must be performed and obtained respectively to allow the HMO to engage the most competent physician
   assistants available.
2. Prior practice in primary care after formal schooling is desirable, but
   not always available to the HMO recruiter because the pre-paid plan
   has traditionally had a salary schedule below FFS practice. Even though
   this may be compensated by "corporate benefits" including a pension
   plan, this may have little appeal for the young man or woman in his
   mid-twenties eager for professional and monetary success.
3. However, the prime factor which allows the physician assistant to proceed smoothly is education of the HMO membership *in advance,* to wit:
   A) In an HMO, publicize the coming of the physician assistant and
      outline the benefits described above to the membership.
   B) Make available in each office pamphlets or leaflets describing the
      education, duties and abilities of the physician assistant.
   C) Emphasize that the member has a choice, and if desired, may also
      stipulate that he prefers to see or will only see a physician. This bit
      of reverse psychology seems to satisfy the "first timer" that he can try
      the physician assistant but still see the doctor if he is not satisfied.
   D) The new physician assistant must be cautioned regarding the legal
      limitations set by law as defined in his state. For example, in Cali-
      fornia the physician assistant is currently forbidden to prescribe
      medicines or write prescriptions. Therefore, the supervising physi-
      cian must be consulted for such orders.

Assuming the physician assistant has been properly recruited, is competent,
is able to meet the public, and conducts himself in a professional manner, I
can think of only two major disadvantages to the HMO. Firstly, the supervising physician must spend some time in supervising the physician assistant
and in discussing cases and methods of treatment. This is readily accepted by
some but is considered a chore by others. Secondly, an HMO is usually a
"training ground" for the new physician assistant. Once trained, he often accepts employment in FFS clinics at a much higher salary. Therefore, "turnover" is great.

As Medical Director for a medium sized HMO, implications for the long-
term are clear to me. Physician assistant programs are continuing to improve

their "finished product." If we are to remain competitive with other HMOs, and continue to compete positively with FFS, and still offer complete medical and ancillary benefits, the physician assistant will be an ever increasing component in our primary care practice.

Chapter 22

THE PRIMARY CARE PHYSICIAN ASSISTANT IN THE OCCUPATIONAL CLINIC

JOHN MCELLIGOTT, MPH, PA-C
T. GUY FORTNEY, M.D.

Occupational medicine is probably one of the more exciting and progressive specialties within the physician assistant profession. Occupational medicine is still one of the few frontiers that has remained untouched by the expansive growth seen in private medicine. The opportunities afforded the physician assistant in the occupational setting are only limited to his knowledge and aggressiveness, coupled with the ability of his supervising physician. The occupational setting affords the physician assistant a very rewarding practice which also offers the stability of a corporation versus the often unstable base of a private practice.

There are some one hundred corporations which utilize the services of physician assistants. Some of these corporations are Dupont, Union Carbide, U.S. Steel, Transworld Airways, ALCOA, and Atlantic Richfield Company. The advantages offered to the corporation are obvious. The physician assistant can deliver quality health care under the supervision of a licensed physician which can reduce their cost for health care delivery while enabling them to service a large population of employees.

Employment information collected by the American Academy of Physician Assistants (AAPA) shows that although the total number of physician assistants in industry are small, it has grown faster than any other specialty group within our profession. AAPA studies show that in the late 1960's and early 1970's, less than one percent of the physician assistants were employed in an occupational health setting. In the last five years, this trend has shifted and the occupational setting has become more attractive to the physician assistant. Likewise, industry—under the pressure of management to control costs and the ever increasing pressure from OSHA to provide preventive medicine as well as active treatment programs—has found that the physician assistant is a viable profession to accomplish this task. Presently, four to six percent of the total population of physician assistants are employed by industry.

The American Academy of Physician Assistants in Occupational Medicine, a chapter of the AAPA, has described the characteristics of this individual. The average physician assistant in occupational medicine is 34 years old, and is married with two children. The physician assistant in the occupational setting is also very active within professional organizations. Sixty-two percent have held at least one state or national office. There is a mean of 6.8 years of health care experience prior to entering the occupational health field.

Salary ranges for the physician assistant have been well established. The occupational health setting is now competitive with the private sector. The benefit packages offered by corporations are very attractive and typical work responsibilities are not unlike those found in private practice. The incentives in occupational medicine are built into the system and apply to all employees. Raises are based on performance which is evaluated on a yearly basis in most corporations. This elimination of crises negotiation for monetary gain adds to the stability of the relationship between the occupational physician and physician assistants, since there is no direct or indirect financial pressure on the physician for the yearly increase in salary.

Utilization of the physician assistant varies from one industrial clinic to another. It is very difficult to develop a job description for a physician assistant based on what one does in comparison with another. It is safe to say that the physician assistant in the occupational setting often reflects the attitudes and practice concepts of his supervising physician. If the physician assistant is supervised by one or more physicians, he or she develops the good points from each and molds them into a protocol which satisfies all physicians involved.

Exemplifying the success of a physician assistant in occupational medicine, one only has to look at a Duke graduate of 1974, Edmond J. Wise, Jr., PA-C. Mr. Wise has been employed by the Nuclear Division of Union Carbide Corporation since 1974. He is presently the senior physician assistant within that corporation which employs the largest number of physician assistants in industry today. Although Mr. Wise's duties have varied over a period of time, he has developed a very outstanding preemployment assessment protocol which is very sophisticated, and has ultimately saved Union Carbide's Nuclear Division untold problems by virtue of his ability to identify underlying medical problems. He has developed what we consider a model cardiopulmonary resuscitation program within the Oak Ridge National Laboratory (ORNL) facility that is second to none. It is virtually impossible for anyone within the ORNL facility to suffer a cardiac arrest without being attended by at least four or five people nearby who are trained and certified in CPR. The employees who participate in the CPR program have an ongoing continuing education program which is coordinated and directed by Mr. Wise. He is also highly regarded by specialists in the area of audiology and in the areas of hearing conservation and screening. Mr. Wise has also developed a very adept psychological assessment which on many occasions has alerted the medical personnel to potential problem employees. On the other hand, if you compared the work of Mr. Wise to Charles Clark, PA-C, another Duke graduate also working in Union Carbide's Nuclear Division, it would be a totally different job description. Mr. Clark is utilized for his ability to manage trauma and his minor surgery skills, not to mention his physical assessment capabilities. However, the trend of all industry to use the physician assistant as an educator for plant personnel has been fairly consistent. Nationwide surveys by the American Academy of Physician Assistants in Occupational Medicine, show that physician assistants, in addition to their educational responsibilities, perform the following tasks on a rather routine basis:

1. Preemployment physical examinations,
2. Return to work examinations,
3. Annual examinations,
4. Assessment and treatment of individual accidents,
5. Assessment and treatment of acute medical problems,
6. Interpretation of audiograms, pulmonary function tests, and electrocardiograms,
7. Performance of proctoscopies and sigmoidoscopies,
8. Teaching cardiopulmonary resuscitation and development of employee education programs, and
9. Basic psychological counseling.

The above list, although not intended to be complete or used as a job description, outlines the functions performed by the occupational physician assistant. The occupational setting is not unlike that of a private practice, however, although the extent of treatment and ability to make definitive diagnoses sometime fall short of what would be done in private practice. This limitation is due chiefly to the fact that the occupational patient has his own family physician who must be considered in any treatment rendered to that patient. This factor leads to the premise that no chronic or prolonged illness is a responsibility of the occupational physician unless it relates to the safety or welfare of the patient while performing his own job.

The overall direction of the occupational practice is still based on the role of physician assistants as that of a dependent practitioner under the supervision of a licensed physician. The occupational physician assistant's scope and role is limited *only* by his supervising physician and the boundaries of the state law. Fortunately, the state laws which exist today provide enabling legislation which provides for "responsible" supervision. This eliminates the implication of continuous on-site or "over-the-shoulder" supervision. Most medical directors who utilize physician assistants agree with the fact that the first year of supervision is very active. Thereafter, the physician assistant more or less predicts which cases need active, immediate supervision from the physician. In the case of an emergency, most states allow very generous leeway for the physician assistant to prevent death or disability until a patient can be transported to the nearest medical facility or a physician is contacted. These implications of the state law make the occupational setting an ideal arena for team medicine.

The question to be answered in the occupational setting is "How can the physician assistant function to expand his or her role within the occupational setting?" With the advent of postgraduate training in occupational health at such schools as the University of Oklahoma and the University of Tennessee, physician assistants have obtained advanced degrees which will enable them to function in an expanded role in the occupational setting. It has come to our attention that the physician assistant with a Master of Public Health degree in Occupational Health would be an ideal person to bridge this gap that exists between other health related fields and industries. It is not difficult for one to surmise that going from medicine into such areas as industrial hygiene, health physics, and safety would be much easier from the physician assistant's standpoint than for these health professions to try to bridge the gap into medicine. With the ever increasing regulations from OSHA for more active monitoring of employees, plants not large enough to employ a full-time physician could utilize the physician assistant as a surrogate medical director under the supervision of a contract physician in a local community.

It is very necessary that early in the physician assistant's employment, he or she should be allowed the opportunity to visit and examine the work site. With a good working knowledge of the plant and the work that is accomplished, the physician assistant will be in a much better position to serve the employees. Time must be allocated for training in company policies and procedures. If a union is present, there must be an understanding of how the medical department interfaces with the union and management. When evaluating the physician assistant it is important to determine his knowledge and also to evaluate the skills and judgments which result from the application of that knowledge. As the physician supervisor completes this evaluation, there can be a review of the original duties and limitations and a new set drawn up to show what the supervisor feels the physician assistant can perform with only minimal supervision.

The question to be answered in the occupational setting is "How can the physician's assistant function to expand his or her role within the occupational setting?" With the advent of postgraduate training in occupational health at such schools as the University of Oklahoma and the University of Tennessee, physician assistants have obtained advanced degrees which will enable them to function in an expanded role in the occupational setting. It has come to our attention that the physician assistant with a Master of Public Health degree in Occupational Health would be an ideal person to bridge this gap that exists between other health related fields and industries. It is not difficult for one to surmise that going from medicine into such areas as industrial hygiene, health physics, and safety would be much easier from the physician assistant's standpoint, than for these health professions to try to bridge the gap into medicine. With the ever increasing regulations from OSHA for more active monitoring of employees, plants not large enough to employ a full-time physician could utilize the physicians assistant as a surrogate medical director under the supervision of a contract physician in a local community.

From the physician assistant's viewpoint, industrial medicine offers great vertical mobility not found in private medicine and yet a very stable and enjoyable specialty. From the physician's viewpoint, the use of physician assistants in occupational medicine is a perfect example in which the blending of training, availability, and need of industry produces an optional use of resources. The motivations for hiring a physician assistant include a lack of availability of medical doctors and budgetary restrictions that would make it advantageous to use a physician assistant.

Once the decision has been made to use the services of a physician assistant, it is necessary that some rules and regulations be formulated to outline the duties and define the limitations of the physician assistant so that optimal utilization will be obtained. It is understandable that each physician will have different ideas governing duties and limitations. Some of the areas covered should be: types of physical examinations allowed, types of treatment of occupational and nonoccupational conditions allowed, the ordering of appropriate laboratory test and x-ray studies, the prescribing of drugs (both stocked at the facility and by prescription), emergency procedures, the placement and lifting of restrictions, types of procedures such as minor surgery, assisting in educational training, and guidelines as to when the physician assistant is to discuss findings with a staff physician. As a physician supervisor I found such an outline of duties and limitations very helpful in informing physicians and nurses alike of what to expect from the physician assistant. In this way the nurses know that I expect them to extend courtesy and assistance to the physician assistant in the duties that I had assigned. It was then the duty of the physician assistant to obtain their respect through his ability and capability of performing the assigned task in a professional manner.

The role of the physician supervisor should include training. The supervisor must be prepared to spend time training the physician assistant to have the skills necessary to operate in the occupational medical setting. There are many things peculiar to occupational medicine that are not taught in the usual curriculum of either medical schools or physician assistant programs. Examples include hearing conservation, pulmonary function testing as it relates to occupational exposures or the ability of an employee to wear a respirator, visual acuity as it relates to safe job performance, and most importantly, the evaluation of an employee's total physical health so as to determine the employee's ability to perform assigned work safely.

It is very necessary that early in the physicians assistant's employment, he or she should be allowed the opportunity to visit and examine the work site. With a good working knowledge of the plant and the work that is accomplished, the physician assistant will be in a much better position to serve the employees. Time must be allocated for training in company policies and procedures. If a union is present, there must be an understanding of how the medical department interfaces with the union and management. When evaluating the physician assistant it is important to determine his knowledge and also to evaluate the skills and judgments which result from the application of that knowledge. As the physician supervisor completes this evaluation, there can be a review of the original duties and limitations and a new set drawn up to show what the supervisor feels the physician assistant can perform with only minimal supervision.

The final role of the physician assistant in the occupational medical setting will be decided by the ability and knowledge the physician assistant brings into the occupational setting and also by the assistant's willingness to learn new skills as outlined by the physician supervisor. Some of the duties common to all occupational medical programs are:
1. Required physical examination,
2. Assisting in emergency situations,
3. Treatment of employees as allowed by each individual corporation,
4. Education of employees, and
5. Rehabilitation of the injured.
This list could be expanded as the physician assistant gains more skills, either from post-graduate education or experience.

A well-trained physician assistant can extend the sphere of influence of the physician supervisor tremendously. I have found my association with a physician assistant to be most rewarding. I have been able to teach him many things I have learned through 30 years of experience and he has brought to me many of the new, modern concepts in medical practice. My physician assistant has been eager to learn and to lend assistance to myself and the other physicians on my staff. I can recommend the use of physician assistants in most all occupational medical programs.

Chapter 23

THE PRIMARY CARE PHYSICIAN ASSISTANT IN A MILITARY AMBULATORY CLINIC

DOUGLAS E. STACKHOUSE, PA-C
PAUL R. CHENEY, M.D., PH.D.

The clinical experience obtained by a physician assistant in this type of setting is typical of family practice. The population as a whole, of course, is generally a "healthy" one, with less of the elderly group seen in most communities. The military clinic setting serves particularly well as an introduction to the clinical problems and physician assistant role problems one would encounter in any family practice settings.

Of the four U.S. military branches utilizing physician assistants, each differs slightly in its perception and regulation of the physician assistant role. These differences are minimal, however, when considering ambulatory care settings. The following discussion is considered representative and describes a clinic setting in a small Air Force hospital serving a patient population of 20,000, including active duty, dependent and retired groups.

From the physician assistant's viewpoint, there are numerous positive aspects to this practice setting. As in the civilian sector, ambulatory care clinics offer stable hours, set schedules, and generally good working conditions. Roles and procedures are usually well defined.

Other advantages are specific to the military structure. Military pay and benefits are quite competitive with civilian, especially to a PA with minimal experience. The benefits of free medical and dental care, 30-day paid annual leave, exchange and commissary privileges tend to keep pace with civilian sector pay increases. Overall financial security is more than solid and retirement benefits are excellent.

The clinical experience obtained by a physician assistant in this type of setting is typical of family practice. The population as a whole, of course, is generally a "healthy" one, with less of the elderly group seen in most communities. The military clinic setting serves particularly well as an introduction to the clinical problems and physical assistant role problems one would encounter in any family practice settings.

If there is one all-encompassing theme to the structure and role of the military ambulatory care clinic, it is to serve as the entry point for all medical problems into the military health care delivery system. In institutions where there are no family practice modules, the "primary care clinic" performs this function alone. In this sense it acts as the narrow end of a funnel through which all patients enter to be evaluated. In most cases treatment occurs here as well. If the patient has a specialized problem, he or she is then referred to the appropriate specialty clinic.

Where there are family practice modules, these can exist alongside the above system or in place of it. In either case the main differences are that whole families are assigned to specific physicians who assume the additional roles of family pediatrician, obstetrician and gynecologist.

Physician assistants serve a very vital, integral role within the military structure. They are, quite frankly, needed. The military physician assistant serves generally to supplement the non-specialized functions of the physicians in order to provide quality health care to the maximum number of patients. In addition, the physician assistant serves to provide a basis for referral to local physicians, specialty clinics and regional military medical centers.

Most military clinics follow Monday to Friday schedules, with hours usually from 7:30 AM to 4:30 PM. Appointments with physician assistants are ten to fifteen minutes in length and are appropriately subdivided into military acute, dependent acute and routine categories.

Military physician assistants work directly under one or two specific physicians who are replaced periodically through normal turnover. Though well supervised, the physician assistant works fairly independently on a daily basis. The physician assistant usually has a scheduled load of 27-31 patients per day, and it is up to the physician assistant to initiate a consult with a supervising physician. If a physician assistant's assigned preceptor is not available, there is always at least one alternate to take his place. On any given day, a physician assistant will see, examine, treat, and discharge or refer most of his patients on his own, seeking consultation for duty excuses, admissions, specialty referrals and complex cases.

At some institutions, the ambulatory clinic physician assistant spends some of his time away from his clinic covering the hospital emergency room. In addition, when an outpatient is admitted, the physician assistant may follow the patient's course along with the physician preceptor. Other miscellaneous activities include staff meetings, grand rounds and professional conferences.

In most military settings, there are elaborate, specific lists of authorized drugs which the physician assistant may prescribe within his own facility. Other medications, including all controlled drugs, require physician endorsement.

The military physician assistant is generally well accepted by his superiors, colleagues and patients. The proverbial clashes with nurses heard of elsewhere are no significant problem in our setting. In most cases, the proven value of the physician assistant and his services has led to the establishment of a work situation in which he can function as independently as possible within his "dependent" role.

At present, all military physician assistants are officers. Those in the Air Force are fully commissioned, while those in other services are warrant officers. While to some this may seem inequitable and suggest some difference between the esteem each service holds for its PA's, such is truly not the case. In all services, military physician assistants are well-trained, highly respected professionals dedicated to one common mission.

If the extent to which physician assistants are utilized by the military *now* is any indication, there will always be a place for them. Their role is a vital one and allows each service added flexibility in meeting its health care demands.

Still, there are two major limitations under which military physician assistants now function. The first involves maximum rank achievable. The highest Air Force rank available to a physician assistant is Major. In the other services, it is Commissioned Warrant Officer, grade 4 (CWO4). The reasons behind this are largely administrative and economic and beyond the scope of this discussion.

The other limitation centers around professional advancement. At present, the vast majority of positions for military physician assistants are in primary care, family practice or emergency settings. The extent of this varies among the services, but generally, physician assistants are assigned the same role regardless of rank or years in service. One hopeful note, however, is that the services are exploring, via trial training programs, ways to expand the physician assistant's role in more specialized areas for the future.

From the physician's point of view, the physician assistant is clearly in his element in the military ambulatory clinic setting. He is considered indispensable in the delivery of quality health care to a population in which the structured aspects of military life, combined with the relatively youthful age of most military members, generate large numbers of essentially benign medical problems. In this unique environment, individuals may be required by superiors to seek medical evaluation for minor illnesses. Dependent spouses, moreover, often young, far from home and spurred by free and accessible medical care, regularly present themselves and their children for medical evaluation.

To these unique aspects of military medicine are added the usual ailments and injuries, which are often first seen by the physician assistant. Here, as mentioned, he serves as the entry point into the medical system — referring as necessary to physicians in various specialties. The physician assistant may occasionally choose to manage a non-routine problem himself with active and step-wise consultation of his supervising physician.

Patient acceptance of the physician assistant in the military setting is not a serious problem. While occasionally some patients balk at seeing the physician assistant, most see this professional as part of a team of care providers and come to trust and appreciate his judgment.

Physician responsibility for physician assistant decisions and treatment creates, in contrast, a potentially greater problem in the military setting. Physician productivity demands often distract him from his supervisory role and place the physician assistant in a role parallel to, rather than under, the physician. This gives the physician assistant more latitude and freedom of action but also makes physician accessibility for advice more difficult. This isolation from attentive physician guidance is more pronounced in facilities without general medical officers solely in charge of the primary care clinic. The acceptance of the primary care clinic by the physician as his first responsibility is probably the key to optimum supervision.

The indispensability of the physician assistant, as military medicine is now practiced, is probably the major distinction between military and civilian physician assistant utilization. This situation sets the stage for a certain autonomy of action, the limits of which are vague in practice. It certainly produced demands and rewards not normally seen in civilian settings.

Chapter 24

THE PRIMARY CARE PHYSICIAN ASSISTANT IN A GERIATRIC PRACTICE

REIN TIDEIKSAAR, Ph.D., P.A.

This century is witnessing an unimagined increase in the proportion of elderly people. At the turn of the century, four percent of the population were over 65. At present, approximately 11 percent of the population is 65 years or older, which translates into 22 million people. It is projected that by the year 2020, the over 65 age group will increase to 20 percent of this country's population (1). Of greater significance are the "old-old," those 75 years and older. They represent the fastest growing segment of the elderly population. The estimate is that in the near future this group over age 75 will outnumber all those elderly who are over 65 years of age today (2).

This unprecedented increase of elderly in our society is creating at the present time a heavy burden on our health care system. This is reflected by the following facts:

- The elderly account for 29 percent of total health care expenditures (3).
- The elderly comprise approximately 30 to 60 percent of patients in the acute care hospital (4).
- The elderly make up 30 percent of an internist's practice and 17 percent of a family medicine practice.
- The elderly have twice as many hospital admissions, and stay in hospitals twice as long per admission as do younger patients (5).
- The elderly utilize 95 percent of the long-term care beds in this country (6).
- The elderly account for 10 percent of the mental disorders seen in the community, which rarely receive psychiatric evaluation (7).
- The elderly receive 25 percent of all prescriptions written for and consume a larger percentage of over the counter medications (8).
- 5 percent of the elderly are in long-term care institutions, another 5 percent are homebound, 13 percent not homebound have difficulty in ambulation, and over 80 percent report having some chronic condition (9).

- The major causes of death for the elderly are diseases of the heart, cancers, and cerebro-vascular disease (10).

Thus, future demographic changes in the aging population will be forecast by an increased utilization of visits to the physician's office, periodic institutionalization, drugs, rehabilitation, and the special considerations that are needed for the achievement of daily living by the elderly.

This helps to underscore the fact that older people need a wide range of health services at affordable costs to stay healthy. Unfortunately, the health care services available at present are largely inaccessible to the aged because of a lack of health facilities, professionals with appropriate training to care for the unique biopsychosocial needs of the elderly, and the fragmentation of our health care delivery services. It is estimated that over a million elderly may not be receiving adequate health care, and that for every person residing in a nursing home, as many as two or three persons who live in the community require an equivalent amount of care (11). In addition, it is documented that physicians unfortunately do not properly monitor the conditions of geriatric patients in nursing homes and, in fact, avoid visiting their patients on a regular basis (12). Physicians, even the well intentioned, do not always know how to treat the old, and an interest for the elderly tends to deteriorate during the process of medical education (13). Kane *et al.* reported that only 0.2 percent of physicians responding to a survey indicated care of geriatric patients as one of the three areas of emphasis in their practice (14). The reasons for this are multiple, but several reasons may be conjectured: (1) negative attitudes towards the elderly; (2) inadequate geriatric training and (3) the frustration of dealing with multiple problems that are not acutely reversible. An added burden is the observation that we will be faced with geriatrician manpower shortages in the face of a doubling of age-related health care utilization in the next decade (15). The sum total adds up to basic inadequacies of health service to the aged, which results in an inappropriate reliance on costly acute hospitalization for the elderly and helps to perpetuate a system of care which concentrates upon treatment of illness rather than on preservation of existing health status. Thus, it is evident that there is a need for improved delivery of health care services which are both cost effective and focus on methods which identify and prevent illness. Changes in delivery of health care with an emphasis of encouraging older people to obtain an access to medical care before they become severely ill would be helpful in maintaining the health status of the elderly and might play a role in controlling spiraling health care costs.

The response to improve the system of health care delivery in an attempt to better meet the health needs of the elderly needs to be addressed within the framework of existing health manpower available, especially in the light of limited health care dollars available in the future and the predictions of a physician over supply as dictated by the recent GMENAC Report.

Naturally, there can be no single approach to planning and delivering health services to the aged. Efforts to remedy the deficiencies in health care for the elderly cannot be dealt with solely by forcing physicians to care for the aged or by increasing the number of physicians. In view of the shortcomings of physician manpower and interest in geriatrics, the physician assistant is beginning to emerge as a viable alternative to the needs of the elderly. What may well be a landmark study of this country's need for geriatricians, states that there is an urgent need to accelerate training and service preparations for the future elderly of this country. More importantly, the exact numbers of health professionals needed will depend largely upon the degree of delegation of care to physician assistants. One example cited indicates that instead of the 38,000 geriatricians needed by the year 2030, without non-physician assistant delegation, that 22,000 geriatricians with maximal physician assistant delegation may suffice in caring for the future elderly (16). An important point to keep in mind is that the purpose of physician assistants in the field of geriatrics is to provide adjunct care for physician directed services in conjunction with physicians and is not intended to indicate that physician assistants will solely fill a gap in physician manpower resources.

As a primary care practitioner with appropriate clinical experience in the field of geriatrics, the physician assistant can be the key in improving the quantity and quality of care delivered. By being physically present and seeing patients on a regular basis within senior community centers, long-term care facilities and other settings where both the ill and well elderly congregate, the physician assistant is increasing the number of elderly that can be cared for by physicians and is preventing the acute manifestations of chronic illness.

In an expanded role of a geriatric specialist, the physician assistant would be able to assist the geriatrician in his or her responsibilities toward elderly patients by:

1. Initially performing a geriatric evaluation, which includes detailing and updating the older patients' medical, psychological and social condition. This would include a formulation of a geriatric problem list gathered from patient history and examination, family interview, contact with prior physicians and past medical records.

2. Providing home care visits if necessary as part of the initial assessment and followup of care. This is especially important within rural and some urban areas, where the homebound elderly have the dual problem of inadequate health services available and social isolation adversely affecting their health. The home visit has the added benefit of assessing family support structures, patient performance in the ADL, (activities of daily living), nutritional status, home safety and accessibility of care

within the patient's living environment. The physician extender within the community system of home visits would be able to follow up individuals absent from medical, nutritional, and social activities so that appropriate contacts, evaluation, and referrals for services can be initiated before severe complications arise. Within this role, the physician extender is focusing attention on the early detection of existing health and social problems when remedial steps in treatment are relatively simple or of great consequence in maintaining the elderly patient within the community. In this way, there is a preventive plan for medical and social intervention as needed in order to improve or stabilize the elderly person's functional capacity to remain in the community in an effort to postpone or eliminate institutionalization.

3. The physician extender can also be utilized to develop community outreach programs that focus on health screening activities that consist of nutritional assessment, dental evaluation, vision and hearing screening, screening for high blood pressure, breast examinations, and colonic cancer screening. In addition, the physician extender can develop educational programs designed to cover such issues as crime prevention, accident safety in the home, proper physical fitness activities, the use and abuse of medications, preventing hypothermia, understanding the myths and realities of the aging process, and promoting self care approaches to the improvement or preservation of existing health.

4. Providing geriatric education to other health care providers such as physicians, nurses, nursing aides, social workers, dieticians, and physical therapists, in order to acquaint them with the unique needs and management issues of treating the elderly. To assist health professionals in crisis situations, plan health management for patients with complex medical regimens and act as support persons for staff members working with terminally ill patients.

5. Pursuing an active involvement of the elderly patient and family in the decision making process of care provided by being available as a resource person. By answering questions, meeting the psychological needs of patients and/or family, and acting as an advocate to represent the best interests of those patients who lack the expertise or help families who are unable to seek solutions to their medical problems without some assistance. This effort will help in increasing the length of time an elderly person will remain in the community and increase the satisfaction of health care delivery.

In assessing the prospects for physician assistants in the field of geriatrics, it is necessary to consider the barriers towards effective role employment. These include a lack of third party reimbursement for the physician assistant, a lack of exposure in training to geriatrics, and lack of role acceptance by physicians and other health care professionals.

RECOMMENDATIONS FOR REMOVING BARRIERS

- A secure position within the reimbursement system must be established to assure that the expanding pool of physician assistants will be able to provide geriatric services. The physician assistant leadership is pressing for a change in reimbursement practice so that third party payers will reimburse physician assistants in the same fashion as they now reimburse physicians on a fee for service basis. The recent exceptions written into federal legislation enabling physician assistants in federally supported rural areas to be reimbursed for services would be a step in the right direction.

- With respect to the educational preparation of physician assistants in geriatrics, I favor a marked need to increase both didactic and clinical courses in geriatrics for physician assistant students. In addition, steps are needed to insure the teaching of geriatrics to graduate physician assistants who have been working for a number of years but who have not had any formal introduction to geriatrics.

- There needs to be a fundamental change in the attitude and behavior of physicians, nurse practitioners, administrators, and other health professionals in their concept towards physician assistants. With progress towards a role definition which provides for the physician assistant's contribution to the care of the elderly, the physician assistant will be considered as a colleague who can contribute professionally, within a team approach, towards deciding, implementing, and managing an elderly person's therapeutic regimen.

REFERENCES

1. Statistical Abstracts of the United States: 1980. Washington, D.C., U.S. Department of Commerce, Bureau of the Census, 1981.
2. Somers, Ann, and Fabian, Dorothy: *The Geriatric Imperative.* New York, Appleton, Century, Crofts, 1981, p. 4.
3. Developments in Aging: 1978. A report of the Special Committee on Aging. United States Senate, Washington, D.C., 1979, U.S. Government Printing Office, pp. 6, 19.
4. Somers, H.U., and Somers, A.R.: Medicine and the Hospitals. Washington, D.C., 1968, The Brookings Institute, p. 57.
5. Brotman, H.: Every ninth American. In Developments of Aging: 1978.1. A report of the Special Committee on Aging, United States Senate, Washington, D.C., 1979, U.S. Government Printing Office, p. 20.
6. National Nursing Home Survey, 1977: Summary for the United States, Vital and Health Statistics Series B., No. 43, DHEW Pub. No. CP 145, 79-1794, July 1979, U.S. Department of Health, Education and Welfare.
7. Kayson, R: Drugs and the Elderly, 1978, Ethel Percy Andrus Gerontological Center, Los Angeles, CA, U.S.C., Press, p. 13.
8. Rabin, D.W.: Use of Medicine: A review of prescribed and nonprescription medicine use, 1972 Reprint Series, DHEW Pub. No. HSM 73-3012, U.S. Department of Health, Education, and Welfare.
9. Brotman, H.: *op cit.* page 5.

10. Fact Book on Aging: A Profile of America's Older Population. Washington, D.C., 1978. The National Council on the Aging, Inc.
11. Long-Term Care: Background and Future Directions, unpublished discussion paper. Washington, D.C., Health Care Financing Administration, June 1981.
12. C. Carl Pegels: *Health Care and the Elderly.* Rockville, Md., Aspen Systems, 1981.
13. Bergen, S.S.: "Foreword," in Somers, *op cit,* page xvii.
14. Robert Kane, David Solomon, John Beck *et al.*: Geriatrics in the U.S.: Manpower Projections and Training Considerations. Lexington, Ma., D.C. Heath, Inc., 1980.
15. Kane, R.; Solomon, D., et al.: *op cit,* page 7.
16. Kane, R.; Solomon, D., et al.: *op cit,* page vi.

Chapter 25

THE PHYSICIAN ASSISTANT
IN A PRISON HEALTH PROGRAM

EARL V. ECHARD, PA-C

The concept of high quality health care as a right of all prisoners is relatively new in correctional policy. Prisons themselves are a fairly new concept, dating back only to 1820 in North America. At that time, prisons were conceived as a more humanitarian way of dealing with offenders than capital punishment, public harassment or torture. The early prisons, however, were designed to separate the offender from all contact with corruption. This was to be accomplished by isolation with little thought being given to prisoner's mental or physical well-being. Indeed, as the concept of isolation (including silence) took hold, prisons became extremely violent places in which prisoners were physically and mentally brutalized in order to enforce obedience to the rules which were established presumably to enhance rehabilitation. It was an easy jump from the idea of penance through isolation and silence to the idea that prisoners should be taught good work habits. Thus was born the notation of prisoners as laborers. This may have at least set the stage for concern about prison health care, but it was purely an economic concern since sick prisoners were less productive than healthy ones. Prison health care was introduced as a social control mechanism. That is, if health care services could keep the prisoners healthy, productivity would be higher. Even so, prison health care was given low priority in terms of resource allocation or administrative interest. By the 1960's, however, an increased awareness of the importance of prison health care came about partly as a result of efforts of a small number of highly committed people and organizations. The civil rights movement of the 1960's resulted in the incarceration of a number of political prisoners throughout the nation. These prisoners and their attorneys began filing legal briefs and forcing prison administrators to recognize prisoner's rights to adequate medical, dental, and mental health care. The dilemma for prison administrators was that prison health care programs did not measure up to any standard set up in the community-at-large, nor were there adequate standards within the criminal justice system itself that might serve as guides to good practice. As the public became aware of serious deficiencies in prison health care, prison officials found themselves facing serious challenges from the citizen action groups and the press about the quality of services offered. The American Correctional Association, The Law Enforcement Assistant Administration, The American Medical Association, and The American Public Health Association have all prepared statements on minimal standards of health care in prisons. As a result, prison officials have become increasingly concerned with improving the availability and quality of prison health services.

When one enters most correctional facilities and observes the high walls, the chain link fence topped with razor sharp barbwire, and guards armed with .44 magnum pistols, it is most difficult to realize that providing medical services is one of the integral parts of the correctional system. The first priority is, understandably, to provide adequate custody of the individuals incarcerated in this system. However, due to the numerous legal suits that have been filed against state correctional facilities, medical care has achieved parity with the custody aspect of the facilities.

Historically, the medical provider in the correctional setting was initially a local physician who provided the service as an adjunct to his service to the local community. Nursing care was usually provided by an inmate who had had some medical experience as an orderly or nursing assistant prior to being incarcerated. Today, a number of facilities are making a concerted effort to employ registered nurses, licensed practical nurses, and physician assistants with proper and adequate supervisory backup from a physician. The care provided by the physician assistants is either on a part-time contractural basis in association with their supervisory physician or on a full-time basis with the backup of a contractural supervisory physician.

One generally considers prisons as dark, primitive, poorly-ventilated, pre-twentieth century buildings. My practice setting, however, is a well-lighted, well-ventilated, newly renovated structure. The treatment room is well-stocked with modern equipment from everyday stethoscopes to a cardiac defibrillator. The routine day begins with sick call and routine follow up care. The nursing personnel take responsibility for the management of the more common complaints such as colds, rashes, mild strains, sprains, abrasions, toothaches, and so forth. I am referred the persistent headaches, dizziness, chest pains, and chronic diseases such as diabetes mellitus and high blood pressure. Those inmates with severe problems are referred to my supervising physician. With the average age of the inmates being 25–28 years, chronic illnesses are somewhat limited. One of the most important functions in the prison system is the need to perform physical exams on all inmates who enter the prison. We presently average 8–20 physical examinations per day, but at times we perform 20–30 per day.

I am the senior medical person located full-time at the unit. With the backup services of my supervising physician, I am responsible for all the medical decisions regarding the treatment of an inmate. I am also responsible for the medical staff which totals approximately 47 individuals, including registered nurses, licensed practical nurses, medical records personnel, correctional health assistants, and supervisors.

My administrative duties as section head require most of my time. In this capacity, I interact on a daily basis with individuals from the dietary department, custody department, psychology department, and other sections within the unit that deal with the activities of the inmate. For example, if an inmate has received an injury, it is necessary that I confer with the Programs Department (which handles recreation activities) to insure that this inmate does not participate in any type of activity that could exacerbate his injury. If the inmate has a dietary problem and it is necessary that we place him on a particular diet regimen, then I confer with the staff in the dietary department to be certain this is done. If an individual is placed on complete bed rest, it is necessary that I relay this information to the custodians who insist that all inmates participate in the routine cleaning of the dorm. Administrative duties of a section head also involve staff problems, scheduling of staff, performance evaluation, planning activities for inmates, and planning health programs for the inmates.

The delivery of health services in prisons is complicated by many problems not found in the "free world" health system. Inmates frequently feign illness in order to avoid unpleasant work assignments. Referrals to specialists for diagnostic or therapeutic services must be coordinated with the custody personnel. Many medical providers practice medicine with an inadequate knowledge and understanding of the culture of their patients. Having the ability to understand the inmates, their needs, their background, and their day-to-day problems is paramount if one wishes to practice good medicine and deliver high quality health services. At times, it is difficult for the health care providers to treat an inmate's medical problems without thinking of the crimes that he may have perpetrated prior to his incarceration. It may be easy for one to feel that an inmate does not deserve good medical care except in an emergency situation.

The complaints of many inmates are frivolous and burdensome to say the least. However, these problems are not any different from those encountered in a "street" practice. One must always keep in mind that the purpose of medicine is to care for the medical needs of patients. In order for the physician assistant to do this in the prison setting, the relationship between the patient's environment and his health must be totally understood and appreciated.

One of the most common problems encountered in the prison system is seizure disorders. These are usually alcohol-related secondary to trauma. An inmate with this problem has to be monitored closely to ascertain that he is taking his medication as directed and that he is not assigned a job that would result in serious injury if he had a seizure while in the performance of his duties (painting on a scaffold, operating dangerous equipment, and so forth).

Juvenile diabetics are frequently encountered. At times, this can present problems other than trying to maintain their glucose at a low level. With the knowledge that most juvenile diabetics are at times very immature acting, it is necessary to protect these individuals from the more aggressive inmate. This is done to avoid assaults or homosexual attacks. Medically, these inmates usually do well, mostly because we are able to control their dietary habits and monitor their urine and blood glucose levels often.

The practice of medicine in the correctional environment can be most rewarding to a physician assistant, providing one is aware of the restraints and potential problem that one has to cope with. For many years, prisoners have received inadequate medical care. Pressure from the courts is providing strong incentives to improve prison health care services. Even with increased supply of physicians, recruitment will likely remain a problem in the prison setting. However, new health practitioners such as physician assistants represent a health manpower resource which has demonstrated an ability to expand the services available to patients and improve patient care. Correctional health care and administrators should evaluate the potential for employing such personnel as one of the available alternatives for alleviating the problem of medically underserved prison populations.

Chapter 26

THE SURGICAL PHYSICIAN ASSISTANT IN A SMALL COMMUNITY

JAMES A. BOUTSELIS, PA-C

I went to school at a small Catholic college in Manchester, New Hampshire called St. Anselm College. My intent upon going there was to achieve a broad education but leaning toward a career somewhere in the vast field of medicine. During summers, I would come home to Georgia and work as an orderly at a local hospital. This was my first exposure to surgery and it fascinated me. I decided that surgery would somehow fit in the picture of my future plans.

It was about this time that a lot of publicity was being given to the physician assistant profession. I looked into a list of physician assistant programs and noted that in Birmingham, Alabama, the University of Alabama School of Medicine offered a physician assistant program geared primarily toward surgery. I applied and was very pleased to be accepted. After attaining a Bachelor of Arts degree in biology in 1974, I enrolled in the Surgeon's Assistant program in Birmingham.

The Surgeon's Assistant program at Birmingham, Alabama, as previously described in this book, is a two-year intensive period of study. The first year is didactic work, and the second year consists of several surgical rotations. Never in my life have I studied as hard as I did that first year. The vast quantity of information would, at times, be overwhelming. The studies required every available free moment and the only breaks attained were in between quarters and final exams. The twelve members of my class became very close and the friendships made are strong and lasting ones.

The second year my rotations included peripheral vascular and thoracic surgery, head and neck surgery, orthopedics, emergency room, general surgery, first assisting, cardiovascular medicine, and pediatrics. Usually, there are two junior residents and one senior resident on each service plus an occasional medical student and myself. I was assigned to work with one of the residents and we took in-house call every second or third night. Duties included dressing changes, obtaining histories and performing physical examinations and clinic coverage. Usually, the resident would first assist and my exposure in this role was limited until I got to my rotation of first assisting a general surgeon in private practice in a local hospital. As can be seen, quite a lot of time is spent in the hospitals and the pressures on marriage can be quite intense. I was married just before my clinical rotation year and, fortunately, my wife Sheila was very understanding throughout the whole program.

Somewhere about the middle of the second year job hunting began. The name and reputation of the Surgeon's Assistant Program at the University of Alabama at Birmingham had produced a number of names of surgeons desiring the service of a surgery oriented physician's assistant.

A person working for two general surgeons in Rome, Georgia was sent for recruitment purposes and I responded. My wife and I are both from the middle Georgia area and decided that we would very much like to remain in this general area of the country.

In August of 1976, we moved to Rome, Georgia. I signed on with Dr. Boyce Brice, a general surgeon. Since then, incidentally, the other general surgeon in the clinic, Dr. Bannester Harbin, has hired a surgeon's assistant, Mr. Paul Lamprey.

Technically, I have a contractual agreement with the Harbin Clinic but work specifically for Dr. Brice. The Harbin Clinic is a multi-specialty clinic, having over thirty doctors including peripheral vascular surgeons, neurosurgeons, cardiologists, orthopedists, general practitioners, pediatricians, opthalmologists, urologists, and, of course, general surgeons.

Rome, Georgia is a town of about 45,000 population. Main industries are textile; however, General Electric, Georgia Power Company and Georgia Kraft Paper Company have large installations here. This small city is very picturesque in its setting nestled in the foothills of the Appalachian Mountains, and serves in health care delivery to an area including all of Northwest Georgia and parts of Northeast Alabama.

Two hospitals are located in Rome. Floyd Medical Center has 314 beds and Redmond Park Hospital has 200 beds. We operate in both hospitals.

In accordance with the law, I submitted a job description to the state and was interviewed along with my employer by the State Board of Medical Examiners. Job descriptions were also supplied to both hospital staffs in accordance with procedure for privilege application. These were approved without incident.

As first assistant to a busy general surgeon in a rather small town, my job is fast paced and challenging. Typically, I make rounds in the mornings prior to surgery, writing orders and discharges as needed and discussing these with my employer as we prepare for surgery. I act as first assistant on all our cases. As in all general surgical practices, the procedures vary. Ours include head and neck procedures, mastectomies, thoracic procedures, and, of course, abdominal surgery including colectomies, hysterectomies, cholecystectomies, hernia repairs, gastrectomies, and so forth. After surgery is completed, usually Dr. Brice and I round together and, while he is in the office in the afternoons, I perform and dictate the histories and physical exams on patients due for surgery the following day. Other dictation duties I help with include discharge summaries and operative notes.

We are responsible for emergency room coverage on a rotating basis approximately six or eight times a month, and I come in only after Dr. Brice has evaluated the patient and has deemed surgery to be necessary. I carry a beeper and, while in town, am subject to call. I field a lot of phone calls from the nursing staff and feel perfectly free to refer any situation to my employing physician that I feel I should not handle.

In the operating room, as previously stated, I am Dr. Brice's first assistant. Basically, this covers anything from helping to get the patient on the table and in proper position, answering any questions the scrub nurse may have concerning the specific items (certain clamps, sutures, and so forth) to draping the patient, traditional first assistant duties (clamping, tying and retraction), sewing the subcutaneous tissue and skin, and making sure the next case is premedicated, allowing for smooth and quick room turnover.

Since I have worked with the same doctor for five and one-half years, I have come to know his procedural routines well, and the scrub nurses seem to appreciate the fact that if I notice a certain item is not prepared on their Mayo stand, I will quietly advise them of this in plenty of time for them to make ready whatever may be needed.

I also like to accompany the patient to the recovery room. There, I write the postoperative orders and dictate the operative note. The nurses feel free to ask me any question and I am glad to oblige whenever I am able. I have gotten along well with the nursing personnel at both hospitals, and do not recall any major conflicts between a member of the nursing staff and myself. I appreciate how hard they work and they appreciate any help I can give to them.

All in all, I find the physician assistant profession to be a challenging and satisfying one. I feel that the horizons are wide open for continued growth. As more surgeons graduate from their residency programs, having worked with surgeon's assistants and knowing what they can do when properly utilized, the opportunities for us as professionals becomes greater.

Chapter 27

THE SURGICAL PHYSICIAN ASSISTANT IN THE ACADEMIC MEDICAL CENTER

PAUL HENDRIX, PA-C

In the academic medical center, the surgical physician assistant is a relatively new and unique member of the heath care team. Increasing manpower requirements due to the reduction or termination of surgical residency training programs and the rapidly increasing patient loads at teaching institutions have created an increased demand for personnel at the junior resident level. Also, passage of Public Law 94-484 and the 1976 Health Manpower Assistance Act, has reduced the inflow of foreign medical graduates to residency training programs (1). These increased manpower requirements have stimulated interest in the utilization of surgical physician assistants who have been found to improve the quality of residency training, improve surgical patient care, and provide a means to compensate for the reduction in the number of surgeons being trained (2).

Under the supervision of licensed physicians, surgical physician assistants can be utilized in numerous patient care settings and can carry out a variety of delegated tasks. This permits staff physicians and residents to focus their skills where the need is greatest. These surgical physician assistant responsibilities include but are not limited to the following:

1. Assisting in the operating room.
2. Assisting in the management of preoperative and postoperative patient care.
3. Obtaining medical histories and performing examinations on patients being admitted to the hospital.
4. Assisting with outpatient clinic visits.
5. Providing night-time coverage of hospitalized surgical patients.
6. Assisting in of the emergency room.
7. Providing education and counseling.
8. Assisting with ongoing research projects.
9. Assuming administrative responsibilities.

Surgical physician assistants are also trained to initiate hospital admission orders, to write preoperative and postoperative orders, and progress notes; to prepare patient discharge summaries; and to react appropriately in life threatening situations. Usually, orders given by surgical physician assistants under the delegated authority of a physician are carried out as though given by the physician. Deviations from this procedure may exist due to state laws or to a particular hospital's general institutional, or physician assistant guidelines.

There is a considerable amount of work done on surgical services daily that is not necessarily educational in nature but which must be accomplished in order to achieve satisfactory levels of patient care. Surgical physician assistants are particularly valuable in performing these patient services which may have minimal educational benefit for the resident staff. For example, acting as first or second assistant during operations which are done very frequently on some services, making dressing changes of greater magnitude than those usually delegated to the nursing staff, providing emergency care for minor trauma, and assisting with follow-up care in the surgical outpatient clinic (3). In providing routine preoperative and postoperative care, surgical physician assistants function at the level of junior surgical house officers; this relieves residents from some of the more routine ward work. In the operating room, the utilization of surgical physician assistants can reduce the number of residents needed for each case thus maximizing teaching and training opportunities. Thus, the surgical physician assistants help the surgical residents to become more efficient and less harried, and they enable the residents to spend more time pursuing reading and research activities. Surgical physician assistants have been found to function very effectively in large teaching hospitals and can alleviate a portion of the need for a large house staff (4). With long-term job commitment, the surgical physician assistant's technical skills become refined and they develop into excellent assistants to staff surgeons and surgical residents.

IMPROVED PATIENT CARE

One important point to emphasize is that surgical physician assistants provide continuity of care in the academic medical center when the residents rotate from service to service within the hospital. Interaction with nursing personnel has not constituted a major problem. Surgical physician assistants are true professionals and complement the health care team of registered nurse and surgical resident.

Patient care can be improved by the addition of surgical physician assistants to the hospital staff. More personnel on the surgical service means that each patient is seen more often by members of the health care team. Surgical residents can devote more time to anticipating and preventing problems since they have fewer routine duties to perform.

Releasing surgical residents from routine chores and from the second assistant slot in the operating room (often a position of minimal educational value) has improved resident morale and thus favorably influenced patient care. Nursing personnel have also seen an advantage with the addition of surgical physician assistants due to the increased ease with which another team member can be contacted in the event of a patient problem.

HEALTH CARE COSTS

Surgeons acting as assistants in the operating room constitute a significant factor in the cost of health care. This expense may be apparent in direct billing by the assistant surgeon or as reflected in higher hospital costs where large house staffs are maintained to provide patient care. The utilization of surgical physician assistants as second and third assistants can thus decrease hospital costs.

SUPERVISION

In most cases, the surgical physician assistant is responsible to a primary supervising physician. However, in an academic medical center, the chief resident may make the daily assignments in the operating room, recovery room, hospital wards, and outpatient clinic.

It should be emphasized that surgical physician assistants must be well trained, properly supervised, and be willing to work within well defined limits. Because surgical physician assistants are an integral part of the surgical team, supervision and daily countersigning of orders pose no problems.

AMERICAN MEDICAL ASSOCIATION VIEWS

The AMA supports the use of surgical physician assistants to provide services to hospitalized patients under physician supervision. The physician assistant may be an employee of the hospital who is supervised by a hospital-salaried staff physician, or employed and supervised by a private physician who is a member of the hospital attending staff. The AMA feels that a physician assistant should be the employee of a licensed physician affiliated with a hospital rather than the employee of a hospital on the grounds that the former arrangement better assures the quality of P.A. services. The American Hospital Association (AHA) calls only for the designation of a physician supervisor. The AMA and the AHA both recommend that physician assistants be utilized under the supervision of licensed physicians and that they be integrated into a single medical staff governed by a single set of bylaws. They also recommend that the extent of functions, responsibilities, and privileges for each P.A. be determined by individual credentials, qualifications, and competency.

The AMA has adopted a statement on the "status and utilization of expanding and emerging health professions in hospitals" in order to assist hospital medical staffs in regulating and guiding the use of physician assistants. This statement calls for the medical staff to recommend to the hospital governing authority the extent of the functions that may be delegated to physician assistants. This usually entails amendments or changes to existing hospital bylaws. Sample amendments to hospital bylaws that recognize physician assistants are available through the American Hospital Association and the American Academy of Physician Assistants. The utilization of physician assistants should be based on an individual's professional training experience as well as on the demonstrated competency of the assistant and his employing physician. Employment of a physician assistant is usually subject to the approval of a credentials committee or other appropriate hospital committee. Some of the minimal credential requirements are as follows:

1. Successful completion of a two year AMA-approved training program.
2. Successful completion of the national certification examination and maintenance of certification by merit of obtaining 100 hours of CME biannually.
3. Proper registration with the State Board of Medical Examiners.
4. Job description and standing orders which adhere to hospital bylaws and state regulations.

REIMBURSEMENT FOR
SURGICAL PHYSICIAN ASSISTANT SERVICES

Under existing public and private insurance plans, reimbursement for a surgical physician assistant's services goes to the employer, whether it is a hospital or a physician. Medicare policy considers the services of hospital-employed assistants as allowable costs under Part A. Physician employers are reimbursed under Part B when the physician is directly involved with the patient services, and if the patient services are normally furnished in the physician's office and are commonly included in the physician's bills. In both cases, surgical physician assistant activities must be under direct and immediate physician supervision in order for reimbursement to be given. Medicaid policy varies from state to state. Generally, recognition is given for a physician's right to employ surgical physician assistants within legal parameters, and to bill and be reimbursed through Medicaid in accordance with prevailing regulations for their services when performed under the physician's direct supervision. Most private third-party carriers consider reimbursement for services rendered by hospital-employed and supervised surgical physician assistants as part of the hospital's general service expenses. Reimbursement for the services of physician-employed surgical physician assistants assumes the existence of direct physician involvement.

LEGAL CONSIDERATIONS

Most states consider the surgical physician assistant to be an agent of a specific licensed physician or of a specific group of licensed physicians. The surgical physician assistant is not independently licensed to perform medical acts but is approved to perform such services *only under the license of the responsible physician or group of physicians.* A physician may delegate to a surgical physician assistant the authority to perform a medical act when the physician is physically present and actually supervising his performance; or the physician may give oral or written orders to an assistant to perform a medical act for a particular patient. When the surgical physician assistant is expected to make independent medical judgments, disease-specific or problem-specific standing orders are required by most states and should be on file at each site in which the assistant is permitted to make such independent medical judgments. Prescription privileges are now available for surgical physician assistants in 13 states and legislation for prescriptive privileges is pending in two states.

Many hospitals establish a special associate medical staff membership category and require that any assistant desiring to function within the hospital must first apply for and be accepted to such membership. The usual process is that the application for such associate membership is filed both by the surgical physician assistant and the supervising physician, reviewed for personal and professional qualifications by the Credentials Committee, and presented for approval by the medical staff. This process serves two purposes: assuring the medical staff that the assistant meets professional and ethical standards, and publicizing the presence of the assistant to the medical staff and the hospital administration (6).

The Joint Commission on Accreditation of Hospitals (JCAH) supports the concept that physician assistants can "exercise judgment within their areas of competence, participate directly in the management of patients under supervision, and write orders." The JCAH recommends that each hospital establish rules and regulations regarding the utilization of surgical physician assistants.

Both HEW and AMA legal advisors have indicated that there is no evidence that utilization of surgical physician assistants leads to an increase in liability. Professional liability insurance is available for surgical physician assistants and their employers.

CLOSING STATEMENTS

One of the unanswered questions is *how long will a surgical physician assistant be happy in this role?* All around him people are moving up the ladder. Medical students become interns, then junior residents, and so forth. *Undoubtedly, surgical physician assistants will travel different paths.* Some will become physicians, some will devote increasing amounts of time to teaching prospective physician assistants and possibly even to teaching certain procedures to medical students or junior house officers. Some will assume administrative responsibilities along with their patient related duties. Some will accept increased responsibilities in research and a few will carve out new and unique niches in the academic medical center setting (4).

Senior staff, residents, and medical students have accepted the surgical physician assistant concept whole-heartedly. Some of the obvious benefits have been improved patient care, more accurate order writing, improved record keeping, and better continuity of service policies and procedures through generations of house staff. The increased utilization of surgical physician assistants will allow a decrease in the number of surgeons required in the United States and will alleviate some of the pressure to train larger numbers of sub-specialty surgeons.

Surgical physician assistants have generally been well accepted by all members of the hospital staff and have become an integral functioning part of the academic medical center. Working together, surgeons, nurses and surgical physician assistants can function in harmony to provide excellent and comprehensive medical care.

REFERENCES

1. Moore, F.D., Zuidema, G.D., and Ballinger, W.F.: Surgical Manpower and Public Policy. *Surgery, 83*:116-20, 1978.
2. Perry, H.B., Detmer, D.E., and Redmond, E.L.: The Current and Future Role of Surgical Physician Assistants: *Annals of Surgery, 193*:132-137, 1981.
3. Laws, H.L., Kirklin, M.K., Diethelm, A.G., *et al.:* Training and Use of Surgeons Assistants. *Surgery, 83:*445-50, 1978.
4. Hatcher, C.R., and Fleming, W.H.: The Role of Physician Assistants on a University Teaching Service. *Journal of Thoracic and Cardiovascular Surgery, 678:*750-756, 1974.
5. Miller, J.I., and Hatcher, C.R.: Physician's Assistants on a University Cardiothoracic Surgical Service. *Journal of Thoracic and Cardiovascular Surgery, 76:*639-642, 1978.
6. Commentary of the Board of Medical Examiners of the State of North Carolina regarding Physician Assistants and Nurse Practitioners, 1980.

Chapter 28

THE SURGEON'S ASSISTANT IN A PRIVATE CARDIOVASCULAR SURGICAL PRACTICE

DEAN F. BLIETZ, S.A., PA-C
LUIS A. TOMATIS, M.D.

The main goal of any health care delivery group is the ultimate well-being of patients. To facilitate the achievement of that goal, a relatively new, highly trained group of medical professionals has emerged: the surgeon's assistant. Employed largely, but by no means exclusively, by thoracic-cardiovascular surgeons to meet the intricate and technical demands of pre-operative, intra-operative and post-operative patient care, the surgeon's assistant has become an invaluable asset to the kind of teamwork essential to efficient cardiovascular-thoracic practice.

Since its advent a decade ago, the role of surgeon's assistant has become attractive as well as creditable field. For example, while providing patients with the same standards of service that the surgeons would normally render, surgeon's assistants nevertheless need not succumb to a life of absolute dedication to their employer's practice which requires exclusion of all other activities. Thus, surgeon's assistants are free to arrange their lives to suit their private needs while still receiving the fulfillment that accompanies their professional responsibilities. In their lifestyles, then, as well as in the quality of their skills, surgeon's assistants should be able to honestly recommend their chosen profession to others. After all, they—like their surgeon employers—have selected not merely an occupation but a lifetime profession.

One of the main advantages of this field from the surgeon's viewpoint is that it frees him from having to rely completely on a labor force of M.D. surgical residents (post-graduate physicians) in various stages of training, as his assistants. Like the surgeon himself, surgeon's assistants are hired already trained in a specific area. This invaluable specialization enables them to carry out many important duties with efficiency and competency while easing the surgeon's burden of concern over the quality of care his patients receive. In order to illustrate the diverse roles and responsibilities of the surgeon's assistant, an extended description of a single practice is presented below.

Granted, no two practices or employer-employee relationships are identical. Yet, what follows may well serve as a model to help clarify the versatility that the surgeon's assistant potentially contributes to a practice. In this case, the setting consists of a private cardiovascular-thoracic surgery team in a midsize U.S. city. Three cardiovascular-thoracic surgeons and one vascular-only surgeon comprise the employing group. Additionally, one of the cardiac surgeons is trained in pediatric cardiovascular surgery. Overall, then, the practice generates a composition of patients quite varied in age, size and extent of illness. The surgeons practice in an office across the street from the hospital where their surgery is performed. The hospital, a community hospital of approximately 550 beds, is affiliated with the state university post-graduate surgery training program. The hospital is also designated as the regional trauma center. In 1981, this group performed 692 pediatric and adult open heart procedures, 191 vascular procedures, and approximately 144 pulmonary resections in addition to approximately 600 other miscellaneous surgical cases not listed in the above categories. But the volume of work is not the important feature in the description of this practice. On the contrary, the highest goal to which the team dedicates its efforts has traditionally been low mortality and morbidity at low cost. Over the past fifteen years these goals have consistently been achieved, with mortality and morbidity rates well below the national average and lower overall net costs to the patients.

Prior to the arrival of the first surgeon's assistants in the mid 1970's, the team received most of its support in the care of non-cardiac patients from post-graduate, general surgery residents. But this left a serious gap in continuous, in-house, twenty-four hour a day care for the cardiac patients. Furthermore, the uneven interest of post-graduate, general surgery residents, during their rotation in cardiac surgery prompted the group to fill that gap by employing first two, and eventually six, surgeon's assistants. These surgeon's assistants were found competent by training and ability to fulfill the requirements of consistent, top quality, in-house coverage for cardiac surgery patients as well as for pulmonary and vascular patients during those months in which there was a void of post-graduate physician coverage for the service.

SERVICE MAKE-UP

The services that surgeon's assistants provide are as many and varied as those provided by the surgeon. To avoid a "grocery list" approach, a typical

stay of an elective surgical patient will serve as a model. As a preliminary re-
mark, however, it is essential to emphasize that the patient's relationship to the
surgeon is in no way diminished by the services of a surgeon's assistant. On the
contrary, the patient-surgeon rapport is enhanced by the continuous presence
of an assistant. A surgeon's assistant is not in the profession to provide independent medical services. The role of an assistant, by definition, is totally dependent upon the surgeon. To have it any other way destroys the original
intent of the profession, which is to serve as an extension of the physician.

PRE-OPERATIVE ROLE OF A SURGEON'S ASSISTANT

Unique to the patients with coronary artery disease, who comprise the majority of patients in this practice, is that diagnosis and definitive work-up can
be nearly completed on an out-patient basis. Once surgical eligibility is determined by the cardiologist and the referring physician, the patient is seen by
the surgeon for evaluation. If the surgeon and cardiologist determine that the
patient is a surgical candidate, the patient is scheduled for admission to the
hospital the night before surgery. Prior to this time, the assistant's only knowledge of the patient is through discussion with the surgeon and/or a brief review of the office chart data which accompanies the patient to the hospital.
Once the patient arrives in his hospital room, the surgeon's assistant makes his
first encounter introducing himself as the surgeon's assistant, being careful to
use the traditional title, "Mr.," before his name.

The assistant's first role with the patient is accepting, in professional confidence, accurate data; recording the chief complaint, the history of the present
illness and the past, family and social history; and conducting a pertinent review of systems. A thorough and complete physical examination follows, with
the surgeon's assistant careful to note any physical findings which might alter
the time of the surgery or the procedure to be performed. For example, the
discovery of a suspicious prostatic nodule, abdominal aortic aneurysm, carotid
bruits or lower extremity venous varicosities may require further medical
work-up or an alternate surgical strategy.

The surgeon's assistant then must accurately record the history and physical
examination on the chart and write an admission note. Next, a set of established printed, open heart admission orders is inserted in the chart and signed
by the assistant to be implemented by the nursing staff for the appropriate
pre-operative laboratory work-up. The medications taken by the patient at
home are reviewed by the assistant, and the appropriate ones continued.
Other non-essential medications are either discontinued or the dosage discussed with the attending physician. A subsequent pre-operative visit is made

by the attending surgeon who examines the patient. The history, physical examination and orders are reviewed and countersigned. Later in the evening, the pre-operative laboratory values, chest x-ray, and electrocardiogram are checked by the assistant and appropriate electrolyte supplements are ordered or lab studies repeated to ascertain an accurate, proper and safe preparation for the following day's surgery. Remaining questions, concerns, or anxieties expressed either by the patient or the family, after the pre-operative preparation class by a clinical nurse, are, if necessary, clarified by the assistant. In this practice, however, most of the patients are mentally and psychologically well prepared through a detailed explanation of the procedures by the surgeon, the clinical nurse and the surgeon's assistant. More accurate data and routine instructions can be relayed to the patient by consistent, long-term employees who are responsible for the patient than by short-term, rotating, medical personnel (such as surgical residents).

INTRA-OPERATIVE ROLE OF THE SURGEON'S ASSISTANT

When the patient is taken to the operating room, the surgeon's assistant accompanies the surgeon. The surgeon makes the pre-operatively medicated patient aware of his presence while the assistant prepares and supervises the monitoring devices and final positioning of the patient in the operating suite. Included in these procedures are the insertions of the arterial and intravenous lines and the Foley catheter as well as the collaboration with the anesthesiologist in controlling the patient's vital signs. Surgical prepping and draping are also done or supervised by the assistant, freeing the surgeon to take care of last minute communications or a quick review of the cardiac catheterization data.

While performing a cardiac revascularization procedure, one assistant first aids with the sternotomy, cannulation and anastomosis of the veins, while the second assistant harvests an adequate supply of saphenous veins. Once the leg incisions are closed, the second assistant is free to take care of other tasks outside the operating room or to assist with another surgery. The first surgeon's assistant continues with the remaining decannulation and closure. If an unusual circumstance arises intraoperatively where the need for a second surgeon is essential, one of the attending surgeons is readily available. Once the incisions are closed, the responsibility of transporting the patient to the Surgical Intensive Care Unit is shared by the anesthesiologist and the surgeon's assistant, who takes over the care of the patient in the Intensive Care Unit.

POST-OPERATIVE ROLE OF THE SURGEON'S ASSISTANT

Once the patient is resting in the Surgical Intensive Care Unit, the overall monitoring and interventions are controlled and ordered by the surgeon's assistant. Many hours of discussion between the surgeon and the assistant, along with a written procedural protocol, makes treatment of hypokalemia, hypovolemia, oliguria, arrhythmias, as well as interpretation of laboratory data, chest roentgenograms, chest drainage volume, and ventilator management, uniform and consistent. In the event of an extraordinary occurrence, the surgeon is always available for consultation by telephone or personal intervention. Meanwhile, the assistant stabilizes and extubates the patient within two or three hours after arrival to the Surgical Intensive Care Unit and relays the patient's progress at regular intervals to the surgeon who, perhaps, has started another surgical procedure or is seeing patients in the hospital or office. In general, over the course of several hours following surgery, the assistant and surgeon exchange a series of suggestions, evaluations and concerns about the patient's condition and care.

The surgeon's assistant continues his surveillance of the patient during the evening and night of surgery. Early the following morning, after being on call throughout the night, the assistant evaluates laboratory data and fully assesses the patient. If his or her progress is within the standards of predetermined, written protocol, the assistant removes the monitoring devices and chest drainage tubes and orders an appropriate diet and range of activities. The patient is then transferred to a more intermediate care area. When the surgeon returns to the hospital in the morning, a prompt report is given to him by the surgeon's assistant and the day's plan established. Later, the surgeon is free to countersign the progress notes and orders written in the chart during the night by the surgeon's assistant.

Daily subsystem assessments are recorded in the progress notes of the patient's chart. Appropriate, pre-approved interventions concerning pulmonary therapy, physical activity, diet, laboratory studies and consultations are carried out by the surgeon's assistant until the time the patient is discharged from the hospital on the fifth to seventh post-operative day.

OVERVIEW OF ACTIVITY

As mentioned earlier, one criterion of a rewarding profession is that it can be honestly recommended to others. The apparently vast amount of assistant coverage detailed above seems overwhelming. The surgeon's assistant role has expanded and evolved into a twenty-four hour a day role. Also mentioned earlier was the fact that this particular practice employs six surgeon's assistants. With this number the above-mentioned tasks may be shared by several assistants for any given case, since each highly trained assistant's abilities are identical; moreover, each assistant's role at any particular time, whether pre-, intra-, or post-operative, is interchangeable with that of any other assistant.

CALL

In this practice, there is a term which designates an assistant who is ultimately responsible for a given period of time to know all the patients and the activities of the other assistants better than anyone else. The person "on-call" is responsible for a twenty-four hour period beginning at 8:00 a.m. Prior to accepting responsibility for the patients in the Intensive Care Unit and various other patient care units of the hospital, a review referred to as "card rounds" is held prior to 8:00 a.m. each day. During this time, the list of patients is reviewed scrupulously and individually by all of the assistants. After the pertinent data, events of the previous day and night are reviewed and four assistants proceed with the day's surgery schedule. The "on-call" assistant and another evaluate all the patients in the units for their daily assessment and interventions. Once the surgery schedule is covered by adequate assistants for the day and the post-operative patients are stabilized, the assistant who was on first call is free to leave and use the rest of the day for personal activities and enjoyment until the following morning. The remaining five assistants will complete the tasks of the day. They are available to assist the surgeries, write the admission histories and physical examinations, dictate discharge summaries, re-evaluate the more critical patients, insert chest tubes, or be available for the emergencies which may arise during the day.

If it is necessary to remain into the late afternoon and evening hours, a second assistant is designated "on second call" at a compensated rate. The responsibilities include remaining to assist on the surgical cases which might run into later hours, after which he may go home. The second on-call assistant remains available through the use of a beeper pager system during the night and returns whenever supplemental help is needed.

COMPLETION OF AWARENESS

The true value of employing surgeon's assistants lies in the capability of the surgeons to be free of the mundane, more routine tasks in the daily patient evaluation process. Assistants by no means are a substitute for the daily presence of an attending physician at the patient's bedside; rather, the ideal surgeon's assistant should be the intelligent extension of the eyes, ears and hands of the surgeon. Still, with the large number of in-house patients, more than one assistant attending the surgeon in the operating suite, and the many and varied duties performed by the surgeon's assistant, it is frequently impossible for the assistant to see the same patient daily with the attending surgeon. To assure thoroughness and continuity, this practice employs two full-time clinical nurses, adding another dimension to surgeon-assistant-patient communications and relationships.

The role of the clinical nurse is one of patient education and communication. First, pre-operative classes are held with the patient and family. Prior to going home, the patient's activities, diet and exercise program are reviewed following the protocol of instructions of the surgeon. These reviews are also done in minute detail by a registered physical therapist who instructs the patient on a cardiac rehabilitation program, and by a registered dietitian who instructs the patient on an appropriate low cholesterol and/or any other suitable diet. Any remaining questions and concerns regarding physical activity and diet are relayed to the clinical nurse and the assistants prior to discharge of the patient.

On a daily basis, the nurse clinician's role is that of total availability. The nurse clinician is available to coordinate both the flow of information and the activities of the patients, families, surgeon's assistant and surgeon. Referring physicians and consultants may always reach or contact a nurse clinician if the surgeon is unavailable for discussion, such as during the time of surgery or while in the office. Upon completion of daily rounds by the surgeon's assistant, he relays a detailed report of each patient to the nurse clinician. Hence, if the assistant is busy at the time the surgeon makes his daily rounds and evaluations, the nurse clinician has the pertinent data and significant findings readily at hand for reference. The nurse clinician can reciprocate by relaying the surgeon's suggestions and management program to the assistant, thus increasing communication and efficacy.

OPENNESS AND UPDATING

Again, with the large number of personnel involved caring for a large number of inpatients, it is necessary to hold some time apart for communication and updating of patient management protocols. This is accomplished through an early morning, weekly, one hour conference designed for discussing topics pertinent to the specific specialty of cardiovascular-thoracic surgery. At other times, morbidities are discussed. Reports of continuing medical education meetings are presented both by assistants and attendings for the purpose of keeping abreast of the current thoughts in the field. Finally, monthly mortality

conferences are an on-going project so that all areas of management are reviewed as learning experiences.

PROTOCOL AIDS

As mentioned earlier, a written protocol exists for the daily procedures.
When in doubt of a particular surgeon's preferred treatment, the assistant can
review the manual to check specific details. Examples of management problems include levels of hemoglobin replacement, criteria for oliguria, hypoten-
sion, hypertension, and arrhythmia treatment, as well as other daily routines.
If doubts remain after reviewing the manual, the assistant will contact the surgeon, either in person or by telephone, to discuss all the unusual management
problems.

Printed orders are also a standard in the armamentarium of this practice in
order to maintain and ensure continuity and standardization. These orders
are to be completed by the surgeon's assistant at various stages in the patient-
care process: upon admission to the hospital, upon post-operative arrival at
the Surgical Intensive Care Unit, and upon transfer to the Intermediate Care
Unit. The countersigning of these orders within twenty-four hours, in keeping
with state law and hospital policy, presents no problem since the attending
surgeon can perform this duty making his daily rounds.

RELATIONS WITH THE
POST GRADUATE SURGICAL RESIDENT

As is evident from the above description, the utilization of surgeon's assistants in a private cardiovascular-thoracic surgery practice has many advantages. Continuity and standardization of patient care is the utmost goal of
such employment and is accomplished by the technical reliability and sound
medical evaluative judgements on the part of the surgeon's assistant. The principal reason for employing a surgeon assistant is that the manpower of the entire service lies within a single, continuous, stable organization. Continuity,
quality and standardization of patient care are maintained, whether at the beginning or the end of a rotation of the surgical resident. For example, the surgeon's assistant is available to supervise and help the resident when necessary.
It is an asset to the organization that "strangers" to the service feel, at all times,
comfortable with the routine of the attending surgeon. On the other hand, the
surgeon at all times feels comfortable and confident, since the service has the
ability to function independently of any temporary assistance. Moreover, surgical resident-surgeon's assistant relationships are based on mutual respect. No
threats are felt by either individual because each has a role: the surgeon's assis-

tant is well trained and experienced in cardiovascular surgery; the resident is obtaining a valuable educational experience during the rotation.

TABLE 28.1
JOB DESCRIPTION FOR SURGEON'S ASSISTANT
CARDIOVASCULAR SURGERY

The role of the surgeon's assistant in cardiovascular surgery is to help the surgical care team provide top quality, in-house, twenty-four hour a day care to cardiothoracic and vascular patients. Working under the direction and supervision of surgeons, the surgeon's assistant can perform a variety of activities throughout the patients stay in the hospital. These activities are divided into three phases of patient care as follows:

I. Pre-operative Care Activities
    A. Obtain and record complete medical history on all patients admitted to surgical service.
    B. Perform thorough physical examination and record findings on chart, present significant findings to surgeons.
    C. Write admission notes.
    D. Present nursing staff established, preprinted orders for appropriate pre-operative laboratory test including chest x-ray, electrocardiogram, and routine laboratory studies.
    E. Collaborate with surgeons to order supplemental laboratory test, consultations, and other needed services.
    F. Help nursing staff answer remaining questions, address concerns, or reduce anxieties expressed by patient or family members.

II. Intra-operative Care Activities
    A. Prepare and supervise arrangement of monitoring equipment and positioning of patient on operating table.
    B. Supervise surgical prepping and draping of patient.
    C. Assist surgeons with insertion of arterial and intravenous lines and Foley catheter.
    D. Assist anesthesiologist in maintaining and monitoring patient's vital signs.
    E. Serve as first or second assistant in operating room.
    F. Assist anesthesiologist with transportation of patient to the Surgical Intensive Care Unit (SICU).

III. Post-operative Care Activities
    A. Following protocols, monitor, write orders, and note progress of patient in the SICU.
    B. With consultation, write transfer orders, order or discontinue routine laboratory test, fluid replacement, post-operative medications and diet.
    C. As predetermined, remove monitoring devices, chest drains, and arrange or discontinue respiratory therapy.
    D. Provide wound care and follow daily progress of patient.
    E. Collaborate with nursing staff to prepare patient for discharge, home care, and return visits to surgeons.
    F. Dictate appropriate discharge summaries.

SUMMARY

The surgeon's assistant, as a member of the health care delivery team, is a viable profession with many assets to the practice of cardiovascular-thoracic surgery. This area of endeavor can fulfill the surgeon's assistants professional and personal ambitions. Mutual respect, maturity and a well-defined surgeon-surgeon's assistant relationship is essential to maintain a lifestyle in the "other-than-medicine" world. Proper respect of time management as a factor of the employer/employee relationship is mandatory. Above all, a teamwork approach results in improved care of the cardio-vascular-thoracic surgery patient.

The usefulness of surgeon's assistants has, indeed, been proven. The longevity of an assistant's employment in thoracic and cardiovascular surgery remains to be seen. The profession is young, growing, maturing and not without some growing pains. Yet despite the essentially dependent role of the surgeon's assistant, it is vitally important that they maintain a completely open approach to any problem that might arise; for surely such an honest relationship is the main ingredient for the successful utilization of surgeon's assistants in practice. Bearing the above in mind, a very workable environment does exist and the profession can, indeed, be recommended to those seeking a fulfilling life-time career in which we can envision learning, maturing and retiring as a thoracic and cardiovascular surgeon's assistant.

Chapter 29

THE SURGICAL PHYSICIAN ASSISTANT AS A MEMBER OF THE CARDIOTHORACIC SURGICAL TEAM IN THE ACADEMIC MEDICAL CENTER

WILLIS H. WILLIAMS, M.D.
JOHN KOPCHAK, PA-C
LEMUEL G. YEARBY, PA-C
CHARLES R. HATCHER, JR, M.D.

INTRODUCTION

The specialties of cardiovascular and thoracic surgery were historically among the first areas of institutional medical care in which the value of physician assistants was demonstrated. Today, these paramedical specialists are accepted and essential members of the cardiovascular and thoracic team. In 1973, two physician assistants were first employed by the Division of Cardiothoracic Surgery of the Emory University School of Medicine, Emory University Clinic, and Emory University Affiliated Hospitals. Fifteen physician assistants are now employed full-time in the Division of Cardiothoracic Surgery alone. It is impossible to imagine the continuing function of this program, in which more than 3,000 patients undergo cardiac and thoracic operations each year, without the physician assistants and their services.

THE SURGICAL PHYSICIAN ASSISTANT'S DAILY DUTIES

The care of patients undergoing thoracic and cardiovascular operations can be categorized as: 1) preoperative, 2) operative, 3) immediate postoperative intensive care, 4) general postoperative care, and 5) late postoperative out-patient care. Depending upon specific institutional needs and individual preferences, physician assistants participate in all or several of these phases of patient care (see Table 29.1).

All physician assistants are involved in *preoperative evaluation* and *preparation* of the patient for cardiac and thoracic operations. Histories are obtained and recorded. Physical examinations are performed. Laboratory data and blood samples are collected. Consultations are requested. Special studies are ordered. Explanations are given to patients and their families and their questions are answered.

Many of the cardiothoracic physician assistants are extensively involved in the *operating room,* preparing the patient for the operation, assisting the surgeon, excising and preparing saphenous veins used for coronary bypass grafts, establishing cardiopulmonary bypass, controlling postoperative bleeding, and closing the incisions at the completion of the operation. Physician assistants aid in the *transport* of critically ill patients and supportive equipment to and from the operating room, coronary care unit, intensive care unit, and cardiac catheterization laboratory.

Participation in patient care decisions, early postoperative management, and data collection in the *intensive care* areas is variable. In some hospitals, physician assistants assume major responsibility for postoperative intensive care, remaining in the hospital throughout the night to make minute-to-minute decisions based upon direct observations of patients in the intensive care unit. This is particularly true for the continually demanding pediatric patients. In other institutions, this critical early postoperative care is provided by cardiothoracic surgical house officers, "intensivists" (usually anesthesiologists or trainees in anesthesiology), cardiologists, and cardiology trainees.

General postoperative care beyond the intensive care unit environment is provided by physician assistants working in close cooperation with the cardiothoracic residents, supervising surgeons, cardiologists, and consultants. Physician assistants work closely with the hospital nursing staff in all phases of perioperative care.

Out-patient care and management of the patient after discharge from the hospital is a relatively small but rewarding part of the cardiothoracic physician assistant's job. A great deal of satisfaction is derived from involvement in the long-term convalescence and rehabilitation of the child or adult with critical cardiothoracic disease, especially when one has come to know the patient and family in the hospital during the critical phases of perioperative management.

To some extent, an individual physician assistant may select areas for concentrated personal activity, although a certain degree of flexibility and interchangeability is expected of all cardiothoracic surgical physician assistants. Some physician assistants are involved primarily in the care of critically ill infants and children in the intensive care setting. Others work only with adult patients. Still others perform a wide range of services for adults with cardiac and thoracic disease and older children with relatively simple congenital cardiac problems. The variables of *patient age* (newborn, adult, and elderly), *diagnosis* (multiple congenital and acquired cardiac, pulmonary, and esophageal diseases), and *severity of illnesses treated* (life-threatening emergencies, semi-elective surgery for valvular heart disease and coronary arterial occlusive disease, and elective correction of simple and complex congenital heart defects) provide limitless challenges for the cardiothoracic surgical physician assistant.

Cardiothoracic surgery is a technologically sophisticated discipline depending for its success today upon the application of many advanced diagnostic and therapeutic modalities. In addition to the usual methods of physical diagnosis, radiology, electrocardiography, and laboratory assessment, the cardiothoracic surgical physician assistant will become familiar with cardiac catheterization, angiocardiography, echocardiography, pacemakers, hemodynamic monitoring, telemetry, cardiopulmonary resuscitation, cardioversion, percutaneous transluminal balloon angioplasty, intra-aortic balloon counterpulsation circulatory assistance, bedside insertion of Swan-Ganz pulmonary arterial catheters, the use of the heart-lung machine for cardiopulmonary bypass, and the pharmacological management of arrhythmias and low cardiac output. Depending upon the specific responsibilities of his position, he will use these and other methods in his daily practice. His professional versatility is thus progressively enhanced.

THE ACADEMIC MEDICAL CENTER MILIEU

Most large cardiothoracic surgical services are based in academic institutions associated with medical schools and residency training programs. Many smaller private practice groups also deliver excellent care to patients requiring cardiac and thoracic operations. Opportunities for physician assistants exist in both of these environments.

The academic *milieu* of a large medical school-affiliated hospital and training program offers some unique opportunities for continuing medical education, career development, teaching, and research. Consultants representing virtually all medical and surgical specialties are readily available as a resource for both patient care and personal education. House officers in surgery, medicine, anesthesiology, and supporting specialties are both "student" *and* "teacher" for the cardiothoracic physician assistant working in an academic medical center. Conferences, postgraduate courses, laboratories, rounds, and libraries are valuable sources for continuous personal and professional development. Supervising attending surgeons are frequently generating new information through their clinical and basic research. Collaborative multidisciplinary patient care and research are encouraged. Extensive computer-based data pools encourage long-term patient follow-up and evaluation of new treatment modalities. The presence of medical students and house officers in training stimulates an attitude of intellectual curiosity and honesty. Support services such as medical illustration, graphics, computer technology, and continuing medical education encourage academic productivity. In such an environment, the likelihood of professional stagnation and "burn-out" are minimized while opportunities for the continued enhancement of one's professional career are optimal.

Many of the opportunities just described are also present in the smaller private practices of cardiothoracic surgery in fine hospitals throughout the country. In these non-academic practices, the physician assistant may enjoy a somewhat closer personal working relationship with the supervising physician and a variety of day-to-day responsibilities and activities. More time may be spent seeing out-patients in the office or directly assisting in the operating room. Responsibility and authority need not be shared with house officers in training or with medical students on rotation. Usually, however, greater flexibility and availability for "on-call" or emergency coverage are required. The competent and versatile cardiothoracic surgical physician assistant is a highly respected and valuable member of the team in either of these two described practice settings.

FUNCTIONS OF THE SURGICAL PHYSICIAN ASSISTANT

Physician assistants in an academic institution play a vital role in the *education* of patients, families, nurses, and house officers in training. They are depended upon to teach procedures, routine protocols, and the logic of patient care to less-experienced personnel including medical students, nurses, rotating house officers, and other physician assistants.

Administrative functions of the physician assistants include the planning of admissions, scheduling of operations and special procedures, arranging and presenting information to patient-care conferences, and maintaining records required for quality assurance, long-term patient evaluation, and clinical research.

Physician assistants constitute an important link in the process of *communication* between cardiothoracic surgeons, cardiologists, and other consulting specialists. Many hours are spent providing information and emotional support to parents and families of children on the pediatric cardiothoracic service where the problems are often complex, the risk to life is high, the emotional involvement is intense, and the hospitalizations and operations are often prolonged or multiple.

Even a cursory glance at the "job description" (see end of chapter) used for employment and credentialing of physician assistants in one of our institutions — the Henrietta Egleston Hospital for Children — will reveal the wide variety of skills required and services performed. During the past four years, three graduates of the Duke University Physician Assistant Program have fulfilled the expectations of this "job description" in an exemplary manner to the mutual benefit of patients, their families, the nursing staff, our house officers, and their surgeon-supervisors. Many other physician assistants have served equally well in the somewhat different roles required in our hospitals providing primarily adult care. In adult care, greater emphasis is placed upon the physician assistant's technical performance in the operating room where they assist in the preparation of the patient for surgery, excise and prepare the saphenous veins for coronary arterial bypass grafts, directly assist the operating surgeon, manage the intra-aortic balloon pump circulatory assist device, facilitate the safe transport of the patient to the intensive care unit when the operation is complete, and inform the intensive care unit staff of factors critical to the patients' postoperative management.

ISSUES IN ACCEPTANCE

As might be expected, all has not been ideal during the evolution of the physician assistant as a member of the cardiothoracic team. In fact, the "learning curve" has been somewhat tumultuous and at times the entire concept of paramedical involvement in this technologically sophisticated field seemed in jeopardy.

To be effective, physician assistants must be accepted for their value and recognized both officially and unofficially by the state licensing board (usually the Board of Medical Examiners or their subsidiary board), the hospital administration, the nursing service and individual nurses on the hospital staff, house officers in training, physician members of the medical staff, patients, families, other paramedical professionals, and, of course, the supervising physicians themselves. The latter group usually have little problem in accepting physician assistants as part of their team since they have seen the need for these important services in the first place. These problems of acceptance and recognition are certainly not unique to the cardiothoracic surgical physician assistant. They have been discussed elsewhere in this monograph in greater detail. In fact, the cardiothoracic surgical physician assistant's role in this high-technology discipline usually assures him of respect, admiration, and appreciation from the institutional staff because of his unique knowledge of pathophysiology, pharmacology, methods, devices, and procedures not often familiar to others.

We have found that cardiothoracic surgical physician assistants have quickly established themselves as a valuable resource to our nurses and house officers seeking new information or the solution to a patient-care related problem. Nonetheless, a few words of caution are in order. Both the state licensing board and the hospital administration, the latter responsible to the hospital governing board, must be assured that the physician assistant will be properly supervised and will not be permitted to function beyond his level of training, competence, and officially approved job description. Proof of such supervision and "back-up" support must be evident to the hospital administration and the nursing staff. Even an occasional incident in which the supervising physician is not available when needed by the physician assistant can severely jeopardize institutional acceptance.

A gradually expanded job description is usually more desirable than a "standard" list of responsibilities. Individual physician assistants are given permission to perform increasingly sophisticated procedures and services as their skills and abilities evolve. Successful fulfillment of simple responsibilities continues to be the best assurance of likely success in future expanded responsibilities.

Conflict of authority and responsibility will undoubtedly occur as physician assistants are introduced into any program or institution where their anticipated role is not already familiar to nurses and house officers. The supervising physician must be careful to recognize and to maintain traditional and existing lines of communication and authority. It is inevitable that the physician assistant will play an intermediary role, serving as "middle-man" between the supervising physician and the nurses, house officers, patients, families, and other physicians. On the other hand, it is absolutely essential that a reasonable degree of *direct* communication continue between the supervising physician and these important groups of individuals. The cardiovascular surgical physician assistant must realize the delicacy of this balance, working toward improved communications and facilitating decision-making while avoiding becoming a "shield" to protect his supervising physician from those who wish to communicate directly with him. This sounds simple and idealistic, but in fact it is quite difficult in the day-to-day practice of a specialty in which the surgeon is involved for long hours in the operating room and in which the patients in the intensive care unit may be gravely ill. We have found that daily "rounds" conducted by the physician, regularly scheduled teaching conferences for nurses and house officers, and plans for a special time each day during which conferences can be arranged among patients, their families, and the surgeon solve many of these concerns about communication and authority.

The surgeon should explain to patients and families the role of the physician assistants and house officers in their care and reassure them of his supervisory role and availability. Periodic conferences with the supervisory nursing staff and responsiveness to their concerns will virtually assure nursing acceptance of a competent physician assistant. The physician must recognize that most nurses still expect to have some opportunity to speak directly with the responsible physician regarding their concerns and plans for their patients' care.

In general, our cardiothoracic surgical residents view the physician assistants as a very positive component of our training program and our surgical care delivery system. They respect the physician assistants for their skill and knowledge. They appreciate the fact that the work done by the physician assistants allows them more freedom for intellectually productive use of their own time. Resident "on-call" time is also reduced. Each resident is able to participate to a greater extent in the operating room than would be possible if many more residents and fellows were required and utilized for the non-operative aspects of patient care. This greater operative experience is obviously viewed by the residents as a distinct advantage. We believe that this approach allows us to train a resident possessing superior technical skills and operative experience while in no way jeopardizing patient care. The resident must continue, however, to participate in preoperative and postoperative care in order to assure his understanding of the problems encountered in these areas. He should conduct daily rounds and accept responsibility for decisions not requiring direct intervention by the supervising surgeon or cardiologist.

SPECIAL REQUIREMENTS OF THE
SURGICAL ASSISTANT ROLE

The responsibilities of the cardiothoracic surgical physician assistant are emotionally stressful, intellectually taxing, physically challenging, and technically demanding. Critical illness and "life-or-death" crises are commonplace. Long hours of responsible concentration are required. Cardiothoracic surgeons tend to be personally intense and perfectionistic; their expectations are high. They may be relatively inaccessible during long hours in the operating room. The potential exists for conflicts in authority and responsibility to arise among the many members of an effective cardiothoracic team. Duties and expectations must be kept within the range of the physician assistant's training and experience. Working hours and availability for emergency coverage must be consistent with a high level of physical and intellectual performance and emotional stability. Professional income must be appropriate for the skills applied and hours worked. Policies for "on-call" coverage and lines of authority must be clearly established. Professional advancement must be encouraged. We urge the cardiothoracic surgical physician assistants supervised by the surgeons on our staff to participate in conferences and research projects and to attend at least one major national medical meeting or postgraduate course each year.

CONCLUSIONS

Physician assistants are vital and effective professional members of our team. Trends in the evolution of cardiothoracic surgical care and training nationally indicate an increasing demand for services which can be efficiently and effectively provided by properly trained and supervised physician assistants. Academically-based cardiothoracic surgery surely offers the physician assistant one of the most challenging, rewarding, and versatile careers available with an unequaled opportunity for continuing "on-the-job" professional development.

TABLE 29.1
JOB DESCRIPTION
PHYSICIAN ASSISTANT
PEDIATRIC CARDIOTHORACIC SURGERY
HENRIETTA EGLESTON HOSPITAL FOR CHILDREN, INC.
AND
EMORY UNIVERSITY CLINIC

The cardiothoracic surgical physician assistant is expected to promote and maintain the highest possible quality of perioperative care for pediatric cardiothoracic patients. In so doing, he or she may . . .

A. Collaborate with the thoracic surgeon, the thoracic surgical resident, and cardiology staff in planning and implementing the patient's surgical care.
   1. Assess the patient's progress daily and records pertinent information in the record.
   2. Communicate any deterioration in the patient's status to the thoracic surgical resident, the attending thoracic surgeon, or the cardiologist.
   3. Recognize personal limitations and when in doubt informs the thoracic surgical resident, the attending thoracic surgeon, or the cardiologist without hesitation.
B. Obtain information and record admission history.
C. Perform and record admission physical examination.
D. Write routine admission orders.
E. Write routine orders agreed upon by the responsible physicians including . . .
   1. Progression of the patient's diet.
   2. Progression of the patient's level of activity.
   3. Establishment of intravenous and oral fluid limits.
   4. Routine lab work, chest x-rays, and EKG's.
   5. Change blood replacement as needed.
   6. Discontinue CVP, RAP, LAP, direct arterial blood pressure determinations, and continuous EKG when no longer indicated and removes the appropriate monitoring devices.
   7. Write transfer orders when patient no longer needs intensive care.
   8. Change IV medications to IM or PO route.
   9. Request blood type and cross match.
   10. Order and/or discontinue chest physiotherapy as indicated.
   11. Guide respiratory support and the process of weaning.
   12. Discontinue antibiotics.

13. Administer emergency drugs such as:
    a. Potassium
    b. Lidocaine
    c. Sodium Bicarbonate
    d. Atropine
    e. Epinephrine
    f. Dextrose
    g. Calcium
    h. Isuprel
    i. Dopamine
14. Order medications routinely used in pre- and postoperative care of cardiovascular surgical patients, i.e., antipyretics, antiemetics, analgesics, and antibiotics.
15. Discontinue intravenous infusions and change IV's to heparin lock.
F. Perform minor procedures such as suture removal, dressing changes, venous and arterial cannulation, wound debridement, chest tube insertion, thoracentesis, emergency pericardio-intubation, urinary bladder catheterization, arterial and venous punctures for laboratory blood work, and initiation of temporary cardiac pacemaking.
G. Is available to the hospital staff as a resource person.
H. Provide continuity of care for the child and his parents.
    1. Provide information regarding the child's hospitalization to the parents.
    2. Assess the family's strengths and weaknesses in order to anticipate the problems the family may have during the child's hospitalization.
    3. Participate in preoperative teaching of the child and his parents to prepare them physically and emotionally for surgery.
    4. Is available to the child and his parents during hospitalization.
    5. Provide the family with discharge instructions.
I. Explain the details and risks of operative procedures and may obtain the signature of the parents on the operation permit. However, this signature must be witnessed by a responsible physician.
J. Assess the need for written patient educational material and collaborate with others in its development.
K. Facilitate the development of interdisciplinary cooperation and rapport in providing comprehensive patient care.
L. Participate in clinical research under the supervision of the responsible thoracic surgeon.
M. Serve as a first or second assistant in the operating room.
N. Communicate with referring physicians and other medical personnel at the request of the sponsoring physician or with his approval.
O. Dictate appropriate narrative summary at the time of patient discharge.
P. Arrange follow-up plans including time and place of appointment with appropriate physician.

GENERAL REFERENCES

1. Hatcher, C.R., Jr., and Fleming, W.H.: The role of physicians' assistants in a university teaching service. *J. Thoracic. Cardiovasc. Surg.*, *68:*750756, 1974.
2. Miller, J.I., Craver, J.M., and Hatcher, C.R.: The use of physicians' assistants in thoracic and cardiovascular surgery in the community hospital. *Am. Surg.*, *44:*162-164, 1978.
3. Miller, J.I., and Hatcher, C.R., Jr.: Physicians' assistants on a university cardiothoracic surgical service. *J. Thorac. Cardiovasc. Surg.*, *76:*639, 1978.

Chapter 30

THE SURGICAL PHYSICIAN ASSISTANT AS A MEMBER OF THE RENAL TRANSPLANT TEAM

MICHAEL G. PHILLIPS, PA-C
JOHN D. WHELCHEL, M.D.

Since 1954, clinical transplantation of kidneys has become an accepted modality for the treatment of many patients suffering from end stage renal disease. Many medical disciplines are involved in transplantation, such as nephrology, surgery, and immunology. A team approach is usually necessary to adequately support a transplant program. This concept has previously been successful in other areas of medicine such as trauma, cardiac surgery, and extremity reimplantation teams.

The number of individuals in need of kidney transplantation is increasing yearly. Approximately nine thousand patients were awaiting a kidney transplant in 1981 in the United States. However, only about four thousand transplants were performed. The majority of patients were not transplanted due to the shortage of cadaver kidneys. Thus, there is a critical need to increase the recovery of suitable kidneys for transplantation. Only through the development and expansion of effective organ procurement programs can the need for cadaver kidneys be met. In conjunction with the development of these procurement systems and the increased commitment to transplantation by transplant centers, many opportunities for the participation of the surgical physician assistant are available. These opportunities will be discussed in this chapter.

A surgical physician assistant may elect to work with a procurement team or with a clinical transplant team. As a member of the procurement team, the individual will have the opportunity to interact with both medical and lay groups. Opportunities exist for the development of managerial, educational, and technical skills. An individual who accepts the position of organ procurement coordinator must become familiar with the physiology and anatomy of the renal system and its relationship to other systems. Under the direction of the physician, the assistant must be prepared to participate in the medical and pharmaceutical support required for potential cadaver donors in accordance with the protocols of the procurement program. The individual must understand the concept of brain death and the associated legalities of this concept in the community. In addition to responsibilities in donor management, donor retrieval, and donor family counseling, the assistant may be requested to assist in the cadaver donor nephrectomy procedure. Frequently, the assistant will flush the surgically removed organs, which is the initial phase of ex-vivo preservation. The assistant may also participate in the surgical dissection of the kidneys for identification of the anatomy and preparation for prolonged preservation.

Preservation for viable organs outside of the human body is an exciting and developing science. The assistant will become familiar with the techniques and physiology of ex-vivo preservation. Through his experience and observation, he will have the opportunity of contributing to the growth of this science.

The surgical physician assistant in an organ procurement program will become familiar with the importance of the histocompatibility (HLA) typing system. The assistant will understand the interpretation of this information and its utilization in recipient selection. Once the histocompatibility information is available on the donor or potential recipients, the assistant may be responsible for contacting the potential recipient and arranging the patient's transportation and admission to the transplant hospital. In those situations where a suitable recipient is not available in the local area, the assistant may be responsible for initiating the sharing of one or both kidneys with another transplant center. This usually involves notifying potential receiving centers identified by a computer sharing program. When another center accepts a kidney for transplant, it may be necessary for the assistant to arrange the logistics of the sharing procedure and even travel with the organ to monitor its preservation.

After the kidneys are either transplanted locally or shared with another transplant center, the surgical physician assistant has completed the renal procurement and preservation responsibility for that particular donor. However, the task of follow-up and data collection to evaluate the success of the procurement preservation technique usually continues for months or even years.

On occasions, the assistant may participate in research, as well as procurement and preservation. He may assist in the writing of protocols for experiments, performing the experiment, and summarizing the data for interpretation by his physician supervisor. The assistant may also be involved with his physician supervisor in grant and scientific writing responsibilities.

A surgical physician assistant may choose the responsibility of participating in patient care with a transplant team. This role may include assisting the transplant surgeon in pre-recipient and potential donor evaluation, the transplant surgical procedure, and post-operative and hospital follow-up care. This particular role usually allows the assistant to become involved in the follow-up of transplant patients in the clinic. The clinical assistant might also assist the transplant surgeon with surgical procedures involved in the care of renal failure patients, such as vascular access.

A PHYSICIAN'S VIEW OF THE SURGICAL PHYSICIAN ASSISTANT'S ROLE IN ORGAN TRANSPLANTATION

Advancements in organ transplantation offer many new opportunities for the surgical physician assistant to participate as a member of the transplantation team. The scope of participation and responsibilities will usually depend on the program's level of activity in transplantation and organ procurement.

Transplant programs performing twenty-five or less transplants per year may require the involvement of the surgical physician assistant in all aspects of the transplant effort. A position of this description might include broad base responsibilities in patient management both prior to and following transplantation. The assistant may be required to assist the transplant surgeon in surgical procedures, and may also be required to assume both technical and administrative duties in organ procurement and preservation.

The responsibilities of the surgical physician assistant in a program performing more than twenty-five transplants per year will probably be oriented to more specific areas. The development of the assistant's expertise in areas such as patient management, surgical procedures, coordination of the transplant support services, or patient follow-up increases the effectiveness of the physician in an active transplant program. Since most transplant programs are based in institutions with residency training programs, the assistant can also provide stability of personnel in the transplant effort.

Career opportunities for surgical physician assistants have been significantly increased with the development of hospital-based and independent organ procurement agencies. The medical background and technical training of the assistant is ideal for the positions of organ procurement coordinator or officer. Positions in these agencies allow the development of public and professional education, surgical procurement, isolated organ preservation, and administrative skills. Since the future of organ transplantation will be closely related to the development of improved organ procurement and preservation techniques, the expanded opportunities for assistants in this area appear promising in the future.

A PHYSICIAN ASSISTANT'S VIEW
OF HIS ROLE IN ORGAN TRANSPLANTATION

The job opportunities, career development, job satisfaction, and personal gratification are excellent as a member of the transplant team. A surgical physician assistant with experience in all aspects of kidney recovery, preservation, dissemination, and transportation may wish to become an administrator or a director of an organ procurement program. An independent organ bank frequently offers director's positions to physician assistants who have had significant experience in transplantation. These positions include administrative, clinical, technical, and supervisory roles. The salary ranges are usually above average to excellent. However, the work schedule is demanding. It is not unusual for a surgical physician assistant to work sixty to sixty-five hours a week as a member of the transplant procurement team. Because of the necessary dedication and job demands of this position, an assistant must be totally informed and willing to accept these conditions in order to enjoy a rewarding career in a transplant or organ procurement specialty.

Tables 30.1 and 30.2 provide typical job descriptions for a surgical physician's assistant procurement coordinator and a transplant clinical surgeon physician assistant. These job descriptions are not intended to be all encompassing, but rather an outline representative of the responsibility of a surgical physician assistant working as an active and productive member of a transplant or organ procurement team.

TABLE 30.1
JOB DESCRIPTION SURGICAL PHYSICIAN ASSISTANT
ORGAN PROCUREMENT COORDINATOR

I. *ACTIVITIES*

All activities of the Surgeon's Assistant Procurement Coordinator will be under the supervision of the Medical Director through the Assistant Director of the Regional Organ Bank in accordance with the organization structure of the University, Department of Surgery and will include two areas:

A. *RETRIEVAL ACTIVITIES* The Procurement Coordinator will be responsible for all retrieval and distribution activities of the Regional Organ Bank. This will include, but not necessarily be limited to the following:

1. Evaluation of potential cadaver donors:
   a. Notify the transplant physician on call for the Regional Organ Bank
   b. Assess adequacy of renal function with appropriate physician consultation
   c. Coordinator participation with local physicians involved in donor management and procurement
2. Family Consultations (as appropriate)
3. Pre-nephrectomy Tissue Typing:
   a. Establish transport routes for potential donor sera to the Central Typing Lab
   b. Coordinate arrival with the Regional Organ Bank and Tissue Typing Lab

TABLE 30.1 (continued)

    4. Coordinate Nephrectomy:
- a. Notify on call personnel at the Regional Organ Bank of planned nephrectomy schedule
- b. Notify nephrectomy team (local physicians)
- c. Insure appropriate notes are written and consent for organ donation is properly obtained
- d. Accept kidneys at nephrectomy, package for shipping and coordinate transport to UAB

    5. Be available to assist the donor surgeon on his request.

    6. Obtain adequate donor and harvest information for subsequent kidney distribution and utilization

B. *ORGAN PRESERVATION:*
    1. *Renal (Kidney Preservation Laboratory):*
- a. Understanding and preparation of various complex records
- b. Review and report quality control status of laboratory histological solutions

    2. *Ice (static) storage of organs (kidneys) for transplantation:*
- a. Prepare sterile wash and solutions
- b. Prepare sterile solutions for static storage
- c. Prepare sterile packaging material for ice storage
- d. Package kidneys for ice storage

    3. *Perfusion:*
- a. Preparation of preservation solution
- b. Quality control of preservation solutions
- c. Preparation of perfusion apparatus (Water's preservation pump)
- d. Placing of kidneys on pulsatile perfusion pump
- e. Quality control of pump
- f. Monitoring of pump
- g. Transport kidneys on pump to O.R.
- h. Transport kidneys on pump to other transplant centers as directed by Medical Director and Assistant Director

C. *EDUCATION ACTIVITIES:*
    1. *Public Education:* The Procurement Coordinator will be responsible for the maintenance of an effective public education effort initiated by the Regional Organ Bank within the designated geographic service area. This will include, but not necessarily be limited to the following:
- a. A selection of key individuals in the community that could be beneficial to such an effort
- b. Notification of Kidney Foundation members of activities in their particular region
- c. Use of local media outlets to support public educational efforts (radio, TV, newspaper, local magazines)
- d. Civic group presentations
- e. Distribution of appropriate literature within community

    2. *Professional Education:* Upon the direction of the Medical Director, through the Assistant Director, the Procurement Coordinator will be responsible for contacting key physicians and health care professionals in the local retrieval area regarding the goals and needs of the Regional Organ Bank and the renal failure patients in the state. A

continuing education program should be established at each hospital to provide a liaison between the Regional Organ Bank and personnel at the local retrieval centers. An effective professional education program should include, but not necessarily be limited to the following:

    a. Establish initial contact and maintain liaison with administrative personnel at participating medical centers

    b. Offer inservice programs to intensive care, emergency room and operating room personnel at participating medical centers

    c. Maintain a rapport with key nursing personnel at all participating medical centers

    d. Establish contact with key physicians in the local retrieval area

    e. Maintain a close liaison with local nephrologists and inform them of any *potential problem area*, i.e., potential donor family, physician participation, etc.

II. *QUALIFICATIONS:*

  A. For employment the Procurement Coordinator must, as minimum, meet the following criteria:

    1. Must have successfully completed an approved P.A. or S.A. program

    2. Must be approved by the Board of Medical Examiners as a Surgical Physician Assistant Procurement Coordinator

    3. Must be a strongly self-motivated and responsible individual with organizational ability

III. *GEOGRAPHICAL SERVICE AREA:*

  A. Local and referral regions of the Regional Organ Bank

  B. Other regional areas: Out of state procurement when requested and directed

IV. *SUPERVISION:*

  A. The coordinator will receive direct supervision from the Medical Director through the Assistant Director of the Regional Organ Bank or a local physician or physicians designated by the Medical Director.

  B. A bi-monthly on-site review will be made by the Assistant Director of the Regional Organ Bank regarding all of the activities mentioned in Section I, A, B, and C.

  C. A weekly expense report will be forwarded to the Regional Organ Bank and this report will include:

    1. Travel:

      a. Professional education

      b. Public education

      c. Retrieval activities

    2. Office expense

    3. Retrieval and/or preservation expense

V. *COMPENSATION:*

  A. Salary:

    1. Low: $18,000

    2. Average: $22,000

    3. High: $26,500

  B. Fringe benefits as set forth in the Non-academic Employee Handbook

  C. Business related expenses:

    1. The Regional Organ Bank will reimburse reasonable and necessary business related expenses in the performance of Organ Bank duties and responsibilities.

    2. Employee professional education entitled to:

      a. One professional meeting per year, with prior Medical Director approval

      b. One technical workshop per year

TABLE 30.2
JOB DESCRIPTION TRANSPLANT CLINICAL SURGICAL PHYSICIAN ASSISTANT

The Surgical Physician Assistant is an Allied Health Professional, who has graduated from an accredited college or university and is nationally Board certified or Board eligible.

ACTIVITIES:
All activities of the Surgical Physician Assistant will be under the supervision of the employing transplant surgeon. Functions under that supervision may include accurate medical history and physical examination, pre-op care for the patient, assisting the surgeon during the operation, participating in the care of the patient during the post-op period, as well as caring for the patients minor illnesses and injuries. Overall, the assistant is involved with the patient care for the transplant surgeon in any medical setting for which the surgeon is responsible. These settings include operating room, recovery room, intensive care unit, emergency room, and hospital out-patient clinic.

I. *Description of Role and Function:*
    A. Obtain history and perform physical exams on any or all admissions
    B. Write routine admission and pre-op orders for the surgeon's signature
    C. Record progress notes on charts
    D. Make daily pre- and post-op rounds on patients
    E. Perform any routine procedures: Start IVs, draw blood, etc.
    F. Serve as first assistant in surgery
    G. Monitor patients during recovery room
    H. Perform routine lab procedures
    I. Perform EKGs
    J. Screen EKGs for abnormalities
    K. Perform minor office surgery, such as: suture removal, suturing of small wounds, I&D of superficial lesions, etc.
    L. Assist post-op wound care
    M. Assessment of minor illnesses, URI, UTI, HEENT infections, skin infections, and allergic reactions
    N. Perform general counseling to patients and families concerning patient's disease
    O. Write discharge orders and summary for transplant surgeon's signature
    P. Dictate discharge summaries for transplant surgeon's signature
    Q. Respond appropriately to life threatening emergencies when no physician is available
11. Assist in the care of the patient in the intensive care unit or the acutely ill patient in the emergency room:
    A. Administer parenteral fluid or blood infusion by means of venipuncture or venous cutdown
    B. Insert central venous line and measure central venous pressure
    C. Administer oxygen via intranasal catheter
    D. Perform arterial puncture
    E. Manage ventilators
    F. Irrigate and aspirate endotracheal tube
    G. Insert nasal-gastric tube and maintain suction decompression of the stomach
    H. Ureteral catheterization
III. Adjustment of Pre-determined medicines as state and local laws permit.
IV. Participate in research as requested.

Depending upon each individual transplant surgeon's surgical commitment, a Transplant Surgical Assistant may well be involved in other types of surgery and in other areas of patient care. Certainly, each of these specific areas could be listed in a job description.

Chapter 31

THE SURGICAL PHYSICIAN ASSISTANT AS A MEMBER OF THE BURN TEAM

J. JEFFREY HEINRICH, PA-C
BRUCE C. FICHANDLER, PA-C
SALVATORE BARESE, PA-C
CHARLES B. CUONO, M.D., Ph.D.

INTRODUCTION

The development of the formally trained physician assistant has provided burn treatment facilities with a skilled professional, who under the supervision of a licensed physician, may direct and coordinate all aspects of the management of the burn patient regardless of the stage of the illness. The physician assistant has proven to be a valuable addition to the Burn Team by contributing to the tremendous amount of effort needed to care for the burn patient. One need only look at the statistics for burn injuries to see the potential for the expanded use of the physician assistant in this area.

Annually, thermal injuries in the United States result in about 10,000 deaths and cause more than 2,000,000 people to seek medical attention. Of these, approximately 100,000 people will be hospitalized with more than a third of this group requiring intensive care. The average length of hospitalization for thermal injuries ranks as one of the longest of all forms of trauma. Numerous man-hours from a wide variety of personnel are required to provide optimal care.

BURN TREATMENT FACILITY

The Burn Treatment Facility at the Yale-New Haven Medical Center believes the key to burn care is a coordinated team effort focused on overall patient benefit. This has been accomplished without need for a "burn unit" and with the addition of only one person to the existing staff, a physician assistant. The team functions as a specialized subdivision of the Section of Plastic and

Reconstructive Surgery. The team needed an interested and able full time professional to coordinate the activities of the Burn Team. For the past nine years, a physician assistant has been utilized in this capacity, functioning at the level of a surgical resident. The physician assistant is involved in the total care of the patient from the acute stage to the rehabilitative and reconstructive phases of burn care.

The responsibilities of the physician assistant begin in the emergency room, where the patient is initially evaluated. Once it has been determined that hospitalization is required, the physician assistant, together with the attending surgeon and other members of the team, discuss and develop a treatment plan. A history and physical examination is performed, the wounds are cleansed, debrided and dressed, and all the orders are written prior to the patient's transfer to the designated floor or intensive care unit.

From there, the daily involvement in the monitoring of the burn patient begins. The physician assistant helps to gather appropriate data, writes progress notes, makes appropriate changes in the therapy by writing orders and closely observes all of the clinical parameters. Each day, all dressings are changed by the physician assistant, which affords him the opportunity to cleanse, debride and evaluate all of the wounds. This is generally done in the whirlpool facilities of the Physical Therapy Department, but is occasionally done at the bedside when the patient's condition is unstable. Wound biopsies for quantitative bacteriology are routinely obtained by the physician assistant to determine the level of bacterial growth within the wound.

The advantages of a physician assistant as an integral part of the team are numerous. In addition to ongoing daily care which he is able to provide, the physician assistant helps to improve communications among all of the people taking care of the patient. The physician assistant makes daily rounds with the other members of the team at which time they discuss how well that patient tolerated physical therapy, the appearance of the wounds and the current treatment, the results of laboratory data, the nutritional status of the patient, the results of the quantitative cultures and the like. By gathering, assimilating, and organizing this important information and presenting it succinctly to the surgeons and other members of the team, the physician assistant plays a key role in patient care. The attending surgeon is thereby constantly apprised of the patient's status. Most days this is the only time the busy attending surgeon is able to see the patient; therefore, the physician assistant improves communication between the surgeon and the patient.

In addition, the physician assistant can improve communications between the surgeon and the nursing staff, since the attending surgeon spends most of his day in the operating room or clinic. It is difficult for the nursing staff to relate to the attending surgeon the problems which arise from hour to hour or in the case of a patient in the intensive care unit, from minute to minute. The physician assistant is always available to answer any questions, write appropriate orders, and care for the patient's needs. If he does not have the answer to the problems, he has the mobility to go directly to the operating room to discuss it with the surgeon. The physician assistant generally communicates with all three nursing shifts, since the team makes early morning and late afternoon or early evening rounds. Therefore, the physician assistant can improve communications between the nursing staff and the surgeon in a manner far superior to writing orders, or having nurses pass messages on from one shift to the next.

The physician assistant works closely with the physical therapist each day and coordinates the patient care, both in physical therapy and on the nursing floor. Generally, while the physician assistant is cleaning and debriding the patient's wounds, the physical therapist is assessing relevant joint mobility and conducting an active and passive exercise regimen. Together they perform the necessary dressing changes.

Since the physician assistant's whole day is aimed specifically at taking care of burn patients, he naturally spends a great deal of his time with the patients, giving him a chance to develop a closer relationship with them. Thus, the physician assistant often learns of those matters which frequently concern the patient, such as what their final appearance and function will be, when they might return to gainful employment, or any financial problems which have developed as a result of the injury. The physician assistant can then begin to effectively deal with some of these problems by orchestrating the various ancillary personnel, such as the social worker and psychiatric nurse. Furthermore, the physician assistant can call upon the specialized services of the dietitian and the occupational therapist as needed.

The only time the physician assistant is not usually readily available to go to the intensive care unit, the floor, or physical therapy is when one of the burn patients requires a major operative procedure. The physician assistant actively participates in all surgical debridement procedures, as well as in the harvesting and application of skin grafts. The physician assistant is an integral part of the team in coordinating the perioperative care of the burn patient.

Upon discharge, the patient is followed by the physician assistant and the attending surgeon in the burn clinic where his progress is assessed and appropriate adjuncts, such as the use of pressure garments, or increased physical therapy are employed. All necessary consults to ancillary personnel during the rehabilitative phase continue to be coordinated by the physician assistant. The majority of severely burned patients require multiple hospital admissions for reconstructive procedures. During these admissions, the physician assistant provides the thread of continuity since there is a high turnover of housestaff and other personnel on the burn service.

Chapter 32

THE SURGICAL PHYSICIAN ASSISTANT AS A MEMBER OF THE ANESTHESIA-CRITICAL CARE TEAM

SHEPARD B. STONE, M.P.S., PA-C
TERRANCE D. RAFFERTY, M.B.

By tradition, anesthesia services in the United States have been furnished by the anesthesiologists and nurse anesthetists. The role of nurse anesthetists in the health care system has been questioned (1, 2). Furthermore, it has long been recognized that the total number of anesthesiologists is well below that necessary to supervise or provide all of the anesthetics administered in the country (3, 4). This problem has been compounded in areas of low population density by the demographic distribution of anesthesiologists who, as a group, tend to locate in urban areas (4). A solution which has been proposed to resolve these issues has been the training of physician assistants in anesthesia (1,5,6). The pioneer in this field has been the School of Medicine of Case Western Reserve University where, in 1971, an under-graduate program was initiated, designed specifically for the discipline of anesthesiology (1, 7). Graduates of this program receive certification from the Ohio Society of Anesthesiologists following successful completion of a written and oral examination (1). A similar program exists at Emory University School of Medicine. Here, the subspecialty training is at the graduate level, a B.S. degree in science or technology being a prerequisite for acceptance into the program. In addition, the student is awarded a masters degree (M.M.Sc.) following successful completion of the course of study (5). It is anticipated that the Case Western Reserve program will be upgraded to graduate level in 1982 (8).

The practice at Yale with regard to non-physician specialty training in anesthesia differs from both of the above programs. It was felt that the broad primary care background of the physician assistant would serve as a more firm foundation for specialty training. Indeed, physician assistant education, in many respects, models the physician's own training with a grounding in the basic and clinical sciences and graded clinical responsibility in terms of bedside clinical care. Accordingly, in 1978, it was elected to train a physician assistant in anesthesiology. There were several reasons for this action. Firstly, there was a concurrence with the view that a great number of tasks in anesthesiology need not be performed by physicians (9, 10). Secondly, there was confidence in the training and performance of other subspecialty physician assistants in this institution (in the care of burn patients, and in cardiothoracic surgery, emergency services, neurosurgery, oncology, pathology, plastic surgery and psychiatry). The final impetus for implementation of such a program was facilitated by the occurrence of an unexpected vacancy at the first year resident physician level. One of us (SBS), then a surgical physician assistant, was selected to enter the anesthesiology residency program. Parenthetically, this physician assistant-anesthesiology resident was known to the members of the department of anesthesiology as he had previously spent a ten week rotation there during his post-graduate surgical residency program. It was decided that he be exposed to the same range of clinical training and didactic instruction as the physician anesthesiology residents. This included participation in preoperative care, regional and general anesthesia, invasive intravascular monitoring techniques (pulmonary and systemic arterial cannulation), postoperative-management and sub-specialty rotations. An exception to this resident physician-physician assistant parity was dictated by perceived medicolegal considerations (11). The physician assistant did not take call at a supervisory level. (Subsequent departmental reorganization has modified this system somewhat.)

Although implementation of such a program required adaptation to the special milieu of a department of anesthesiology, the administrative groundwork had been established by the prior utilization of physician assistants in other specialties at Yale. The problems that arose with implementation of portions of the program resolved themselves with time as the nurses and physicians saw that the physician assistant was associated with no detrimental effect on patient care, and, indeed, his enthusiasm and zeal brought commendation from many.

The experience proved eminently satisfactory to the physician assistant himself. An additional group also reaped benefits, namely, members of the physician assistant surgical residency progam who were informally assigned to him during the course of their surgical residency. Upon completion of the base two-year residency, the physician assistant requested additional exposure in cardiac anesthesia and critical care medicine. With completion of this "fellowship year," the physician assistant had attained considerable experience as a cardiac anesthetist and intensivist and was appointed to the hospital medical staff, the medical school faculty and the physician assistant surgical residency faculty.

At present, his duties are primarily clinical. Four days per week are devoted to clinical anesthesia. The depth of previous training has resulted in broad responsibilities. At the discretion and direction of the attending staff, he may administer anesthesia (regional or general, including cardiothoracic, neurologic, obstetric, outpatient and pediatric anesthesia), assist in the administration of anesthesia by residents, serve as the anesthesiology representative in the various critical care areas and perform anesthesiology consultations. He also participates in the on-call schedule. The fifth day of the week is devoted to continuing education, to fulfilling his role as an effector in the didactic component of the intramural general physician assistant program and postgraduate surgical physician assistant residency program and participation in departmental research protocols. These activities have resulted in several publications, the most noteworthy being a composite review of closed circuit anesthesia (12). Audiences for presentations have included emergency services personnel, graduate nursing students, physician assistant students, physician assistant surgery residents, graduate physician assistants, residents and attending physicians. This versatility in utilization is of value to the department of anesthesiology. The anesthesiology residents accept the physician assistant-anesthesiologist as a colleague with broad clinical experience. Faculty can devote greater supervision and educational efforts to the resident staff without diminishing clinical patient care. In the face of resident unavailability (illness, examinations, and so forth), the physician assistant-anesthesiologist may, with attending backup, fill any of a number of clinical slots. Typical activities during operative anesthesia and critical care assignments are detailed in Tables 32.1 and 32.2.

TABLE 32.1

TYPICAL ACTIVITIES DURING AN OPERATIVE ANESTHESIA ASSIGNMENT

1. Chart review
2. Obtaining a history
3. Performing a physical examination
4. Discussion with patient regarding:
   a. pre-operative preparation
   b. anesthetic induction technique
   c. post-operative events
5. Writing of preanesthetic orders
6. Discussion with nursing and responsible physician staffs of special preoperative evaluation or preparation as necessary
7. Equipment preparation including that of invasive monitoring
8. Attachment and insertions of appropriate monitoring aids prior to induction of anesthesia
9. Induction of general and regional anesthesia
10. Maintenance of anesthesia
11. Transportation to post-anesthesia recovery room or critical care unit, as appropriate
12. Postoperative care as indicated

TABLE 32.2
TYPICAL ACTIVITIES DURING A CRITICAL CARE UNIT ASSIGNMENT

1. Routine airway management in the recovery room area and surgical intensive care unit (SICU).
2. Emergency airway management as a member of the cardio-pulmonary resuscitation team.
3. Interpretation and management of mechanical ventilation and respiratory care procedures in the SICU.
4. Intra-arterial, central venous and pulmonary artery catheterization; attendant in-depth cardiovascular and respiratory data acquisition and synthesis; delineation of appropriate hemodynamic (intropic support, vasodilatory therapy, fluid management) and ventilatory interventions (oxygen therapy, endotracheal intubation, positive end-expiratory pressure [PEEP], optimal compliance and "best PEEP").
5. Diagnostic and therapeutic nerve blocks.
6. Elective anesthesiology consultations.

While the role of the physician assistant in anesthesiology and critical care medicine is controversial (6), the experiences at Case Western Reserve, Emory and Yale have been positive. However, the ultimate fate of the Yale Anesthesiology-physician assistant program is uncertain. This is due, in part, to the reluctance of the department to undertake the responsibility of furnishing this particular subspecialty training to others without the immediate local availability of long term career opportunities in this field. An additional consideration is a change in departmental needs brought about by a recent marked increase in highly qualified physician applicants being available for residency positions.

However, the niche created for this sole graduate of the program is consistent with his personal goals in that he has both the clinical responsibility and educational role which he desires.

REFERENCES

1. Rhoton, M., and Gravenstein, J.: University education for nonphysician health professionals in anesthesia. *In: Review of Allied Health Education.* Hamburg, J., editor, 1976. Louisville, Ky., University Press. pp 1-18.
2. Homi, H.: Correspondence. *Anesth Analg (Cleve),* 54:820-821, 1975.
3. Keown, K.: Status of anesthesiology. *JAMA, 195:*761-763, 1966.
4. Carron, H.: Anesthesia manpower in the United States. *In: Public Health Aspects of Critical Care Medicine and Anesthesiology.* Safar, P., editor, Philadelphia, Pa., F. Davis, Co., pp 246-264, 1974.
5. Steinhaus, J., Evans, J., and Frazier, W.: The physician assistant in anesthesiology. *Anesth Analg (Cleve),* 52:794-799, 1973.
6. McCaughey, T.: Anesthetic technicians in the province of Quebec. *Canad Anaesth Soc J,* 22:106-110, 1975.
7. Gravenstein, J., and Rhoton, M.: Teaching anesthesia to undergraduate college students. *Anesthesiology,* 37:641-646, 1972.
8. Rhoton, M.: Personal communication.

9. Gravenstein, J., Steinhaus, J., and Volpitto, P.: Analysis of manpower needs in anesthesiology. *Anesthesiology, 33:*350-357, 1970.
10. Tomlin, P.: The future. *Anaesthesia, 22:*354-355, 1967.
11. Berger, R.: Irregular assistants and legal risks. *JAMA, 207:*1231-   , 1969.
12. Stone, S., and Greene, N.: Low-flow anesthesia. *Curr Rev Clin Anesth, 1:*114-120, 1981.

The much appreciated secretarial support of Mrs. Marion Bruch, Ms. Gail Norup and Ms. Linda Shiffrin is gratefully acknowledged.

Chapter 33

THE SURGICAL PHYSICIAN ASSISTANT IN UROLOGIC SURGERY PRACTICE

DANIEL T. VETROSKY, P.A.
SIGMUND I. TANNENBAUM, M.D.

Urology is a branch of medicine which is concerned with the medical and surgical treatment of diseases of the male and female urinary tract and of the male reproductive organs (1). Urology spans the age spectrum and includes diagnosis and treatment of congenital anomalies as well as various kinds of hypertension and neoplasms. Urology uses established general surgical principles, as well as advancements made in organ transplantation, fiberoptic endoscopy, and microsurgical technique.

Urologic physician assistant training programs began in 1970 at Cincinnati. However, lack of funding caused closure of this particular training program in 1976 (3, 4). Currently 8% of all surgical physician assistants in large United States hospitals are employed in urologic departments (2). This population has been formally trained by primary care or surgeon's assistant programs, with further instruction by employing urologists.

Reasons for choosing one surgical discipline over another may depend on an individual's life goal, background, or bias. In my own case (D.V.) I enjoy working with patients, and I had worked as a urologic technician for six years prior to entering physician assistant training.

DAILY DUTIES OF A UROLOGIC PHYSICIAN ASSISTANT

A routine schedule for a urologic physician assistant at Duke is as follows:

6:30 a.m. — Ward rounds with residents and interns.

7:30 a.m. — Surgery on Tuesday, Wednesday and Friday.

8:30 a.m. — Clinic (General and Oncology), Monday and Thursday.

12:00 noon — Lunch (if clinic is not heavy or surgery is not scheduled).

1:00 p.m. — Fertility clinic, Wednesday.

3:30 p.m. — Clinic ends (usually), gather laboratory data before rounds.

4:00 p.m. — Ward rounds with supervising physician.

5:00 p.m. — Sign out rounds with residents to pass on information.

5-6 p.m. — Home.

Additional responsibilities include performing admission histories and physical examinations, writing admission orders, scheduling patients for future admissions, and dictating discharge summaries.

State law and hospital bylaws provide guidelines for the surgical physician assistant's role. Within this framework lies a considerable freedom for the urologic physician assistant. Table 33.1 describes the potential capabilities of the urologic physician assistant. The degree to which this capability is attained depends upon both the physician assistant's ability and aggressiveness as well as physician's flexibility in allowing the physician assistant to "grow" with the job.

The advantages of having a urologic physician assistant in a private practice or in an institute with residency training programs are numerous and result from the wide range of duties the physician assistant can perform. A recent study has shown that surgical physician assistants have improved the quality of patient care and, furthermore, have enhanced the quality of training received by surgical residents (2). In contrast to the urologic surgical resident, the urologic physician assistant is a permanent staff person who does not rotate every few months to a different service. Consequently, continuity of policies in patient care is assured. In addition, the urologic physician assistant can perform tasks which may no longer be educational for the urologic resident, thus allowing the resident more opportunities to participate in educational activities such as reading, attending conferences or pursuing challenging and difficult cases (2). The urologic physician assistant can also function as an instructor in the use of specialized instruments and thereby save both time and money for a urology practice or program (see Table 33.2).

Urology offers a broad spectrum of medical knowledge, diagnostic tests and surgical techniques to continually challenge the physician assistant (see Tables 33.2 and 33.3). In an academic medical center, one has the opportunity to attend not only urological conferences by all medical/surgical specialty conferences, time permitting. The opportunity to become involved in research activities such as drug studies, new diagnostic tests, and new microsurgical techniques is another advantage offered by an academic medical center.

ISSUES IN ACCEPTANCE AND ADVANCEMENT

In our own medical center, problems in acceptance or role definition of the urologic physician assistant have not been encountered. However, potential problems for urologic physician assistants in other practice settings include: acceptance by nursing personnel, acceptance by resident staff, lack of recognition of the physician assistant's abilities, severe limitation of job scope, problems with attaining hospital privileges, and problems of "lag time" in obtaining certification or registration with State Board of Medical Examiners.

The problems offered are by no means an exhaustive list and may vary from practice to practice. However, these are problems often considered by most beginning physician assistants in any specialty.

Important considerations in any field of endeavor is its career potential. For the urologic physician assistant, avenues of advancement include involvement in research projects, learning microsurgical techniques, and involvement with kidney transplantations. Other responsibilities might include a position with a private practice group, pursuit of a graduate degree and a teaching position, or involvement in another medical or surgical discipline.

The beauty of being a physician assistant is the breadth of knowledge one has. A physician assistant knows "a little about a lot." Hence, employment possibilities need not be hampered by not having options for pursuing any of the medical or surgical fields. It is reassuring to know there are other subspecialties for which a physician assistant could qualify.

In conclusion, the role of the physician assistant in subspecialty practices has expanded since its inception in 1965. Physician assistants bring expanded technical capabilities to the practitioner's office, allowing better coverage between multi-hospital and office practices. Additionally, the physician assistant working in a private practice setting can decrease the administrative demand upon the physician by dictating discharge summaries, completing insurance forms, and monitoring changes in Medicare and Medicaid regulations.

ADVANTAGES TO THE UROLOGIST

The physician assistant offers many advantages to the physician in the office. The physician assistant can perform routine diagnostic and therapeutic office procedures including history and physical examinations, dressing changes, urethral calibrations, dilations, urodynamics, radiography, and patient education. Patients spend less time in the office waiting room, and relatively more time attending to their health care needs. After having been evaluated by the physician assistant, the patient is more organized when discussing the problems with the physician, allowing for more in-depth discussion of significant health care questions.

The successful introduction of the physician assistant into the private practice setting depends upon the acceptance by office personnel, local hospitals, and, of course, by the patient. The chances of malpractice suits in the private practice setting are actually decreased with the addition of a physician assistant (5). Malpractice action against the practitioner is frequently the result of poor chart documentation, as well as patient demand for more physician time. Physician assistants facilitate complete and accurate chart documentation, allow the physician to establish a stronger physician-patient relationship, and help to avoid patient misunderstanding while gaining better patient compliance.

Although the urologic physician assistant offers the urologist greater latitude in office practice, the latter continues to be responsible for each patient, for the supervision of the physician assistant, and for communicating directly with referring physicians. The urologic physician assistant's role should expand over time within the limitations of the expertise of the responsible physician.

Used in this manner, the physician assistant can make an important contribution to the care of the urologic patient.

TABLE 33.1

CAPABILITIES OF A SURGICAL PHYSICIAN ASSISTANT IN UROLOGIC PRACTICE

Administrative
  Evaluation of new urologic instruments
  Organization of research laboratory
  Organization and implementation of research protocols
  Instruction of interns, medical students and allied health personnel
  Supervision of allied health personnel
  Office dictation: Histories, physical exams, discharge summaries, letters
  Organization and maintenance of cystoscopy suite
Clinical
  Perform office evaluations, history and physical examinations.
  Perform preoperative and postoperative care
  Participate in ward rounds
  First assistant in both open and closed cases
  Perform patient education and counseling, i.e.: vasectomy, penile prosthesis, urologic surgical procedures, catheters and their care, urologic appliances, chemotherapy.
Procedures Performed
  Urethral catheterization, calibration and dilation
  Suprapubic aspiration and insertion of suprapubic catheters
  Cystometrograms
  Laboratory data: urinalysis, culture and sensitivity
  Retrograde urethrograms, cystograms
  Bladder barbitage and catheter (urethral and ureteral) irrigation

TABLE 33.2

KNOWLEDGE OF UROLOGIC INSTRUMENTS NECESSARY FOR A
SURGICAL PHYSICIAN ASSISTANT IN UROLOGIC PRACTICE

Catheters
  Foley, Robinson, Coude' Tip, Malecot, Ureteral, Suprapubic Stamey, Bonano, Cystocath
Dialators and Sounds
  Filiform & Followers, Bougies a boules, Van Buren, McCrea, Kollman Dialator
Cystoscopic and Urethroscopic Instruments
  McCarthy Panendoscope, Lenses, Wappler Cystourethroscope, Stern McCarthy, Iglesias, Nesbit and Baumrucker Resectoscopes, Ellik Evacuator, Bigelow, Lowsely and Hendrickson Lithotrites, Biopsy forceps, Cold cup forceps, resection loops and knives, Otis Urethrotome, Ureteral stone baskets, Brodney clamp.
Miscellaneous
  Biopsy needles: Vim Silverman Franklin, Travenol True Cut
  Types of penile and testicular prosthetic implants and artificial sphincters
  Microsurgical instruments and sutures
  Kidney stone forceps
  General surgical instruments and sutures

TABLE 33.3
OTHER FIELDS WITH WHICH A UROLOGIC PHYSICIAN ASSISTANT
WILL BE ACQUAINTED

Nephrology—Congenital renal diseases, dialysis, transplantation
Endocrinology—Stone disease, hypertension, fertility
Immunology—Transplantation, chemotherapy
Hematology/Oncology—Chemotherapy, metastatic genitourinary cancers
Radiology—Intravenous pyelograms, CT scans, ultrasound
General Surgery—Trauma, ileal loops, transplantation
Neurology & Neurosurgery—Spinal cord anomilies/injuries
Obstetrics & Gynecology—Female incontinence, urinary tract infections during pregnancy
Infectious Disease—Renal TB, urinary tract infections: bacterial, viral, fungal
Pediatrics—Congenital anomilies, neoplasms
Pulmonary—Metastatic genitourinary cancers
Orthopedics—Metastatic genitourinary cancers
Vascular Surgery—Transplantations/reimplantations
Plastic Surgery—Reconstruction of penile anomilies/injuries, prosthetic implantations, microvascular techniques
General Medicine—Hypertension, hematuria, infections

REFERENCES

1. Tanago EA: Anatomy of the genitourinary tract. In: *General Urology*, DR Smith (ed), 10th edition, p. 1–14, 1981.
2. Perry HB, et al.: The current and future role of surgical physician assistants. *Ann Surg, 193:*132–137, 1981.
3. Church RT, and Mellinger GT: The urological assistant: New aid in growing manpower shortage. *Hosp Topics, 48:*89–92, 1970.
4. Blackard CE, and Church RT: Urological assistant: A preliminary report. *J Urol, 108:*188–189, 1972.
5. Vanderbilt CE: Physician Assistants in a Surgical Practice. *Medical Law and Practice Management.* Vol 1, No. 5.

Chapter 34

THE SURGICAL PHYSICIAN ASSISTANT FUNCTIONING IN THE ROLE OF THE JUNIOR SURGICAL HOUSE OFFICER IN A COMMUNITY HOSPITAL

CYNTHIA L. CARSON, PA-C
MALCOLM S. BIENFIELD, M.D.

Faced with cutbacks in surgical residency training programs and the curtailment of foreign medical graduates' entry into the United States, community hospitals across the nation have been hard pressed to recruit sufficient personnel appropriately qualified to help maintain the necessary standards of excellence in surgical patient care. To meet this growing need, a group of physicians and physician assistants at Norwalk Hospital and Yale University School of Medicine envisioned a program in which selected graduate physician assistants could be trained to serve as surgeon extenders functioning at the highest level in pre-, intra-, and post-operative care of the surgical patient.

The result was the Norwalk Hospital/Yale University School of Medicine PA Surgical Residency Program, initiated in 1975 to augment the surgical skills of the certified primary care physician assistant through eight months of structured didactic and clinical experience on the surgical service at Norwalk Hospital and four months of laboratory work, gross anatomy and pathophysiology at Yale Medical School.

Upon completion of this postgraduate specialty training, alumni are employed by the Department of Surgery at Norwalk Hospital as staff surgical physician assistants; permanent positions in which they function as house officers under the responsibility and supervision of the attending surgeon on each surgical service. Ultimate responsibility is to the Chairman of the Department of Surgery. At Norwalk Hospital, a 427 bed community hospital in southwestern Connecticut, the entire surgical housestaff is comprised of surgical physician assistants, currently totaling 11 staff surgical physician assistants in addition to 10 physician assistant residents in training. The Norwalk/Yale training program and the resultant utilization of surgical physician assistants by the Norwalk Hospital Department of Surgery may be regarded as a prototype for other community hospitals in need of skilled individuals trained to meet their surgical housestaff requirements.

It is our opinion that the basis for the successful replacement of MD housestaff by physician assistant housestaff is a well-structured and intense residency year. Since the physician assistant surgical resident-in-training and the graduate staff surgical physician assistant follow essentially the same job description, in this chapter only the role of the fully-trained, or staff surgical physician assistant will be described in detail (see Chapter 14 for a discussion of residency training for surgical physician assistants). The use of trained surgical physician assistants to perform history and physical examinations, to assist at operations and with the pre- and postoperative care of patients, and to assist and evaluate the patient in an emergency situation has enabled Norwalk Hospital to continue to meet the needs of surgical patients in a manner compatible with sound medical practice and good patient care.

ORGANIZATION AND RESPONSIBILITY

Each surgical physician assistant is assigned to a "service" or group of attending surgeons whose specialties include general surgery, cardiothoracic, genito-urinary, orthopaedic, plastic and vascular surgery as well as neurosurgery, ophthalmology, and otorhinolaryngology. Training during the residency year has familiarized the physician assistant with all of these specialty areas. A surgical physician assistant may continue to work with the same surgeons for years, and thereby develop an understanding of their individual professional preferences. With time, the surgical physician assistant learns what type of bowel prep will be ordered for the preoperative patient, when nasogastric feeding will be discontinued in favor of oral feeding following sigmoid resection, what laboratory studies are considered appropriate, when should the patient be ambulated or what analgesic agents should be utilized. This continuity of relationship improves patient care.

The surgical physician assistant and the elective surgery patient meet on the patient's first hospital day. At this time, the physician assistant explains in broad outline his role as it impacts on the patient's hospital experience. The physician assistant also elicits a detailed history and performs a thorough physical examination of the patient for the assigned surgeon. In addition, the physician assistant answers questions and addresses concerns expressed by the patient.

Following the initial interview, the physician assistant writes preoperative orders in keeping with the clinical practices of the patient's surgeon. The orders will include appropriate laboratory studies, x-rays, electrocardiograms, preoperative prep orders, diet, medications and specialized studies such as CT scans or ultrasound. If, in the judgment of the physician assistant on the basis of the physical examination the patient requires additional tests, the physician assistant may order them. All orders written by the physician assistant must be countersigned by the attending surgeon within 24 hours.

OPERATING ROOM ASSISTING

The surgical physician assistant functions as first or second assistant during the operative procedure providing retraction for adequate exposure, assisting in dissection, clamping and tying bleeding vessels and assisting with, and often completing, closure of the surgical wound. Frequent work with the same surgeon enables the surgical physician assistant to anticipate the surgeon's needs and contributes to a smoother operating procedure. Never does the surgical physician assistant assume the role of the surgeon. Unlike M.D. surgical residents, physician assistants are trained to function as surgical assistants rather than as independent operating surgeons. Should the surgeon prefer to utilize a surgical colleague as first assistant, the surgical physician assistant may then be called upon to act as a second assistant.

POSTOPERATIVE CARE

During the closure of the wound in the operating room, the surgeon and the surgical physician assistant may review any specialized postoperative needs of the patient. When the surgical procedure is completed, the surgical physician assistant accompanies the patient to the recovery room to further assess the status of the patient and document any problems. Here, the surgical physician assistant writes postoperative orders for fluid and respiratory management, antibiotics, analgesics, diet and special considerations, with particular attention to the requirements of the individual patient. The surgical physician assistant also writes a brief operative summary which includes the operative procedure, pre- and post-operative diagnosis, surgeon, assistants, IV fluids, type of anesthesia, operative findings, drains placed and any intraoperative complications. The surgeon, however, dictates the formal operative note which describes the surgical procedure in detail.

Bedside rounds are made daily by the physician assistant and surgeon (together when possible) and the physician assistant documents the patient's progress on the chart. The surgical physician assistant is responsible for ordering and reviewing appropriate laboratory data, for correlating these data with the patient's clinical status, and for writing further orders according to the patient's needs.

Postoperative duties of the surgical physician assistant include regular checks of the operative wound and removal of clips or sutures at the proper time. Interaction of the physician assistant with the surgical patient continues throughout the patient's entire hospital experience. Patients who qualify may attend the surgical clinic where they are followed by the surgical physician assistant and attending surgeon until further surgical care is no longer necessary.

SURGICAL INTENSIVE CARE

Staff physician assistants and physician assistant residents rotate through the surgical ICU on a regular basis. Staff physician assistants are assigned two month rotations and physician assistant residents one month rotations in the units.

Much of the Norwalk Hospital/Yale University School of Medicine surgical physician assistant residency training is devoted to the understanding of the pathophysiology of surgical disease processes. The 12-month program includes a 17-week dog surgery course at Yale where, under the direction of both surgeons and anesthesiologists, the physician assistant residents learn to insert and monitor Swan Ganz catheters, perform cutdowns and tracheostomies and study cardiac, renal and pulmonary physiology. While at Yale, the physician assistants rotate through anesthesia and the surgical intensive care unit. A course in human anatomy cadaver dissection is taught by clinical surgeons at Yale and emphasizes the clinical significance of surgical anatomy.

The curriculum also includes a series of lectures on such topics as fluid and electrolyte therapy, acid-base balance, hyperalimentation, electrocardiographs and the use of cardiac drugs, surgical complications, major burn care, respiratory care and cardiopulmonary resuscitation.

It is this orientation that enables the physician assistant to function knowledgeably in the intensive care unit. Staff physician assistants rotate through the ICU so that their familiarity with the constantly changing methods of assessing physiological parameters are updated and reinforced.

When on duty in the Norwalk Hospital surgical intensive care unit, the physician assistant relies heavily on the counsel of a full-time intensivist who is a member of the medical staff. At the same time, the training and experience of the surgical physician assistants permit them to exercise broad clinical judgment within the parameters authorized by the attending surgeon who is immediately responsible for the physician assistant's performance.

It is the surgical physician assistant's responsibility to continually monitor and assess the varying conditions of acutely ill patients. When determining a patient's fluid requirements, the physician assistant assesses such physiological parameters as intake and outputs, pulmonary capillary wedge pressure, and serum and urine osmolalities. Stabilization of these patients includes starting IV lines, administering IV medications such as Dilantin, Lidocaine, Dopamine or Nipride, giving IV fluids, inserting arterial or central venous lines and initiating cardiopulmonary resuscitation. Intensive care patients often have multiple system failure and the surgical physician assistant helps to coordinate the various treatment modalities.

When the patient's condition warrants transfer, the physician assistant writes an ICU discharge summary and the transfer orders, which include specialized instructions and care to be provided on the surgical ward.

IN-HOUSE CALL COVERAGE

Two physician assistants (a staff surgical physician assistant and a physician assistant resident-in-training) are on call in the hospital at all times. The staff surgical physician assistants take call on an average of every ninth night and are off duty the day after call. First call is taken by the physician assistant resident with backup provided by the second call surgical staff physician assistant and by telephone communication with the surgeon when necessary. Prior to leaving the hospital the day after call, the physician assistant not only makes rounds on the patients he is following, but informs the appropriate physician assistant of any problems which may have arisen with his patients during the night. Call hours are from 5:00 P.M. to 8:00 A.M. the following day and 8:00 A.M. to 8:00 A.M. on weekends and holidays. The average work week for a physician assistant at Norwalk Hospital is 56 hours.

When on call, the physician assistant is responsible for clinical problems arising on the surgical service and in the surgical ICU. The physician assistant must be the eyes, ears and hands of the surgeon who is on the other end of a telephone line. In addition, the physician assistant is called to act as first assistant in all emergency procedures and may be called by the attending surgeon to the emergency suite where he becomes involved in the initial management of the patient.

PROCEDURES

Physician assistants perform venous cutdowns, insert angiocatheters, Foley catheters, arterial lines, perform percutaneous subclavian and jugular catheterizations and also insert nasogastric tubes, as well as Cantor and Miller-Abbot tubes. Under direct physician supervision, physician assistants execute procedures such as thoracenteses, paracenteses, endotracheal intubation, and insertion of Swan Ganz catheters.

TEACHING RESPONSIBILITIES AND IN-HOUSE CME

A significant responsibility of the Norwalk Hospital staff surgical physician assistant is active participation in all phases of physician assistant surgical residency training. Staff physician assistant contributions to the teaching process and their presence as role models for resident physician assistants provides cohesiveness within the program. The collaboration of surgical practitioners and students in a joint commitment to learning helps develop and maintain the highest levels of clinical skills and knowledge.

In addition to their daily service as preceptors on the job, staff surgical physician assistants give courses for student physician assistants who rotate through Norwalk Hospital on clinical rotations from the physician assistant programs at Yale University School of Medicine, George Washington University, Hahnemann Medical College and other major university medical centers. A 5-week cycle of student lectures organized and presented by staff physician assistants covers topics such as the acute abdomen, pre- and postoperative evaluation, fluids, electrolytes, and acid-base balance.

As members of the physician assistant staff in the Department of Surgery, surgical physician assistants attend and participate in all clinical conferences. At Norwalk Hospital, these include weekly Grand Rounds, a monthly Mortality and Morbidity Conference, and regularly scheduled department lectures, panel discussions, and symposiums.

At Grand Rounds, physician assistants select and present interesting cases for discussion by their peers, the surgical attending staff, and representatives from other disciplines. A single physician assistant is responsible for the content and quality of the presentation and will review it before Grand Rounds. Physician assistants also select from professional journals and distribute copies of current articles which pertain to the presentation in order to enhance discussion and stimulate debate. A combined Medical/Surgical conference for presentation of cases of interest to both medicine and surgery is held monthly. Case summaries and evaluations of complications are written and presented by physician assistants at the monthly Mortality and Morbidity Conference which is attended by representatives from Anesthesiology, Radiology and Pathology as well as Surgery.

Additionally, to promote the development of clear and concise thinking, each Norwalk Hospital surgical physician assistant resident is required to write an independent research paper on a clinical topic. The utilization of resources and organization of material contributes to the physician assistant's ability to present material at surgical conferences. They are encouraged to prepare papers for publication. A voluntary Journal Club, hosted by a surgical attending, is held monthly.

ADMINISTRATIVE DUTIES

Staff physician assistants elect from their membership a chief and an assistant chief to direct the annual and daily activities of the group and to represent them at meetings with the Chairman of the Department of Surgery, to whose approval all physician assistant resolutions are subject. Within this framework, staff physician assistants are responsible for scheduling on-call time, rotation, vacation and specialty appointments and assigning all assistants in the Operating Rooms to meet the specific needs outlined by the individual surgeons. In addition, elected physician assistant representatives serve on hospital and medical staff committees such as the Trauma Committee, Operating Room Committee, and the Infection Control Committee.

INTERACTION WITH NURSING STAFF

Contributing to the success of the Norwalk Hospital physician assistant program has been the excellent relationship between physician assistants and the nursing staff. Members of the Department of Nursing, invited to participate in the development of the Physician Assistant Program at its inception, have had considerable input into the design and implementation of the program and are consistently supportive of the physician assistants who, in turn, welcome the counsel of the experienced surgical nurse. A significant interpersonal dependency permits physician assistants and nurses to exchange knowledge and learn from each other. Such exchanges enhance the communication of patient information and the quality of patient management.

RELATIONSHIP WITH SURGEONS

While Norwalk Hospital policy dictates that the patient is initially seen by an attending physician, the physician assistants are valued by the surgical attending staff as rigorously trained surgeon extenders who, in the hospital at all times, are qualified to cope with emergencies and monitor clinical progress. Through months or years of working together, the surgeons and physician assistants develop a strong rapport.

The high standard of the physician assistants' daily performance, their willingness to learn and their capacity to contribute have led to enthusiastic acceptance of the physician assistant program by the Norwalk Hospital surgical staff. Indeed, after six years experience with surgical physician assistants, the attending general surgeons express no interest in pursuing a renewal of a freestanding surgical residency program. The replacement of M.D. residents by physician assistant housestaff at the Norwalk Hospital has successfully filled the clinical requirements of the Department of Surgery.

Chapter 35

THE ORTHOPEDIC PHYSICIAN ASSISTANT IN A PRIVATE OFFICE-BASED SETTING

HOLM W. NEUMANN, Ph.D., M.D.
MARTIN MISRACK, OPA-C

With the present day busy schedule, the orthopedic surgeon is faced with long office waits for his patients, extended hours and increased preoccupation with minor orthopedic office procedures of a broad variety and types. Fortunately, a new type of specially trained person is now available to help provide some relief from this busy schedule and to increase practice efficiency. The orthopedic physician assistant fulfills this role well.

What are the factors to be considered by an orthopedic surgeon when faced with the decision as to whether or not to employ an orthopedic physician assistant? One must weigh the advantages and disadvantages. A busy schedule, increasing patient care expense, long patient waiting times and the availability of a certified, well-trained, knowledgeable, and reliable assistant are all factors prompting one to seek the services of an orthopedic physician assistant. Recognizing that the patient and physician expense could be decreased, that an increase in patient accessibility to qualified care could be attained and that a decrease in patient waiting time can be achieved, the decision to employ an orthopedic physician assistant can be greatly simplified. It is important to emphasize, however, that such a physician assistant should be highly trained and skilled in his field so that a mutual confidence can be gained between employer and employee. A continuing, ongoing educational and personal "interaction" is vital to the professional development of the physician assistant. The rewards of a satisfactory work relationship are reaped many times over through the provision of a more efficient, enjoyable, and quality patient care program.

One should mention a word about the disadvantages of employing a physician assistant in the field of orthopedics. They are few, indeed, if an ideal relationship is established. One must invest some time initially to "break in" the new employee. The physician must learn to understand the physician

assistant's limitations and capabilities as well as his own. Each must take time
to gain a mutual trust and to define his working role. A financial investment is
required initially, but once a mature working relationship is established, the
physician assistant will "easily pay his way." An orthopedic surgeon who
employs a physician assistant must establish an individual working relationship
with the physician assistant. This will vary with personalities involved, training
background of both the M.D. and the physician assistant, and the establishment of a state of mutual trust and interest in providing quality medical care.

Initially, when engaging the services of an orthopedic physician assistant,
certain barriers and obstacles will arise. These problems will prove to be temporary in nature, however, and fade away in a short time. An orthopedic
physician assistant will need to be accepted by the patient population. A person who gets along well with people and introduces his role or purpose "for
being there" will certainly speed up the acceptance process. Soon, patients will
recognize the value of having someone "extra" to assist them in times of need.

The medical community, likewise, will need to be educated to the role of
the new health practitioner in the "system." With time, they will recognize the
abilities and skills of the orthopedic physician assistant and later insist on his or
her helping. The supervising M.D. and his physician assistant should work as a
team and be available together when times of need arise. Ideally, a one-to-one
working relationship is best for providing uninterrupted continuity of patient
care. Office hours and emergency call time should be taken together. Certain
basic issues are to be faced when setting up a practice with an orthopedic
physician assistant. One must assure that the entire medical community is
introduced to the role being played by the orthopedic physician assistant.
Nursing staff, physical therapy departments, emergency room departments,
other M.D.'s operating room staff, and other paramedicals should all understand what the role of the physician assistant is in the community. These medical associates should be made aware of the physician assistant's training
background, education, abilities and limitations to avoid conflict with "the
unknown." Hospital and office practice privileges should be outlined in depth
and written out in order to avoid confusion. State regulations and local requirements must be met and satisfied. An appropriate continuing education
program should be set up to insure ultimate standards of medical care. Certification should be encouraged and is required in some states. Medical malpractice standards should be established and an accepted contract set up with the
insurance carrier.

What are some of the duties that the orthopedic surgeon can delegate to his
orthopedic physician assistant in the office and hospital practice? Obviously,
these will vary according to the specific physician assistant's training, knowledge, skill level, and nature of the physician's practice. In the hospital, duties

such as rounds, minor debridements, suturing of lacerations, and assisting in surgery can be delegated. The orthopedic physician assistant can assist the nursing and allied health personnel with patient care problems such as setting up and adjusting of traction, dressing changes, and wound elevation. Additional extra time and care can be provided to the patient's advantage, and an improvement in the quality of patient care is provided.

Preoperative information and reinforcement of postoperative instructions to the patient can be provided by the orthopedic physician assistant. Other modalities of patient care instruction such as therapeutic exercises, demonstrations and instructions in gait training and the use of ambulatory aids can be given. The physician assistant may serve as a valuable surgical assistant. His services regularly will provide the operating room orthopedist with an efficient, reliable assistant who can provide services at a lesser cost to the patient. Depending upon his individual skills, cast application at surgery, wound closures, and dressing applications can all be performed by the orthopedic physician assistant. Valuable time can be saved in the preoperative preparation of the patient with setting up a fracture table, diagnostic equipment and in assisting the scrub nurse to select and organize needed surgical instruments.

In the office, the orthopedic physician assistant can save valuable time for the orthopedist by screening phone calls and providing medical and general information to patients in need. Dressing and cast changes can be performed as well as minor surgery such as debridement of wounds and pin removal. Postoperative follow-up care can be greatly facilitated by his or her assistance. The orthopedic physician assistant can also provide assistance with medicine refills and helping with special diagnostic x-ray studies such as stress views and arthograms. Routine problems and follow-up appointments can usually be scheduled with the physician assistant, again freeing the busy orthopedic surgeon from these more routine types of patient visits, thus allowing him to see patients with more complex problems. Preoperative preparation can also be evaluated, and the assistant can alert the M.D. if any laboratory work, preoperative x-rays or history and physical findings are not on the chart and in good order. Supplementary nursing home visits can also be provided helping the patient care services for the busy orthopedic surgeon.

In summary, the well trained, informed orthopedic physician assistant can provide valuable time-saving, efficient assistance to his orthopedic surgeon in the areas of recognition and diagnosis of ailments or complaints, pre-treatment evaluation, treatment modalities and orthopedic follow-up care. In our opinion, the advantages make utilizing an orthopedic physician assistant essential in a medical practice today.

PART THREE

PERSONAL, INSTITUTIONAL, AND NATIONAL ISSUES RELATED TO THE ROLE OF PHYSICIAN ASSISTANTS

Chapter 36

JOB SATISFACTION AND CAREER PATTERNS FOR PHYSICIAN ASSISTANTS

HENRY B. PERRY, M.D., Ph.D.

Issues of job satisfaction and career fulfillment have been of major concern since the creation in 1965 of an entirely new health profession with uncertain role responsibilities and uncertain career opportunities. Although it is still too soon to address these issues definitively, the accumulated evidence supports the concept that physician assistants remain satisfied with their work and find meaningful careers in their new health profession.

PREVIOUS STUDIES

In a 1974 national survey of the physician assistant profession, ratings of the Hoppock Job Satisfaction Scale were found to be quite high, surpassed only by ratings previously reported for physicians, dentists, and lawyers (1). In a survey in 1976-77 of 38 physician assistants, 47% were "very satisfied" with their work. The two most important single influences upon job satisfaction for physician assistants were found to be physician role support (the physician assistant's perception of the professional and personal support provided by the supervising physician) and level of responsibility for patient care (greater responsibility was associated with greater job satisfaction) (1). Others have also observed the importance of level of patient care responsibility for job satisfaction (2, 3).

In a 1974 survey of physician assistants, 58% of the respondents considered their career opportunities to be limited or non-existent and two-thirds had considered or thought they might consider in the future entering a different field (4). Schneller (5) found that 57% of 1,126 physician assistants graduating in 1977 expressed doubts about the physician assistant profession as a career. Such concerns were understandable considering that an upper limit on responsibility for patient care was always envisioned since the supervising physician would hold responsibility for the actions of his assistant. Furthermore, the viability of the entire physician assistant movement was still not certain in spite of considerable early enthusiasm for the concept.

An analysis of documented attrition from the physician assistant profession has provided some useful information on the dynamics of professional satisfaction and career patterns. In the 1978 survey of the physician assistant profession, 13% indicated that they were no longer working as physician assistants (6). We estimate that for the physician assistant profession as a whole, 15–20% of graduates are no longer working as physician assistants. Attrition was considerably higher for women (22%) than for men (9%). Furthermore, attrition for women increased by 3–4% per year following graduation. For men, however, attrition was 7% one year following graduation and showed notable increase thereafter. Only a small number of physician assistants were known to have attended medical school, representing 8% of those not working as physician assistants (6). In a cohort analysis of 727 physician assistants between 1974 and 1978, attrition was significantly greater for physician assistants who graduated at a younger age or who had a higher high school class standing. These individuals presumably left the physician assistant profession to pursue additional education (6).

TABLE 36.1

RATINGS OF OVERALL JOB SATISFACTION BY PHYSICIAN ASSISTANTS, 1981

Overall Job Satisfaction Rating	*Percentage* *(n = 4801)*
5 (Excellent)	21.1
4	47.2
3	24.5
2	5.7
1 (Poor)	1.5
	100.0

TABLE 36.2

MEAN JOB SATISFACTION RATING OF PHYSICIAN ASSISTANTS
In 1981 BY YEAR OF GRADUATION

Year of Graduation	*Mean Job Satisfaction* *Rating in 1981*
1979–1980	4.1
1977–1978	3.7
1975–1976	3.7
1973–1974	3.8
1971–1972	4.0
1970 and before	4.0

RECENT EVIDENCE

The 1981 Association of Physician Assistant Program's national survey of the physician assistant profession provided some recent information concerning the job satisfaction. Two-thirds of the respondents (68%) gave a job satisfaction rating of 4 or 5 (5 = excellent) on a scale of 1–5 (see Table 36.1). It is noteworthy that the mean job satisfaction scale some did not change significantly with year of graduation. Earlier graduates had job satisfaction scores as high as recent graduates (see Table 36.2). Job satisfaction scores were significantly different among physician assistants depending upon their health occupation prior to entering physician assistant training. Those who had been nurses, medical corpsmen, or technicians had higher satisfaction scores than those who had worked in another health occupation or who had had no prior health experience (see Table 36.3). The rationale for these findings may well be that those who had not worked previously in a health occupation may not appreciate to the same extent as those with prior experience the relatively high status of the physician assistant.

Physician assistants working primarily in office settings demonstrate highest levels of job satisfaction (see Table 36.4). As a group, physician assistants working in the following group of practice settings classified as "other" in Table 36.4 demonstrated the lowest levels of job satisfaction:

Community Based Public Clinic
Drug and Alcohol Abuse Clinic
Industrial Clinic
Nursing Home, Extended Care Facility
Military Hospital or Dispensary
Federal Prison
City/County/State Prison
Health Maintenance Organization

TABLE 36.3
JOB SATISFACTION OF PHYSICIAN ASSISTANTS
IN 1981 BY PRIOR HEALTH EXPERIENCE

Prior Health Experience	*Job Satisfaction Score*
Medical Corpsman (n = 1715)	3.85
Registered Nurse or LPN (n = 582)	3.88
Technician/Technologist (n = 1206)	3.81
Other Health Field (n = 672)	3.74
No Prior Health Experience (n = 626)	3.68

$F(4,4796) = 5.83$
$P < .0001$

"Office settings" are characterized primarily by private practices, either solo or group. The findings of Table 36.4 are probably best explained by the difficulty of managing patients encountered in the "other" practice settings listed above together with the relatively lower salaries provided by many of these institutions (See Table 3.6 in Chapter 3). Outpatient care in private practice settings provide physician assistants with opportunities for considerable autonomy (as opposed to inpatient hospital care) without the disadvantages cited for the "other" practice settings.

TABLE 36.4

JOB SATISFACTION OF PHYSICIAN ASSISTANTS
IN 1981 BY PRACTICE SETTING

Practice Setting	Job Satisfaction Score
Office (n = 1751)	3.92
Hospital (n = 1641	3.77
Other (n = 1409)	3.70

$$F(2,47981) = 27.18$$
$$P < .00001$$

TABLE 36.5

SATISFACTION OF PHYSICIAN ASSISTANTS WITH
SPECIFIC JOB CHARACTERISTICS

Job Characteristic	Percentage of Physician Assistants Rating Job Characteristic Good or Excellent (N = 4,822)
Location	69.1
Income	48.9
Benefits	59.1
Hours	68.9
Relationship with Supervising physician	81.4
Recognition for work well done	59.9
Level of responsibility	79.5
Acceptance by physicians	81.5
Acceptance by nurses	78.7
Acceptance by patients	95.7
Opportunity for role expansion	45.3
Opportunity for continuing education	60.7
Opportunity for career advancement	31.3

Satisfaction with specific job characteristics was also assessed in the 1981 National survey of physician assistants. These results, shown in Table 36.5, were obtained by calculating the percentage of respondents who rated satisfaction with the particular job characteristic a rating of 4 or 5 on a scale from

(1) poor to 5 (excellent). The job characteristic with which physician assistants indicated the highest level of satisfaction is patient acceptance. Level of responsibility and acceptance by nurses and physicians received high satisfaction scores from physician assistants as well. Those characteristics receiving notably low satisfaction scores merit special attention. These include income, opportunity for role expansion, and, most significantly, opportunity for career advancement. These items will merit increasing attention in the future if long-term job and career satisfaction of physician assistants are to be maintained.

Data on long-term career trends for physician assistants are still not conclusive. An estimated overall attrition rate of 15–20% does not speak badly for the profession in spite of a perceived lack of career advancement opportunities. Because of the greater attrition observed for women, presumably because of family responsibilities, it can be anticipated that attrition rates for the profession will increase as the percentage of women continues to increase.

CONCLUSIONS

Physician assistants find their work on the whole meaningful and rewarding. The intrinsic satisfactions associated with performing an important role in the medical management of patients are no doubt largely responsible for these findings (7).

Now that the physician assistant movement has become widely accepted and appreciated, the viability of a career as a physician assistant is no longer a major concern (8). Nevertheless, dissatisfaction exists among physician assistants with income, opportunities for role expansion, and opportunities for career advancement. Income levels for physician assistants appear to peak and then plateau at $25,000 within four to five years following graduation (see Chapter 3). Whether professional responsibilities continue to grow as physician assistants advance in their careers can only be answered by ongoing studies in the future. Long term career retention rates can be optimized only by careful attention directed to the dissatisfactions of physician assistants in a serious and substantive manner.

REFERENCES

1. Perry, H.B.: The Job Satisfaction of Physician Assistants: A Casual Analysis. *Social Science and Medicine, 12:*377–385, 1978.
2. Bottom, W.D.: Analysis of Employment Turnover and Job Satisfaction of Physician Assistants Graduated from the Physician's Assistant Program of the University of Alabama in Birmingham, 1972–1975. A thesis for the degree of Master of Public Health, University of Alabama. Birmingham, Alabama, 1976.
3. Engel, G.V.: Social Factors Affecting Work Satisfaction of the Physician Assistant: A Preliminary Report. *The Sociological Review Monograph, 20:*245–261, 1973.

4. Perry, H.B.: Physician Assistants: An Overview of an Emerging Health Profession. *Medical Care, 15:*982–990, 1977.
5. Schneller, E.S. *The Physician's Assistant: Innovation in the Medical Division of Labor.* Lexington, Mass.: Heath, 1978.
6. Perry, H.B.: Career Trends Among Physician Assistants: *Physician Assistant* (in press).
7. Perry, H.B., and B. Breitner: The Vocational Fulfillment and Career Development of Physician Assistants. In *Physician Assistants: Their Contribution to Health Care.* New York, Human Sciences Press, 1981, pp. 158–173.
8. Engel, G.V.: An Evaluation of the Continued Viability of the Occupation of the Physician's Assistant. *Journal of Medical Education, 56:*659–662, 1981.

Chapter 37

INTRODUCING THE PRIMARY CARE
PHYSICIAN ASSISTANT
INTO THE OFFICE SETTING

DAVID A. SYMOND, M.D.
MARY G. WISEMAN, MEDEX

From the vantage point of having a physician assistant incorporated into our practice for the past ten years, I am comfortable in co-authoring this chapter with my present physician assistant. Our experience includes both our first physician assistant, whose initial exploration in medicine came as a Viet Nam corpsman, as well as his eventual successor who was a strong member of our office-based health care team prior to her training. Both of these practitioners were trained at the Utah Medex Program and, indeed, we have had a long association with that program, working intermittently as staff contributors and with students in the program.

A physician assistant was initially sought simply to spread the workload. I needed to gain some time away from my practice, even though I thoroughly enjoyed the challenge and variety of my work. Subsequently, it became apparent that acquiring a physician assistant had been valuable in many other ways.

Quality of patient care had improved. In the hospital, chart work was more current and of better quality because of better attention to details. Throughout the practice there was a perceptible upgrading of practitioner sensitivity and awareness of patient problems and needs. Consequently, more needs and problems were being met and solved. Over the course of even our first year's experience, certain whole new services and procedures had been instituted. At times, the physician assistant's initiative accomplished this. At other times, I was able to delegate to the Medex time and energy toward accomplishment of a special project. Examples include the development of a unit for hyperbilirubinemia of the newborn, and working out procedures and putting into practice a graded exercise testing program for patients with coronary artery disease. While it had not been a goal to increase the quantity of patient care, we found that as additional services were offered and an additional practitioner's skills were available, more patients were being reached and more needs were being met. Because of some increased flexibility with the additional practitioner-time available, the unscheduled crying five year old with a scalp laceration no longer threw our appointment schedule hopelessly behind. We were more consistently on time. We worked with less pressure and enjoyed it more.

An additional significant advantage was provided for me in my small, rather isolated community when it became apparent that I was no longer professionally alone. It has been a great deal of help to be able to consider and talk over difficult patients, interesting cases, and new procedures with a bright and knowledgeable fellow practitioner.

In considering a rural office-based setting, the physician assistant must make some wise and careful decisions. These decisions must involve the assistant's partner or spouse also. Any site visitations, interviews, and social interactions should give ample opportunity for thorough sensing of the medical community, the social community, and the geographical area by both the budding practitioner and his spouse or partner. There must be an opportunity for awareness of a real degree of professional and personal compatability with the supervising physician-to-be. Frequently, on the heels of an extraordinarily demanding university training phase, the physician assistant and his or her family are thrust abruptly into an entirely strange environment, a change of home, a loss of old supporting friends, and possibly even significant cultural changes. The physician assistant's hours probably will be long. The energy requirements for doing the job well, for learning the pre-existing systems, and for negotiating important relationships with paramedical personnel are great. If there is a spouse, she or he must be willing and able to provide a great deal of support while at the same time making all of the adjustments necessary for a successful transplanting. The spouse may well be exploring a new job also. There are genuine hazards associated with this time in a young physician assistant's life. It is our notion that there is probably a great deal of threat to his or her pre-existing marriage. We have seen many divorces in this time. Careful preparation by both the physician assistant and his spouse, as well as by the supervising physician and the welcoming medical community will ease this stress.

If the young physician assistant is not married, the problem of spouse adjustment is certainly not present. A partner may find even more difficulty with adjustments, and an unattached physician assistant finds himself needing to cultivate an entire new support system.

From the point of view of the physician anticipating hiring his first primary-care physician assistant, I need to point out the importance of doing careful and thorough groundwork. In our small community, it was necessary that all the key people in my daily living were agreed that we would intend to make the experience of having a physician assistant work. This included my wife, as well as my office manager, the Nurse Superintendent of our hospital, our Hospital Administrator and Board of Directors, and representative samplings of my patients. For the three months prior to the arrival of our first physician assistant, information was disseminated to the general population through some introductory newspaper coverage, through handout sheets from my office, and most of all by word-of-mouth communication to many individuals in the practice and throughout the community. In meetings with the hospital Board of Directors, additional time and effort was spent explaining the concept of the physician assistant and our hope of its strengthening the health care delivery team. The nursing personnel were contacted individually. In each case we were able to agree that an additional dedicated set of head and hands could only strengthen our team effort. Within a month of the arrival of our first physician assistant, it became apparent that our anticipation of dedicated head and hands was accurate. However, neither this assistant's excellence and sincerity nor our careful groundwork produced a painless transition or an instantly effective practitioner. The smooth running efficiency of our office was frequently disrupted by the sometimes conflicting needs of the physician assistant.

Occasional crises developed at the practitioner/patient interface. Here and there "little things" reared their ugly heads. Nevertheless, the painstaking preparations, the basic needs of the practice, and the sincere dedication of the primary people involved were sufficient to straighten out the periods of confusion. By the time we were six months into the adventure, it was apparent that the long-term goals were reachable and the physician assistant concept was alive and healthy in our practice and town. The patient reaction to the presence of a physician assistant on our clinical staff has always been accepting and positive. It became apparent that the responsibility of the physician extended through the hands of the physician assistant, just as it did through the hands of the other paramedical workers such as nurses, laboratory and x-ray technicians. It also became apparent that both the physician and the physician assistant respected this responsibility and that patients became very comfortable in the hands of this new practitioner.

In fact, patient acceptance, at times, can be too favorable, making it possible for a physician assistant to act relatively independently. This must be recognized and compensated for by communication between the physician and the physician assistant, so that an overextension of authority and responsibility are not expected from the young practitioner. We had no problems of negative professional reaction in our community, although if one practiced in an area with other physicians who did not enjoy working with a Medex or physician assistant or nurse practitioner, one might expect some problems. I would think these could be anticipated to some degree and should be managed by dialogue with the other physicians.

The economics of utilization of a physician assistant should be carefully thought out. The primary goals for us were concerned with resolving the "time bind" while maintaining or improving quality of patient care. From a practical point of view, this simply must be done within the economic structure of the practice. Attempting to manage this without careful consideration of economic expectations of physician assistant and spouse,of existing staff, and of patients can lead to failure of an otherwise successful venture. Probably early specific figure commitments between doctor and physician assistant are better than "ball park" generalizations. The young physician assistant must recognize that it may be as long as two years before he actually pays his way. Long before this, however, there will be real improvements in freeing up the physician from many of his grueling time constraints. The physician assistant must be fairly compensated.

As stated above, his first two years will be a time of significant stress. He must be willing to put in long hours and his physician must be willing to pay him adequately so that serious economic stress is not added to his problems. Additionally, there should be a formula worked out that finds the young practitioner anticipating opportunity for further improvement of his economic circumstances. In our practice, it worked well to establish a guaranteed monthly salary with projected increases. Upon achieving a good level of productivity, it then became apparent to modify the wage scale so that the physician assistant had a monthly guarantee *or* an understood percentage of his gross, whichever was the greater. This resulted in a reasonable incentive for productivity as well as an automatic appreciation for additional services rendered. Our physician assistant also appreciated the opportunity to have a guaranteed income, to allow taking time off when possible for recreation, personal activities, or professional education.

Probably the main message here is to not avoid early specific commitments. There is too much need for working out problems in the complicated business of health care delivery without having an economic basis for discontent. From the physician assistant's point of view, rural office-based family practice probably is one of the most exciting of professional occupations. In our practice, our physician assistant sees every type of patient. Her services consist of complete physical examinations, sharing the making of hospital rounds, and providing the necessary services for any and all patients seen in the acute afternoon clinics. We have found it extremely workable to alternate obstetrical visits and well-baby examinations.

Two pairs of eyes see more than one. Two brains pick up more than one. Our physician assistant assists at major surgery and at deliveries. Her experience is such that she has managed precipitous deliveries competently when the unforeseen need has arisen. She is skilled in minor surgery, laceration repairs, and excisional biopsies. She shares night and week-end call, though of course she is always backed by a physician. We have learned what all practitioners should learn—that some patients are more comfortable with Practitioner A, while others prefer Practitioner B. We have even learned that some patients prefer to discuss certain problems with a male practitioner, others with a female practitioner. We have learned that sometimes a younger practitioner seems more appropriate, other times the older practitioner is the one sought. All of this has been to the advantage of our practice. Our patients know that they have complete choice as to who they see. They know that we share our records, the basic information about their ongoing health care, and they appreciate this kind of practice. Psychosocial problems, particularly, are helped by this flexibility of practitioners and by having the option of either a male or a female practitioner.

It is obviously necessary that there be a very high level of understanding between the doctor and his physician assistant. It must be clear that there is no competition on this team. There must be an absolute level of confidence that the doctor is consulted when the physician assistant knows he needs help. Likewise, the physician assistant must know that his physician will answer his call every time it is made.

I have reported the impact of the acquiring of a physician assistant on our office-based rural family practice. It is appropriate to report the very real personal benefits that have also developed. As the physician assistant has matured toward being a more and more complete practitioner, nearly forgotten experiences reappeared in my life. With my physician assistant backed by a fellow physician, time for vacation became available and visits to distant family members not seen for years took place. In each case, on returning, I found the practice was in order, the needs had been met, and the fellow physician covering my practice had not been run off his feet. Alternating night call and weekends brings many hours of time with my family, enjoyable hours working in my yard, and short excursions into the nearby mountains. Both my physician assistant and I were able to select continuing educational opportunities and to attend them occasionally without concern for the job at home. The usual practice day remained fairly long, but those grueling sessions of stacking emergency surgery and obstetrics into an already full scheduled week were spread and divided, so that fatigue was more an intermittent friend than a constant companion. In some ways, most rewarding of all, has been the opportunity to work with a bright, inquiring physician assistant both as a preceptor and as a fellow practitioner. As most physicians know, teaching does much to keep the pathways of learning open. In this rural family practice, it is my intention to never practice without the help and support of a physician assistant.

Chapter 38

INTERPERSONAL CONSIDERATIONS IN THE INTRODUCTION OF THE SURGICAL PHYSICIAN ASSISTANT INTO THE PRACTICE SETTING

GORDON T. SCHAEDEL, PA-C
MALCOLM S. BEINFIELD, M.D.

Since the inception and continuation of postgraduate training in surgery for physician assistants, both men and women have entered the hospital, institution or private practice settings with varying degrees of success. For the individual who decides to practice in the medical community where he or she was trained and is already accepted as a member of the health care team, the transition from resident to practitioner should not present a problem. The resident who is interested in practicing in the setting where he was trained should be fully appraised of job responsibilities, compensation, and benefits prior to considering a position. Once a contract has been presented and deemed acceptable, the transition from resident to staff member should follow quite nicely.

The process of going from resident to staff member may appear over-simplified if one does not mention the planning and education of all hospital disciplines required in the foundation of any hospital or university based training program. One must remember that great attention was given to provide educational content and scope of practice to the individuals and groups with which the surgical physician assistant would interface. For example, the departments of nursing and pharmacy would be aware that the surgical physician assistant may write orders as long as they are countersigned by an attending physician in the prescribed period of time. Also, the medical staff were made aware that various tasks such as venous cutdowns, first assisting in the operating suite or gastro-intestinal intubation could be performed by the surgical physician assistant.

For the individual who chooses to practice in a private setting or in a hospital setting where no surgical physician assistant has preceded, acceptance can be anticipated if the same careful planning which is the foundation of a successful training program is employed.

This places the major portion of education on the shoulders of the physician assistant. If the surgical physician assistant finds himself moving from one state to another, it is essential that he become familiar with the laws which will be governing his practice. He should not rely on hearsay, but obtain a copy of the legislation pertaining to the practice of physician assistants in the state where he intends to work. If any portion of the law pertaining to practice is unclear, seek clarification through the local medical association or governmental agency, or state Physician Assistant Association.

After all, the necessary prerequisite material has been received and accepted by a prospective employer, it is time for the parties involved to explore the requirements and goals of the position being considered. Cognizance of the state law governing physician assistant practice will enable the physician assistant and physician to define these goals realistically. The capabilities and limitations of the physician assistant should be defined. In this definition, allowance should be made for the expansion of the role as productivity and experience permit. This definition, along with the educational background, will form the foundation for the introduction of the physician assistant to the various departments of the hospital and the private medical community. Now the physician can intelligently address the task of establishing the physician assistant's role with his colleagues and all other hospital personnel. It is imperative that all interested parties are included. Specifically, a detailed job description should be formulated and distributed to the hospital's medical board, all specialty department heads, nursing service, admissions, pharmacy and personnel. The job description should detail the physician assistant's administrative, technical, and legal responsibilities. Incorporated in this document should be a provision for the expansion of the role of the physician assistant as his continuing education and clinical experience will dictate.

If preparation for introducing a physician assistant is carried out in this fashion before the first patient is seen, the hospital community should not be wary of this new health care practitioner. For example, let us consider a physician assistant working on a cardiothoracic service with three surgeons. It is important to be aware of each surgeon's preferences in patient management. This information can be obtained from the individual surgeons and their supporting staffs. In the field of cardiothoracic surgery it is quite common for a patient's care to be shared by the surgery department and the department of cardiology. In this setting it is extremely important to understand the roles of each discipline in patient management. Discussion with the members of the cardiology department with whom the physician assistant will be working is a very straightforward and efficient way of understanding their responsibility in the management of the cardiothoracic patient.

Also of prime importance is the relationship that should be developed between the physician assistant and nursing staff. Much of the physician assistant's time will be spent in the company of nurses from the operating room to the recovery room and finally to the ward. Each party must learn to rely on each other for the satisfactory administration of patient care. Upon initial exposure there will be, understandably, the need for clarification of the role each is to play. This will be done courteously by asking and answering questions. It is important to reserve judgement of any given nursing policy until there is a full understanding of all factors governing that policy. If the necessity arises to suggest a change in a given policy, it is best to consult with the individual most closely associated with its function. A wise physician assistant will also be receptive to alterations in a patient care procedure suggested by the nursing staff. This trio of common courtesy, thoughtful suggestion for change, and a receptive ear will do much to produce harmony between the physician assistant and the nursing community.

If the practice the physician assistant is going to enter includes hospital based resident physicians, physician assistants, or nursing practitioners in training, a recall of his own training period will be paramount in a successful interaction with those involved. The new staff member should look back to his student days, remembering circumstances which led to a less than optimal learning experience and strive to alleviate those practices. Also important to remember is that the polishing of skills is obtained through years of clinical experience and a like opportunity should be afforded the resident. For example, if a mode of therapy has been altered, be sure to communicate this to the house staff with an explanation for this change. Continued communication of this nature will produce an atmosphere conducive to optimal patient care and will perpetuate intellectual growth for all parties concerned. The physician assistant should be receptive to questions arising from any of the personnel being trained at his institution. It is a good practice to include the newcomer in any situation which might promote and enhance his learning experience. If one discovers any unusual physical finding, share it with the house staff and the student population.

Perhaps the single most important relationship is that found between the physician assistant and the surgeon with whom he practices. This is a situation where each involved party must learn to trust and rely on the other's actions. From the onset, an atmosphere of honesty and open communication must be nurtured. It is not uncommon when two professionals are working together that there will be times when they are in disagreement. In resolving these differences of opinion, one should never bring personalities into play. Facts will settle differences, name calling will not. Unhindered communication, along with time, will establish the desired working relationship required in the demanding practice of surgery.

The measurement of success of the physician assistant practicing in surgery is the consistent delivery of the best possible patient care. Upon setting out to achieve this objective, the physician assistant must be well educated in every facet which pertains to his profession. He must be prepared to educate those members of the health care team who are unfamiliar with his function in the delivery of health care. This educational process should be fostered jointly by the physician assistant and the attending surgeon.

It is common belief that a student is only as good as his teacher. To be a good teacher, one must be thoroughly familiar with the subject matter, receptive to questions and courteous enough to listen when others air their views. The physician assistant must be a good teacher, for it is through his teaching that he will be able to establish his position within the medical community. Once this has been achieved, he will be able to pursue his profession in a satisfactory and rewarding manner.

Chapter 39

GUIDELINES FOR THE EMPLOYMENT OF THE PRIMARY CARE PHYSICIAN ASSISTANT BY THE PRIVATELY PRACTICING PHYSICIAN

FREDERICK A. BLOUNT, M.D.
W. WARD PATRICK, M.D., M.S.P.H.
JOSEPH G. DADDOBBO, PA-C
VIRGINIA K. MACFARLANE, ED.M., PA-C
JOHN S. MUELLER, M.D.
JIMMIE L. PHARRIS, Ph.D.

MAKING THE DECISION TO HIRE A PHYSICIAN ASSISTANT

A physician must consider the matter very carefully before deciding to hire a physician assistant because it will certainly have great impact on his practice. Some of the potential advantages of physician assistant utilization include:
1) Improved quality of medical practice (1 & 2).
2) Expanded services such as home visits or patient education.
3) Increased income for the practice.
4) Increased control over scheduling of activities.
5) Greater time for the physician to see complicated patients and less time required for the physician to see routine medical problems.
6) Sharpened clinical skills resulting from supervision and teaching.

There may be disadvantages also. The physician assistant may disturb the traditional relationships between the physician and his patients or the physician and the nursing staff. Although some physicians may be reluctant to have physician assistants treat their patients, studies show that the patients are satisfied (3 & 4).

Nurses and other office staff members may react very emotionally to a physician assistant and he must be skilled at working harmoniously with them. The physician must make a clear statement regarding the role of the physician assistant. This can help to reduce the possibility of dissension. Frequent staff meetings will also increase harmony in the group.

The physician who hires an assistant is breaking with tradition. There is, nevertheless, substantial data to indicate that the action will be successful. Furthermore, since research indicates that 80% or more of routine office care can be delegated safely, it is likely that more physicians will hire assistants.

WRITING A JOB DESCRIPTION

The job description should define precisely the physician assistant's responsibilities. The physician must be familiar with his state laws regarding delegation of medical acts. New Jersey is the only state that forbids the use of physician assistants in medical practice. A list of practice tasks can be expanded into protocols for managing specific clinical problems. Such protocols for the management of common medical problems are now available (5-9). The supervising physician should make all the modifications necessary to fit his practice.

The job description should include professional relationships with back-up physicians, nurses and other staff members. The physician assistant's role can be helped by direct discussions with those who will be working with him. The physician assistant should be introduced to the medical staff and administration of the hospital.

Most physicians require that their assistants be certified by the National Board of Medical Examiners. The National Certifying Examination for Physician Assistants to the Primary Care Physician has been administered since 1973 and many states require national certification to practice.

All aspects of employment should be agreed to: working hours, night call, vacation, opportunities for continuing medical education, insurance coverage, as well as salary. An office manager may be very helpful with a job description, and he can offer valuable advice on specifics.

LOCATING CANDIDATES

A physician may elect to advertise in national publications directed toward physician assistants. *The New Health Practitioner/Physician Assistant,* and the *Newsletter* of the American Academy of Physician Assistants are received by a large number of physician assistants. Most states have professional associations which can help find experienced candidates.

Many physicians find that precepting students during their clinical training is a good way to learn of their skills. By reviewing the *National Health Practitioner Program Profile,* an annual publication of the Association of Physician Assistant Programs, one can become familiar with students in clinical training. Teaching will afford an opportunity to assess the skills of physician assistants and may help in a decision regarding to employment. A nearby physician assistant program will often provide students.

INTERVIEWING CANDIDATES

A candidate's educational experience is an important step in evaluating his abilities. Although training programs vary somewhat, they all include didactic and clinical instruction. Discuss with an applicant how his experience can help a practice. Review the *Profile* to gain information on the curriculum of each AMA approved training program.

Analyze the candidate's professional experience if he or she has been previously employed. Explore professional references — by telephone, if possible. Training program transcripts will provide valuable information about the candidate. A productive addition to an interview is a discussion of various clinical problems and their management.

WORKING OUT THE CONTRACT

The final step in employing a physician assistant is drafting a contract. Precise terms of employment avoids any misunderstanding. The following details should be included.

1) *Professional duties*
   a. Obtaining medical histories and performing physician examinations.
   b. Diagnosing and planning treatment.
   c. Ordering and interpreting ancillary studies.
   d. Providing appropriate emergency treatment.
   e. Performing with proper supervision such procedures as venipuncture, cast application and removal, urinary bladder catheterization, cardiopulmonary resuscitation, nasogastric intubation, suturing, ocular tonometry, urinalysis, complete blood count, and other laboratory tests.
   f. Providing patient education and follow-up care.
   h. Developing criteria for patient referral and a constructive relationship with these specialists.
2) *Compensation.* Salary for a 40-hour week should be explicit with provisions made for additional work.
3) *Fringe Benefits.* The employer must make explicit the insurance programs he will provide for his assistant.
4) *Vacation.* The amount should be made clear.
5) *Continuing Medical Education.* Most physicians allow five to ten days with pay each year.

6) *On-call.* Night and weekend responsibility with the details of supervision for the physician assistant should be agreed on. An alternate supervisor will usually allow the physician assistant to continue to practice when his physician is not available.

7) *Profit Sharing.* This may provide a valuable incentive for the assistant.

A lawyer can help avoid many problems with a contract. A probationary period of 3-6 months before signing the contract may be very prudent. A systematic approach such as the one described here should help to create the best opportunity for a constructive and mutually beneficial relationship between the physician assistant and his or her employer.

REFERENCES

1. Goldberg GA: Quality of care provided by physician's extenders in Air Force primary medicine clinics. A project Air Force report prepared for the United States Air Force. California Rand Corporation, 1981.
2. Sox AC: Quality of patients care by nurse practitioners and physician assistants: a ten-year perspective. *Ann Intern Med, 91:* 459, 1979.
3. Smith CW Jr.: Patient attitudes toward physician's assistants, *JFP, 13:*201-204, 1981.
4. Perry HB. An analysis of the professional performance of physician assistants. *J Med Educ., 52:*639-647, 1977.
5. Greenfield S, Komaroff AL, and Anderson H.: A headache protocol for nurses, effectiveness and efficiency. *Arch Intern Med, 136:*1111-1116, 1976.
6. Greenfield S, Lewis CE, and Kaplan SH: Davidson MB. Peer review by criteria mapping: criteria for diabetes mellitus. The use of decision-making in chart audit. *Ann Intern Med, 83:*761-770, 1975.
7. Greenfield S, Nadler MA, Morgan MT, and Shine KI: The clinical investigation and management of chest pain in an emergency department; quality assessment by criteria mapping. *Med Care, XV:*898-905, 1977.
8. Greenfield S, Friedland G, Scifers S, Rhodes A, Black WL, and Komaroff AL: Protocol management of dysuria, urinary frequency, and vaginal discharge. *Ann Inter Med, 81:*452-457, 1974.
9. Hoole A, Greenberg R, and Pickard G: *Patient Care Guidelines for Family Nurse Practitioners.* Boston, Little, Brown and Company, 1976.

Chapter 40

ISSUES IN OBTAINING HOSPITAL PRIVILEGES FOR THE PRIMARY CARE PHYSICIAN ASSISTANT

JIMMIE L. PHARRIS, Ph.D.
FREDERICK A. BLOUNT, M.D.
JOSEPH G. DADDABBO, PA-C
JOHN C. MUELLER, M.D.
WARD W. PATRICK, M.D., M.S.P.H.

INTRODUCTION

Since hospital privileges are not inherent rights, the condition by which they are conferred is defined by hospital bylaws. These bylaws express the attitude of the majority of the physicians operating under their jurisdiction.

As in similar situations of self-government, some physicians may develop a proprietary interest in the bylaws and require a detailed justification for any changes. Physicians who have granted only to themselves professional privileges may be reluctant to assign any of these to an assistant.

If an employing physician wishes certain hospital privileges for his assistant, he must plan carefully to obtain them. He should first seek from the hospital staff recognition and respect of the physician assistant profession. Then he will seek any necessary amendment to hospital bylaws for this new member of the patient care team (1).

In this chapter are presented several concerns which a physician may need to allay in securing hospital privileges for his assistant. Research of the subject suggests a successful strategy.

OPTIONS

A physician planning to employ a physician assistant has several options regarding the physician assistant's role:

1. He can confine the physician assistant's activities to the office practice. Many important auxiliary tasks can be performed by the assistant in the office while the physician provides hospital services.

2. He can utilize the physician assistant in the care of hospitalized patients. If hospital practice is to be included in the physician assistant's job description, the employing physician must gain the necessary privileges for his assistant. This can become a significant problem when the employing physician uses a hospital which never before has granted privileges to physician assistants. The physician must decide whether the assistant will be introduced into the hospital before or after hospital privileges have been granted. This will be discussed further in the next section.

PAVING THE WAY

A successful plan eliminates many serious problems before they arise and will minimize built-in problems. It is wise to defer all efforts until the best possible plan has been created.

Because hospital privileges for a physician assistant depend on the favorable reaction of hospital administrators, staff physicians, and hospital nurses, these professionals must be informed about the experience of similar groups in hospitals which have granted privileges to physician assistants. The information is most effective when it is credible and personal. Research studies that report favorable personal experiences and conclusions are especially helpful. Encourage the program chairmen of medical and nursing hospital staffs to schedule presentations on physician assistants. State and local associations of physician assistants, physician assistants who practice in nearby hospitals, and representatives of physician assistant programs should be enlisted. Studies on various aspects of the physician assistant profession can be usefully circulated to key personnel. A common error is to over-estimate the number who will read such material and change their attitudes. Personal contacts and informal discussion remain essential!

To mold favorable attitudes toward physician assistants, the employing physician may introduce new members of his team to key personnel before making formal application for hospital privileges. This works particularly well in small community hospitals. Have the assistant accompany the employing physician on hospital rounds. During these visits, the physician shows that the assistant only helps him with his tasks, performing no independent practice acts. The opportunity for others to see the assistant in action under close supervision enhances understanding especially later when formal application is made for hospital privileges.

Gradually, through informal discussions, the physician can identify specific concerns of different professional groups in the hospital setting. Crucial issues for each of these groups are usually the following:

(1) Hospital administrators: legal parameters and insurance

(2) Medical staff: professional prerogative and clinical supervision

(3) Nursing staff: written orders and professional territoriality

(4) Ancillary services staff: services expected by the physician assistant

These concerns are real, appropriate, and must be dealt with.

The physician should be familiar with applicable state laws, local customs of delegation and supervision, and the requirements from nurses to respond to orders written by physician assistants (2). He must have a clear understanding with his assistant about the scope of his authority.

Other issues include: (a) patient acceptance of physician assistants, (b) the quality of service provided by physician assistants, (c) the irrelevant or hypothetical issues often raised by all who are resistant to change, (d) the capability of the physician assistant to see patients of other physicians because he is available in the hospital, and (e) supervision of the physician assistant when his employer is not always available.

Then, too, the physician assistant gradually may gain a status with certain hospital personnel as an authoritative medical figure. In small hospitals, the physician assistant may on some occasions be the only medical provider in the hospital. Can the physician assistant be asked by the nursing staff to make medical decisions in an emergency? In true emergencies, no legal problems should arise. However, professional issues may arise particularly if such an emergency involves a patient of a physician who does not support the use of physician assistants. However, if such an event proves not to have been an emergency, legal issues regarding supervision and responsibility may arise.

PLANNING THE ROLE OF THE
PHYSICIAN ASSISTANT IN THE HOSPITAL

During the period of educating hospital personnel before asking for an amendment to the hospital bylaws, a plan should be developed describing the projected role of the physician assistant in the hospital. The plan must be gradual in its increasing responsibility, and also be very specific. All parties must consider this plan to be a nonthreatening, legal statement whose aim it is to develop a symbiotic relationship that promotes professionalism at all levels and above all—better patient care.

If the physician assistant is a pioneer for his profession in the hospital, the employing physician must not only relate the planned role for the assistant to each of the issues, but also display to any challenger the knowledge of the planned role that will allay the concerns associated with each issue. This is not an easy task, to be sure, but it represents a significant and satisfying step forward for the entire patient care team.

AMENDING THE HOSPITAL'S BYLAWS

Amending hospital bylaws to obtain privileges for physician assistants should be done systematically as discussed in this chapter. The proposed by-laws should serve several specific functions:

(1) To identify the clinicians who are included under the provision of the regulations
(2) To identify the rules authorizing such practice
(3) To identify those who can be responsible for supervision of the physician assistant
(4) To define the legal relationship between the physician assistant, the supervising physicians, and the hospital
(5) To outline the scope of the clinical role of the physician assistant in a way that permits appropriate flexibility.

A sample set of articles is shown below. These are the additions made to the bylaws of a small community general hospital in North Carolina (3), to authorize and regulate the practice of physician assistants:

"*Section 8. Associate Medical Staff—Specified Professional Personnel (Non-Physician Professional)*

"Specified professional personnel (non-physician professional) shall include such categories as physician's assistants, nurse practitioners, and advanced technologists. Non-physician professionals shall not be eligible to vote or to hold office in the Medical Staff organization.

"The specified professional personnel in regard to his performance and responsibilities, shall be assigned to a specific physician or to a service chief. The non-physician professional shall undergo the same appointment and re-appointment process as relating to physicians, dentists, and podiatrists. Administrative consultation is provided for by his ex-officio membership on the Executive Committee of the Medical Staff. In addition, the clinical duties and responsibilities shall be outlined as set forth within the current Rules and Regulations. There shall be kept on permanent file a current resume of the non-physician professional's training, experience, and demonstrated current competence. This shall be placed in such a way to permit their performing the following:

A. The exercising of judgment within their areas of competence, providing that a physician member of the Medical Staff shall have the ultimate responsibility for patient care.
B. For participating directly in the management of patients under the supervision and direction of a member of the Medical Staff.
C. Within the limits established by the Medical Staff and consistent with State Practice Acts, the writing of orders as well as the recording of reports and progress notes in patients' medical record.

D. Specified professional personnel (non-physician professionals) shall be
    individually assigned to an appropriate clinical service and shall carry
    out their activities subject to service policies and procedures in con-
    formance with the applicable provisions of the Medical Staff Bylaws,
    Rules, and Regulations. Cognizance shall be taken where state or
    federal regulations apply."

REFERENCES

1. Green, James Y., Hal T. Wilson: *Acceptance of Physician Extenders by Hospital Medical
   Personnel,* (unpublished, 1975).
2. *Guidelines on the Physician's Assistant in the Hospital.* Approved by the American Hospital
   Association, February, 1975.
3. *Bylaws of the Medical Staff of Valdese General Hospital.* Valdese, North Carolina.

Chapter 41

ISSUES IN THE EMPLOYMENT OF PHYSICIAN ASSISTANTS AS HOUSESTAFF

CLARA E. VANDERBILT, PA-C
RICHARD G. ROSEN, M.D.

Physician interns and residents were not always with us. They are a relatively new development, and residency training programs have become widespread only since World War II. The growth of this method of medical training and medical care has paralleled the growth of specialization and the need for a team approach in managing complex medical problems. An appreciation of the value of housestaff to the patient and to the hospital is now widespread. More recently, a demand has arisen for housestaff at smaller community hospitals which have traditionally never had house officers.

Historically, housestaff have been hired on the basis of a hospital's own need for help in patient care. Hospitals were not compelled to concern themselves with the manpower needs of the larger community, region or nation. Interns and residents were so inexpensive that the cost factor was negligible. No other alternative was available. Much of this has changed over the past decade. Housestaff salaries have increased considerably. Accrediting boards for residency programs have begun taking into consideration the community's need for specialists. Governmental regulations have limited the admission of foreign medical graduates into residency programs in this country.

The advent of the physician assistant offered a viable alternative to the traditional physician resident. We at the Montefiore Hospital and Medical Center felt that our institution would be a good place to test this concept. Montefiore is a large teaching hospital in an urban setting serving to a largely middle class population. We had developed a highly regarded residency training National Intern and Residency Matching Plan some 20 years earlier, and we had a reputation for innovation in the health care delivery system. With this in mind, in 1971 we started hiring physician assistants not in addition to, but instead of, a surgical resident. Each physician assistant was expected to do the same work, follow the same schedule, and fulfill the same responsibilities as physician housestaff at his or her level. This included admitting and working up patients, assisting at surgery, and managing under supervision a group of patients on the service to which the physician assistant was assigned.

Because so many hospitals were being forced to decrease the numbers of housestaff both in general surgery and in the surgical specialties, and because most physician assistant programs were training physician assistants predominantly in primary care, Montefiore Hospital began a formal postgraduate program to train physician assistants in surgery and the surgical specialties. Over the past five years, our graduates have taken positions as housestaff officers or with surgical specialists.

Over the eleven years since we began using physician assistants as housestaff, we have found that we have been able to maintain our high standards of patient care. We have gradually increased the number of physician assistants employed to our current level of 75, one third of which are working in surgery. Physician assistants now account for 20% of our surgical housestaff. The concepts described in this chapter are based on this experience together with our experience in a consulting capacity at other hospitals around the country where physician assistant training has been developed.

There are three main elements in the preparation of a hospital for the introduction of physician assistants: analysis, education, and supervision. Failure to devote proper time and effort to each element will likely result in failure of the program. Important, but subsidiary, concerns in the planning and implementation will also be discussed.

Analysis of the needs and expectations of the institution must precede any other preparation. The following questions should be answered honestly and completely.

1. Why, precisely, are you considering physician assistants? What role are they expected to play? Can that role be satisfied by other types of health care personnel? If so, why choose physician assistants? Who will benefit from the services of the physician assistant—the individual practitioner and his patients, the patients of the institution as a group, or the hospital as an institution?

2. From whence comes the idea to utilize physician assistants? If the impetus comes from the administration, will the medical staff accept them enthusiastically? Conversely, if the impetus comes from the medical staff, is there still a strong group who are vigorously opposed and will endeavor to be an obstruction? Will the administration give the proper support both initially and for the long haul?

3. Is the money available? Physician assistants are not cheap and salaries are not the sole expense. There are indirect costs, particularly associated with supervision, that must be calculated. If physician assistants are used to substitute for housestaff, there will be no financial savings at all, whereas if they are used to substitute for attending physicians, savings may not be as great as first perceived. Obviously, if physician assistants are to be used to improve or supplement services rather than substitute for personnel already providing a service, costs will necessarily rise.

If these questions are answered properly, preferably in an organized and written form, it should be relatively easy for the hospital counsel to determine if the applicable state laws are in conflict with the contemplated role. It may not be so easy, however, to make the next decision, a crucial one on which all further plans will hinge. Who will hire the physician assistants — the hospital or the individual practitioners? Administrative procedures, financial implications, potential benefits and shortcomings, quality control, methods of supervision, effect on the teaching program — all these and more will depend on the answer to this key question.

If the physician assistant is hired by the individual attending physician to help care for his own patients, the benefits to that practitioner and his patients are clear. The benefit to the institution, to the overall patient population, and to the hospital are limited at best. On the other hand, this requires no commitment of hard money from the hospital, no effort at recruiting, no responsibility for a hiatus in service due to illness, retirement or disability, and only minimal involvement by the remainder of the medical staff who may be resistant to the concept. It does pose a problem for the hospital in terms of insuring that this physician assistant is properly supervised, for this implies a closer look into an individual practice situation than is usually the case.

The disadvantages of having all physician assistants hired by the hospital are the converse of the advantages mentioned in the previous paragraph. It is more expensive and more administratively complicated. Most institutions, however, will find that the advantages outweigh the costs, many of which are recoverable in any case. The direct costs for physician assistants are usually fully reimbursable under Medicare Part A, Medicaid, and most Blue Cross plans, while the cost to the practitioner for services rendered by the physician assistant are not, as of yet, reimbursable under Medicare Part B or most Blue Shield plans. A few states will reimburse under Medicaid.

The advantages of the hospital being the employer are now fairly obvious. The physician assistant services can accrue to the benefit of the patient population as a whole, and they can be shifted from one area to another as needed. Uniform standards for qualifications — often exceeding the minimal state requirements — can be required more easily. It is also easier to integrate physician assistant activities into the various quality control programs that have increasingly become a more visible part of the hospital routine.

Lastly, the interaction between the physician assistants and existing house-staff (if present) must be considered when determining employment status. Unless physician assistants are employed only in a very technical role, it is difficult to maintain the proper relationship between the attending physicians (as teachers) and the physician housestaff (as students) when physician assistants are employed by the attendings. The attendings tend to relate to their physician assistants, bypassing the housestaff who then lose a potentially valuable teaching experience. In the few institutions that have tried this arrangement (usually in cardiothoracic surgery or other surgical subspecialty), the teaching program for the residents is incomplete and of less than ideal quality.

Once it has been decided that physician assistants will be introduced into the institution and what their role and status will be, an educational program must be planned. It is presumed that the initial planning and decision-making-stage received input from all significant factions in the hospital community. The representatives of these factions, however, cannot be relied upon to properly educate their constituents.

We would recommend that the Board of Trustees, representing both the overall community and the ultimate responsibility for the hospital, be contacted at an early stage. After a full discussion establishing basic principles, the necessary changes to the hospital bylaws and rules and regulations are then drafted. It is best to put the minimum amount of restrictions into the bylaws, allowing for greater flexibility. The rules and regulations can usually be modified as needed much more easily.

The medical staff are, of course, the key players. There is almost always some suspicions, anxiety, and reluctance to accept change. The physician assistant, however, is unique among health professionals. The physician assistant was designed to be a member of a team — a team of variable size and composition, but always including a physician. A physician assistant is always a dependent practitioner — dependent on powers specifically delegated to him by his supervising physician. Since the physician assistant is to act only as an extension of a physician, he needs the continuing and enthusiastic support of the physician to whom he will be reporting. Since the physician assistant, unlike some physicians who are hired by the hospital, is always an extension of the medical staff with whom he is working, the medical staff should be less suspicious of him than would otherwise be the case in an administration sponsored proposal. A series of meetings, extending over some months, is desirable so that the medical staff as a whole has a chance to give voice to their apprehensions and so that these apprehensions can be addressed.

This is also the forum to discuss the tricky question of clinical consultations.

Can a physician assistant initiate a consult to another service? Can he be the first one to repond to a consult from another service? We have answered the first question in the affirmative, on the theory that he is, in this case, merely the spokesman for his supervising physician. We have answered the second question with a tentative yes. In an emergency situation, the physician assistant might provide faster service for the patient if allowed to be the first responder. When there are multiple simultaneous demands on a physician's attention (a not uncommon situation in a busy acute hospital), the physician assistant might help the physician order his priorities better.

Historically, nursing administrators, or nurses as a group, have been the ones to show the most reluctance to accept physician assistants initially. In part, this is a result of the conservatism of organized nursing but only in part since most nurses are not members of their state or national organizations. The fears of the physician assistant concept that many nurses have are real and substantial and, if not tackled at every level, will prove to be a stumbling block to the smooth running of the program.

It should be made perfectly clear that no matter how nursing or medicine are defined, physician assistants are there to do "doctor-type work," not "nursing-type work." In our hospital, we have found two of our approaches fruitful and transplantable. First, we allow the nurses themselves to define nursing and nursing activities — those activities that they wish to keep in their domain, without encroachment from the physicians or their surrogates. Thus, physician assistants are not threatening their jobs, their independence, or their "turf." Secondly, we stress that nurses are expected, as professionals, to make independent professional judgements. For example, nurses are not only allowed, but expected to refuse to carry out any order which, in the nurse's judgement, is not in the best interest of the patient. This applies to orders written by senior attendings as well as by physician assistants.

Nurses are instructed to call any such order to the attention of their supervisors who are usually able to work out the problem satisfactorily and amicably. In practice, once physician assistants have been introduced to a hospital, the nurses who are most antagonistic are those with whom the physician assistants have the least contact. The concepts, attitudes, and mechanisms for relating to physician assistants should be presented to nurses at all levels, from senior supervisors down to staff nurses in all areas of the hospital. This may require multiple meetings at various times to accommodate all shifts.

The administrative hierarchy must also be considered. The physician assistant will be having numerous contacts with administrators or with people who report to administrators (technicians, housekeepers, dietary personnel, telephone operators, and so forth.) It should be remembered that physician assistants in their professional role must report through the professional rather than the administrative hierarchy. It is better, in fact, if all interaction between the hospital administrator and the physician assistant be channeled through the professional hierarchy. This is not easy for some administrators to accept, but it will do as much as anything to make the program work.

The question of the nature of the supervision is most important, but also one that requires the most variability depending on the local situation. Ideally, every physician assistant should have a single, formally designated supervising physician. Again, ideally, it should be a chief of whatever service to which he is assigned. The day-to-day supervision can then be delegated to a subordinate physician. Where physician assistants are integrated into a system with physician housestaff, that can be the chief or senior resident. Otherwise, some other physician, who is readily available, is designated unless the chief of service is willing and able to take on this responsibility himself.

At the very least, histories, physical examinations, progress notes, and orders of any kind should be reviewed periodically and where appropriate, countersigned. This review need not be done more often than once a day, and in some cases, a few times a week. At our institution, we require daily review.

Lastly, before hiring the first physician assistant, one additional question must be asked and answered. By this time, a thorough analysis has been done as to the advantages to the institution, its staff and its patients, of adding physician assistants to its health care delivery system. But what will the physician assistant get out of it? If the only answer is a salary, the physician assistant will not stay very long and high turnover will obviate one of the major advantages of physician assistants — continuity of care. Will the physician assistant be treated as a professional and as a valuable and valued colleague? Will attention be paid to his needs for continuing education and for professional growth? If, at this point, you can answer yes to these questions, in addition to satisfactorily handling all the other problems — congratulations! You have got a physician assistant program going, and it will probably be successful.

Chapter 42

PERSONAL CAREER CONSIDERATIONS FOR THE SURGICAL PHYSICIAN ASSISTANT

KATHLEEN M. ROONEY, PA-C
LINDA C. BRANDT
MALCOLM S. BEINFIELD, M.D.

The role of the physician assistant in surgery, the variations of that role, and the factors that affect it have been discussed throughout this book. Why any particular physician assistant would want to pursue a career in surgery is a thoughtful personal decision usually arrived at during the course of clinical training. What should be considered in pursuing, developing and maintaining this field of interest will be discussed here. Certainly, the scope of surgery itself is enough to entice the physician assistant wishing to be challenged. Specializing in surgery allows the primary care physician assistant a broader base of knowledge upon which to draw in total patient care. The surgical physician assistant calls upon his primary care training as well as his specialty skills when involved with patient education, the patient's emotional reaction to surgery and pre-, intra-, and postoperative management.

Entry into the specialty field of surgery can be attained by on-the-job training or through an established postgraduate surgical training program. A postgraduate training year provides the primary care physician assistant with a structured environment within which he may gradually increase his responsibility. An additional period of formal education and clinical supervision allows the physician assistant time to acquire specific skills and knowledge as well as to gain confidence prior to undertaking that first position as a surgical physician assistant. A brief student rotation in surgery simply cannot encompass the entirety of the surgical physician assistant's role. Additional training is needed to prepare the P.A. to perform confidently and knowledgeably as a surgeon extender either in a hospital or private group setting.

Currently, there are two well-established surgical residency programs for graduate physician assistants and several others are in the planning stages. The established programs, as detailed in Chapter 14, offer adequate stipends and other benefits such as vacation, medical and malpractice insurance cover-age so that expense is not a consideration when choosing post-graduate educa-tion over on-the-job training. Indeed, these stipends and fringe benefits are often comparable to many first job salaries offered to physician assistants with no prior surgical experience. Bridging the student role and that of confident productive surgical physician assistant, these programs provide clinical ex-posure to all the surgical specialties. This broad experience prepares the physi-cian assistant to work in any surgical area and facilitates an informed choice of employment opportunities. As more and more formal postgraduate surgical training programs develop and continue to turn out well-trained graduates, future employers will increasingly turn to them when seeking qualified surgical physician assistants.

For some, however, the strict admission criteria and limited enrollment of these programs may make it difficult or impossible to attend. For others, family or personal considerations may preclude relocating for a "temporary" one or two year period. Others may find the long hours and strenuous requirements of postgraduate work too taxing. For these physician assistants who still want to pursue an interest in surgery, on-the-job training with a surgical specialty group or in a hospital setting may be an alternate path to a surgical physician assistant career.

The physician assistant who chooses to be trained on-the-job must be well motivated and disciplined in his desire to learn about surgical patient care. If he is hired in a hospital setting where other more experienced physician assistants are working in surgery, they may serve as role models and provide teaching necessary to the inexperienced physician assistant. In a private surgical group, there must be a willingness to provide instruction which pro-vides the physician assistant with increased function and responsibility. De-pending upon the site, the physician assistant may find Continuing Medical Education and didactic teaching readily available as in a university or teach-ing hospital, or he may find that he has to rely entirely on his own outside reading to fill this void. The experience will vary considerably, depending upon the practice setting, how the physician assistant is utilized and the qual-ity of instruction available to him. Certainly, prior to the establishment of postgraduate education, on-the-job training was the only available course for surgical physician assistants to follow and there are many physician assistants working in surgery who are providing quality patient care through their many years of on-the-job experience. However, because of the great variability of this experience, the physician assistant may find himself undertrained and, therefore, underutilized, possibly limiting future career advancement. As more formally trained surgical physician assistants seek employment oppor-tunities, those without surgical experience may find themselves competing for these same positions. As this occurs, the availability of on-the-job training may be sharply curtailed.

Employment for surgical physician assistants is increasing, especially in hospital and institutional settings. A recently conducted national survey, published by Perry and Detmer, predicts an 87% increase in available positions in the next five years (1). Salaries for surgical physician assistants are certainly competitive with those for other physician assistant positions and, in most cases, are considerably higher. However, the hours are usually longer and, in most hospitals, include on-call time which may or may not be compensated. As the trend for hospitals' use of surgical physician assistants continues, many physician assistants will find that they are the first to be hired in a particular institution. They may work alone or along with surgical MD residents. In either case, they are often charged with establishing the surgical physician assistant role in an institution which may or may not understand its full scope. The physician assistant with prior specialty training should be able to work effectively with his employers to develop an accurate job description. If the physician assistant is himself unfamiliar with the surgical physician assistant role, the result may be underutilization.

The surgical physician assistant job description is the great variable of this new profession, and the key to job satisfaction. Employers are looking for assistants over a very broad spectrum of responsibility in patient care. While completion of patient history and physical exams with minor ward duties may suffice in some jobs, a combination of clinic duties, intensive care unit monitoring and first call for in-house emergencies may be expected in other settings. First assisting in the operating room is a significant part of surgical physician assistant training and maintaining those skills might be a large part of job satisfaction and enrichment. Surgical physician assistants in any setting have to be a part of the team, their skills and clinical judgement must be respected, or frustration and boredom are the inevitable results. In looking at a prospective job, the surgical physician assistant should weigh employer expectations with his own to assure compatibility.

Many hospital house staff positions can be a fine experience for a few years, but being a permanent surgical physician assistant house officer is not an ideal situation for some individuals. There may be a frustrating lack of upward mobility as one gains experience and the job responsibilities do not change. This frustration may be eased by increased teaching projects, research papers, rotations through the hospital's intensive care unit or emergency room to vary the duties, reduction of working hours to approximate a forty hour work week, increased compensation, or, if necessary, a change of jobs. To hold surgical physician assistants on a long term basis in a single position, employers must remain sensitive to the professional social and economic needs of highly trained and competetent individuals.

There remains a compelling trend for experienced surgical physician assistants to seek surgical sub-specialty and private practice employment. To work for an individual surgeon or group of specialists with whom one is respected and utilized as a skilled associate is a coveted step in career progression for those wishing to remain in surgical practice. There should also be adequate compensation in a busy practice where surgical physician assistants are a tangible financial asset. The difficulty with this specialization at the present time is the limited number of jobs available in desirable locations. The opportunities are increasing slowly, but one must be prepared to relocate to another area of the country and this may not be practical or desirable for family or personal reasons. Patience and job compromise are sometimes necessary until the right opportunity arises.

Conversely, some surgical physician assistants who leave hospital settings for private practice groups find that they miss the hospital environment and the challenge of inpatient management. These physician assistants usually return to hospital or university based positions after a year or so with a private office group.

There is a lateral mobility among surgical physician assistant jobs that is an asset for career expansion. With a surgical background, it is not difficult to move into emergency rooms, primary care clinics, academic and administrative roles (including developing new surgical physician assistant residency programs), public health and patient education, industrial medicine, research and any of the surgical specialties. If an individual retains a certain flexibility there are many health care areas to explore.

As contemporary medicine becomes more sophisticated and specialized, national certification and higher academic degrees become an accepted measure of competence and of educational achievement. Although some physician assistants hold masters degrees, most hold associate and baccalaureate degrees. Academic degrees may have little bearing on a person's practical abilities, but masters level degrees for surgical physician assistants would demonstrate academic achievement in proportion with their patient care responsibilities. Recognition of the surgical physician assistants' additional training has been made by the National Commission for the Certification of Physician Assistants (NCCPA) which now offers an "add on" proficiency examination in surgery to the primary care certification examination. Obtaining and renewing NCCPA primary care certification is a required professional responsibility for most physician assistants, including those specializing in surgery. Continuing medical education, including attending lectures, reading medical literature and participating in hospital conferences are necessary activities to continue in the mainstream of medical and surgical advances.

In any profession, career problems can arise curtailing advancement and diminishing interest and skills in the job. These problems present new challenges for the individual. Changes in hospital policy, state and federal legislation, malpractice litigation and the death or retirement of a surgical physician assistant's M.D. preceptor, can all lead to major career adjustments. As more M.D.s complete their residencies, with projections of an overabundance of M.D.s by 1990, surgical physician assistants may find themselves competing with doctors for some jobs.

A significant part of a surgical physician assistant job description is order writing, under M.D. supervision, for medications and patient treatments. This responsibility is vital for optimal surgical physician assistant utilization in the hospital setting. Some surgical physician assistants are doing many tasks involved with good patient care but are unable to write orders, or they are greatly restricted in initiating orders without immediate verbal consent from an attending physician. The purpose of the surgical physician assistant is attenuated by this problem with concomitant legal implications if it is not dealt with carefully and constructively.

As individual surgical physician assistants mature and gain experience, a small percentage will feel that the M.D. degree is really their desired goal. If so, it is better to pursue medical school admission rather than remain a frustrated surgical physician assistant. Presently, there are no waivers of premed requirements for physician assistants at medical school and the surgical physician assistant background is not necessarily beneficial for matriculation.

Economic and legal considerations may prove to be deciding factors for the continuation and expansion of the surgical physician assistant profession. The fiscal advantages of employing surgical physician assistants are under constant review by medical groups and, so far, the results have always been strongly in favor of the utilization of physician assistants as a cost effective means for maintaining the quality of surgical care. However, the wide disparity in surgical physician assistant job descriptions from state to state has created regulatory and practice problems. Many states do not yet have the licensing requirements which define professional competency. In some states, lobbying against the profession and reluctance on the part of third party payors to allow reimbursement for surgical physician assistant services in the operating room and in office practice slows acceptance of a practical and valuable concept in surgical health care. Until the profession is universally acknowledged, surgical physician assistants themselves through state and national organizations will have to be active participants in the political lobbying and good public relations necessary to establish it in public opinion as a legitimate and worthwhile service.

One further consideration inherent in the very strengths of the profession is that physician assistants may be overtrained for what the majority of them will be permitted to do in the future, or for what the jobs available will demand of them. As a group, physician assistants are enthusiastic, qualified professionals with resources that can be expanded to the benefit of many present and projected health care settings. The adaptability of the physician assistant role is good in that physician assistants can be productive in many areas of surgery. But, there is also the danger that they may be exploited financially and inappropriately utilized below their ability level. If surgical physician assistants are to fulfill their promise as an effective resource of manpower for more comprehensive surgical care delivery, then both surgical physician assistants and their employers must be aware of the real market value of their practical skills and knowledge in order to reach mutual agreement on job responsibilities and satisfactory compensation.

The surgical physician assistant career has developed from an innovative concept; that a skilled professional may usefully augment the services of the surgeon as a supervised associate, doing many of the routine, necessary tasks of good medical-surgical team care in a busy setting. Patience, competence, perseverance, flexibility, and firmness are all qualities required of the men and women who would make a success of the profession. The contributions surgical physician assistants are currently making to health care delivery are positive and multi-faceted. The potential for professional growth is promising but not assured as the pioneers in this new field move toward the 21st century.

REFERENCE

1. Perry H.B., Detmer D.E., and Redmond E.L.: The Current and Future Role of Surgical Physician Assistants: Report of a National Survey of Surgical Chairman in Large U.S. Hospitals. *Ann Surg., 193:*132–137, Feb., 1981.

Chapter 43

LEGAL PERSPECTIVES
ON HOSPITAL PRIVILEGES

DAVID G. WARREN, J.D.

The legal issues surrounding the utilization of physician assistant services in hospitals include some of the same questions that affect both physicians and non-physicians. For several purposes physician assistants are akin to physicians in their legal rights and responsibilities. Otherwise, however, the legal considerations affecting the employment or privileges of non-physician health care workers, such as clinical psychologists, are more germane. For an understanding of why physician assistants are not entirely parallel to one group or the other, it is necessary to know both the legal powers of the hospital as well as the lawful role of the physician assistant. It is important to begin by examining the legal authorities which have determined the hospital's position in regard to permitting various types of practitioners. Once the relevant statutes, court case law and customary policies are identified and tested against constitutional principles, then the license laws and certification procedures for physician assistants come into play in determining what physicians and physician assistants can expect in seeking hospitals privileges for physician assistants.

It has long been established that hospitals can individually decide which practitioners will be permitted to admit and treat patients within its walls. This institutional right is based on the principle that the hospital is responsible for the quality of care provided there and is liable for the negligent selection or retention of incompetent physicians as employees or agents of the hospital. Under newer legal doctrines, there is also a responsibility for the hospital to screen private physicians who apply for privileges and to monitor their performance in the hospital on the basis of the hospital's duty to protect its patients.

This legal position is reflected in the widespread adoption of the American Hospital Association's "Patients Bill of Rights" by individual hospitals as policy statements. These statements also satisfy the accreditation standards of the Joint Commission on Accreditation of Hospitals. Likewise, policy statements regarding the responsibility of hospitals towards employees and others who work there have been adopted, perhaps for both administrative and legal purposes. One institution has specifically set forth its philosophy about the utilization of physician assistants as follows:

PHILOSOPHY
PHYSICIANS' ASSISTANTS/NURSE PRACTITIONERS

The physicians' assistant/nurse practitioner at Geisinger Medical Center is a skilled member of the health care team who is qualified by academic and clinical education to provide patient services under the supervision of a staff physician who, in turn, is responsible for the performance and clinical evaluation of these persons.

Their education in accredited programs encompasses training in biomedical, behavioral, surgical and clinical skills which are maintained by continuing medical education.

The physician's utilization of these personnel creates a unique health care team dedicated equally to:

- Increasing accessibility to high quality health care,
- Maintaining an atmosphere of caring and trust among the patient, the family and the health care team and
- Improving continuity of patient care within the health care system.

Responsibilities and limitations shall be defined by the by-laws committee and approved by the Board of Governors of the Geisinger Medical Center, conforming to the regulations as set forth by the State Board of Medical Education and Licensure and the State Board of Nurse Examiners. (Geisinger Medical Center, Danville, Pennsylvania, Feb. 8, 1980)

Such statements serve to indicate an institution's adherence to a high standard of patient care and professional performance, but in themselves do not provide protection from liability for misuse or mistakes of physician assistants or other professionals performing services in the hospital.

In the early days, charitable and non-profit hospitals were somewhat protected from liability by the requirement that a patient's lawsuit must be based solely on the claim that the hospital either negligently selected incompetent or careless employees or failed to limit or terminate their activities. Otherwise, the hospital was able to shield itself and avoid liability by the defense of charitable immunity. All other hospitals were fully liable under the doctrine of *respondeat superior* for the negligence of their employees, but not the medical staff. The question of who was an "employee" was determined by who controlled the activities of that person as well as who paid him or her. Thus, physicians were generally not considered "employees" for imposing vicarious liability on the hospital.

Closely related to this policy of limited liability of hospitals for its medical staff was the traditional viewpoint that hospitals were merely the doctor's workshop and he or she, not the hospital, was in control of any patient care rendered there. Thus, in the operating room the physician was considered "captain of the ship" and legally responsible for any actionable mistakes committed there, even by nurses and other hospital employees whom he may have "borrowed" to perform the operation. The hospital was generally free of any direct legal obligation to protect patients from poor quality care by physicians. Thus, for many years hospital management and governing boards exercised little control over which practitioners had practice privileges in the hospital. Although the law has never given physicians an unlimited right to practice in any hospital they choose, there has been little interest by hospital governing boards and management until recently in controlling access to the medical staff. On the other hand, most hospital medical staffs have been restrictive in who they permitted to have privileges, often for economic reasons as much as concerns about quality. Especially noticeable has been the absence of podiatrists, and earlier, osteopaths from medical staffs, as well as strict limitations on dentists.

Much of this climate has changed recently and the expectations of physician assistants about hospital privileges have been directly affected by changes in statutes, case law and accreditation standards. Nevertheless, the legal picture is not entirely clear at this time and some important issues about privilege procedures and policies remain unresolved.

Starting with what is reliably clarified, it must be pointed out that in 1927 the U.S. Supreme Court declared that a hospital does not have to accept every physician who wants to practice there. Other criteria related to quality of patient care can be imposed on applicants even though they are duly licensed. This is so even when the physician points out that he has a license to practice medicine anywhere in the state. It is so, even though the hospital is a public hospital, supported by tax monies and obligated to serve the general public. Thus, the possession of a state license, certification or other "official" approval is not an automatic ticket for obtaining hospital privileges. The case was *Hayman v. Galveston,* 273 U.S. 414, and is the only medical staff controversy the High Court has ever decided. There are nevertheless multitudes of important and decisive cases from state supreme courts and various federal courts which have answered numerous questions about hospital privileges.

A review of these court cases, especially since the decision by the Joint Commission on Accreditation of Hospitals (JCAH) in 1970 to establish medical staff criteria in the accreditation standards for hospitals, provides increasingly clear guidelines about who can apply for privileges, how privileges can be limited or denied, and what review must be provided for adverse determinations. However, some of these cases have raised complicated antitrust law issues about when a hospital is subject to charges of restraint of trade in denying privileges to applicants.

Another set of court cases and various state statutes, coupled with trends in hospital policies, impose rules about hospital liability for the actions of both physicians and hospital employees affecting patients care. Still a third category of court cases, and more importantly, regulations and agency determinations, determine third party reimbursement practices and procedures. The rules about utilization, supervision, documentation, and other matters involved in utilization of physician assistant services in hospitals have an obvious pragmatic effect on hospital privilege considerations.

First, a review of the court cases involving application, denial, suspension and termination of hospital medical staff privileges furnishes some basic principles which also limit any privileges physician assistants may eventually seek.

1. The hospital board is responsible through its medical staff and hospital administrator for quality control of hospital care. "No court should substitute its evaluation of such matters for that of the Hospital Board. It is the Board, not the court, which is charged with the responsibility of providing a competent staff of doctors. The Board has chosen to rely on the advice of its Medical Staff, and the court cannot surrogate for the Staff in executing this responsibility. Human lives are at stake, and the governing board must be given discretion in its selection so that it can have confidence in the competence and moral commitment of its staff. The evaluation of professional proficiency of doctors is best left to the specialized expertise of their peers, subject only to limited judicial surveillance. The court is charged with the narrow responsibility of assuring that the qualifications imposed by the Board are reasonably related to the operation of the hospital and fairly administered. In short, so long as staff selections are administered with fairness, geared by a rationale compatible with hospital responsibility, and unemcumbered with irrelevant considerations, a court should not interfere."
   Sosa v. Bd. of Managers of Val Verde Hosp., 437 F.2d 173 (5th Cir. 1971).

2. All hospitals must grant "due process protection" and act "reasonably" in dealing with medical staff matters. A.F. Southwick in "The Physician's Right to Due Process in Public and Private Hospitals: Is There a Difference?," (*Medicolegal News*, pp. 4–10, February 1981), advocates that constitutional principles and common law requirements for "fairness" have effectively dissolved most distinctions between public and private hospitals. He recommends that both members and would-be members of all hospital medical staffs always be granted the essentials of due process, regardless of several court decisions saying private hospitals have more latitude in denying privileges without cause and do not have to face judicial review of their decisions.

3. The minimal requirements of procedural due process have been articulated as follows:

   The physician is entitled to: (1) *written notice* of reasons for denial of appointment or of the charges against him or her; (2) an opportunity for a timely *hearing* after such notice; (3) a relatively *impartial hearing* body; (4) an opportunity to produce *evidence* and witnesses on his or her behalf and to refute the hospital's proferred evidence; (5) a *finding* by the hearing body based upon substantial, credible factual evidence; (6) *written notice* of the hearing body's recommended decision together with the reasons for the decision; and (7) an opportunity to *appeal* the decision.

   See *Silver v. Castle Mem. Hosp.*, 497 P.3d 564, cert. denied 409 U.S. 1048 (1972).

4. Rules and conditions in medical staff by-laws which are reasonably related to quality of care will be judicially approved, such as the following:

   a. applicants document their training, experience and specialty board certification and eligibility
   b. mandated supervision where applicant's competency needed documentation or where limited practitioner granted privileges
   c. consultation
   d. timely completion of medical records
   e. adherence to medical staff by-laws, rules and regulations
   f. summary suspension in circumstances indicating an immediate threat to safety of patients
   g. documented clinical incompetence as grounds for suspension or discipline
   h. periodic re-evaluation

5. Actions of hospitals in matters of medical staff privileges are subject to antitrust law jurisdiction. *Robinson v. Magovern,* 521 F.Supp. 842 (W.D.Pa. 1981).

While these basic privileges are not inclusive, they indicate the general approach to the privilege application and granting process for physicians. Nevertheless, there are numerous newly developing legal considerations about hospital privileges, such as the application of federal and state antitrust laws to the matter of exclusion of individual physicians from hospital staffs. In addition, both tax and antitrust laws have changing implications for exclusive contracts for specialized services such as anesthesiology, pathology, radiology, and emergency room services. Justification for closing or imposing a moratorium on a particular specialty or an entire medical staff must meet the current tests of antitrust laws and also the state planning laws. Furthermore, various state statutes or regulations may prescribe the minimum content for medical staff bylaws. The significance of these fast-changing legal considerations for practicing physicians spills over onto the aspirations of non-physicians for hospital credentialling, raising both present and possibly future restrictions. It is essential that a physician assistant who is denied approval for hospital practice should thoroughly review the current state of the law about medical staff privileges in general before deciding on any particular course of action concerning his own privilege application.

The next category of legal precedent impacting on hospitals' discretion in employing or credentialling physician assistants is perhaps the most dramatic, yet the most direct in effect: liability suits. As alluded to earlier, the days of charitable immunity and protective application of *respondeat superior,* or the master-servant doctrine, have disappeared. In their places are corporate negligence and more liberal interpretations of vicarious liability. The famous 1965 Illinois case, *Darling v. Charleston Community Memorial Hospital,* 211 N.E. 2d 253 (Ill. 1965), cert. denied, 383 U.S. 946 (1966), established for the first time a hospital's direct duty to a patient for furnishing standard medical care. Since then, numerous states have adopted this doctrine of corporate negligence, the principle that hospitals owe their patients a measure of protection from incompetent private physicians as well as incompetent or negligent hospital employees. This means that hospital governing boards, through their medical staff organization, must carefully screen applicants for privileges and must continue to monitor the performance of individual medical staff members.

The fear of liability being imposed on the hospital for permitting unqualified or incompetent practitioners to injure patients in the hospital has jolted both administrators and board members into active involvement in the privileges review process. The admonition to a hospital in a recent court case on this question serves as a guideline for hospital diligence in protecting patients from physicians' (and other professionals, including physician assistants) malpractice.

That case was a negligence suit brought by a patient against both a Wisconsin hospital and a new private staff physician for injuries received as a result of a negligently-performed surgical operation. At the trial the jury awarded the plaintiff $315,000 for personal injuries, past and future, and $90,000 for impairment of earning capacity, past and future. Not only was the surgeon held liable for his surgical incompetency, but also the hospital was held liable for negligence in granting the surgeon privileges in the first place. The hospital had failed to make any investigation of the doctor's application; if it had done so, it would have discovered that the doctor's privileges had recently been revoked or limited by other hospitals, that seven malpractice lawsuits had been filed against him and that he was not considered competent by many of his peers. The Wisconsin Supreme Court in *Johnson v. Misericordia Community Hospital,* 301 N.W.2d 156 (Wis. 1981) explained the rule that is now being followed in numerous states:

In summary, we hold that a hospital owes a duty to its patients to exercise reasonable care in the selection of its medical staff and in granting specialized privileges. The final appointing authority resides in the hospital's governing body, although it must rely on the medical staff and in particular the credentials committee (or committee of the whole) to investigate and evaluate an applicant's qualifications for the requested privileges. However, this delegation of the responsibility to investigate and evaluate the professional competence of applicants for clinical privileges does not relieve the governing body of its duty to appoint only qualified physicians and surgeons to its medical staff and periodically monitor and review their competency. The credentials committee (or committee of the whole) must investigate the qualifications of applicants. The facts of this case demonstrate that a hospital should, at a minimum, require completion of the application and verify the accuracy of the applicant's statements, training and experience. Additionally, it should: (1) solicit information from the applicant's peers, including those not referenced in his application, who are knowledgeable about his education, training, experience, health, competence and ethical character; (2) determine if the applicant is currently licensed to practice in this state and if his licensure or registration has been or is currently being challenged; and (3) inquire whether the applicant has been involved in any adverse malpractice action and whether he has experienced a loss of medical organization membership or medical privileges or membership at any other hospital. The investigating committee must also evaluate the information gained through its inquiries and make a reasonable judgment as to the approval or denial of each application for staff privileges. The hospital will be charged with gaining and evaluating the knowledge that would have been acquired had it exercised ordinary care in investigating its medical staff applicants and the hospital's failure to exercise that degree of care, skill and judgment that is exercised by the average hospital in approving an applicant's request for privileges is negligence (at pp. 147-75; citations omitted).

This emphasis on the hospital governing boards' legal responsibility, through the medical staff organization, for careful screening and monitoring of medical staff membership signals the importance of full preparation by physician assistants for demonstrating qualifications and competency.

A recent California court case, *Elam v. College Park Hospital,* 183 Cal.Rptr.156 (1982), involving negligent patient care by a podiatrist who had been given staff privileges, determined that the hospital was liable under the doctrine of corporate negligence for failure to insure the initial competency and the *continuing review* of its medical staff. The court noted the relevancy of the procedures for selection and reappointment required by the Joint Commission on Accreditation of Hospitals (JCAH) and pointed out the importance of internal review processes.

Thus, the third category of legal considerations for physician assistant privileges is the accreditation standards imposed by the Joint Commission on Accreditation of Hospitals (JCAH). The 1982 Accreditation Manual does not refer specifically to physician assistants but indicates that hospitals should make provision for physician assistant services. The JCAH Medical Staff Standard III states that the bylaws shall at least provide for:

> . . . the mechanism for delineation of and retention of privileges, and reduction and withdrawal of privileges. This includes the privileges of non-physician . . . practitioners who require medical staff processing because of the patient services to be rendered

Standard I provides more detail about handling non-physician professionals: The medical staff shall delineate in its bylaws, rules and regulations the qualifications, status, clinical duties, and responsibilities of specified professional personnel whose service require that they be processed through the usual medical staff channels. This should be performed in consultation with the chief executive officer on a categorical rather than an individual basis. The training, experience, and demonstrated current competence of individuals in such categories shall be sufficient to permit their performing the following:

- The exercising of judgment within their areas of competence, providing that a physician member of the medical staff shall have the ultimate responsibility for patient care;
- Participating directly in the management of patients under the supervision or direction of a member of the medical staff; and
- Within the limits established by the medical staff and consistent with the State Practice Acts, the writing of orders and the recording of reports and progress notes in patients' medical records.

Specified professional personnel shall be individually assigned to an appropriate clinical department/service and shall carry out their activities subject to department/service policies and procedures and in conformity with the applicable provisions of the medical staff bylaws, rules and regulations. Cognizance shall be taken when state or federal regulations, or the approved bylaws, rules and regulations of the medical staff, require assignment of specified professional personnel to individual staff members rather than to departments/services.

Thus, a physician assistant would be subject to the limitations set forth in the medical staff bylaws and rules that would apply to all physician assistants as a group. It is important to note that the JCAH discourages but does not preclude an individual approval process for physician assistants.

There is some indication that the 1983 standards will deal more specifically with the physician assistant question. Advance information in the July 19, 1982, issue of *Medical World News* reveals that the title of the medical staff section will be changed to "Professional or Medical Staff" and further that modifications will be made to the existing language about medical staffs being limited to licensed medical physicians. This is being done to avoid possible antitrust charges against JCAH for facilitating monopoly practices by physicians against other professional groups seeking hospital privileges.

How should a hospital respond to the current JCAH standards in order to accommodate physician assistants? One suggestion is made by Nathan Hershey in "A Guide for Developing Bylaws Provisions in Hospitals for Credentialing Limited Health Practitioners (including, but not limited to, podiatrists, physician assistants and nurse practitioners)," distributed by the Pennsylvania Medical Society in January 1980. He recommends that granting specific privileges "depends upon the qualifications of each individual who is seeking to provide services" (p. 3) and offers this model bylaw provision and comment:

LIMITED HEALTH PRACTITIONERS

The medical staff may recommend to the board the granting of clinical privileges to limited health practitioners, including, but not limited to, podiatrists, physicians' assistants and nurse practitioners, based upon investigation and evaluation of the education, training, experience, and demonstrated ability and judgment of individuals requesting privileges as limited health practitioners, according to procedures established in the rules and regulations of the medical staff. A recommendation by or on behalf of the medical staff to not grant privileges to an applicant for privileges as a limited health practitioner, or to suspend, to terminate, or to reduce such privileges, or such a decision by the board, shall not give rise to any procedural rights set forth in Article _____.

Comments

The bylaw provision above should appear as a section in the article of the medical staff bylaws relating to the granting and delineation of clinical privileges. The detail of procedures and processes need not and should not be set forth in the medical staff bylaws for several reasons, most prominent of which is that at most hospitals the medical staff bylaws are subject to a more complex and time-consuming amendment process than medical staff rules and regulations, that would have to be followed in order to accomplish relatively minor changes in such procedures as changed circumstances may require.

Another model has been proposed by the American Academy of Physician Assistants in its 1980–81 Policy Manual:

PROPOSED AMENDMENT TO THE MEDICAL STAFF BYLAWS

I. Clinical Privileges

Section 1. Clinical Privileges Restricted for Physician Assistant Staff
A. Definition of the role of the Physician Assistant in the Hospital

The Physician Assistant (PA) is a person qualified by academic and clinical training to provide patient services under the supervision and responsibility of a doctor of medicine or osteopathy who is, in turn, responsible for the performance of the PA. Prior to the granting of hospital privileges, the supervising physician shall provide evidence to the Medical Staff that the PA is qualified to practice his profession under appropriate state laws or, if such laws do not exist, is a graduate of an American Medical Association accredited program training such assistants and/or certified by the National Commission on Certification of Physician Assistants.

A qualified, certified, physician assistant shall be granted hospital privileges by the governing body of the hospital on the recommendation of the executive committee of the Medical Staff. The delineation of their clinical privileges shall be based upon the applicant's academic and clinical training, experience, judgment and demonstrated competence to provide patient service under the supervision and responsibility of the physician licensed by the state and does not include physicians having a temporary license for residency training. The physician employing the physician assistant is responsible for the care of any medical problem that may be present, or may arise during hospitalization. Physician assistants shall comply with all applicable Medical Staff Bylaws, Rules and Regulations.

The initial certification shall be for one year and renewed annually on that anniversary date. Recertification and review of the physician assistant, the employing physician, and his practice shall be made prior to renewal of the certificate.

The physician assistant may be involved with the patients of the physician in any medical setting within the established scope of the physician's practice, not prohibited by law. The physician assistant's service may be utilized in all medical care settings, including the office, the hospital, the patient's home, extended care facilities, and nursing home. Diagnostic and therapeutic procedures common to the physician's practice that may be delegated to the physician assistant are:

Receiving patients, obtaining case histories, performing an appropriate physical examination, and presenting meaningful data to the physician;

Performing or assisting in laboratory procedures and related studies in the practice setting:

Giving injections and immunizations; suturing and caring for wounds;

Providing patient counseling services; referring patients to other services;

Responding to emergency situations which arise in the physician's absence within the assistant's range of skills and experience.

The delineation and granting of clinical privileges for physician assistants shall be accomplished in a manner consistent with the overall procedure established for the Medical Staff.

B. Description of Physician Assistant Duties and Responsibilities

1. Perform history and physical examination on new and return patients in the office, hospital, and extended care facility. Establish presumptive diagnoses, establish the general workup of the patient by ordering appropriate laboratory studies, and be responsible under the physician's supervision for the management of the patients' problems following diagnosis.

2. Assist in hospital and nursing home rounds. Making complete chart entries on patient transaction, writing orders and recording progress notes which will be reviewed and countersigned by the responsible physician within 24 hours.

3. Initiate appropriate laboratory, radiologic, and special examinations or tests required for the evaluation of illness.

4. Communicate with patients by phone and letter regarding their problems, following consultation with the responsible physician.

5. Provide counseling and instruction regarding patient problems.

6. Prepare and dictate patient summaries of patients hospitalization and clinic care.

7. Order oral and parenteral medications, except controlled substances, as specified by established protocols or as directed by the responsible physician.

8. First and second assist on major and minor surgery as directed by the responsible physician in both the hospital and clinic.

9. Manage medical emergencies and initiate appropriate therapy until the arrival of a physician.

10. Provide follow-up and health maintenance care including appropriate adjustments of medications to patients in accordance with established protocols or specific instructions from the responsible physician.

11. Assist the physician as directed in the training of health personnel in certain diagnostic, therapeutic, and clinic techniques.

12. Participate in appropriate continuing medical education programs.

13. Perform clinical procedures under the direction and supervision of the responsible physician, such as: venipuncture and arteriopuncture; electro-cardiogram; administer intravenous medications, fluids, blood and blood components; administer injections; I.M., subcutaneous and intradermal; administer intradermal skin tests; nasogastric intubation; insertion of urinary catheters; clean and debridement of wounds; administer local infiltrative anesthetic; suture minor lacerations that do not involve artery, tendon, or nerve damage; application of dressings, bandages, splints, and traction; application and removal of orthopedic casts under responsible supervision of the physician; incision and drainage; routine lab work such as complete blood counts, urinalysis, and gram staining of clinical specimens; pelvic examination with pap smear; audiometric and tonometric examination; interpretation of routine x-rays prior to reading by the responsible physician or radiologist; basic interpretation of ECG's until read by the responsible physician; and such other tasks as the supervising physician may request and the Medical Staff may approve.

These bylaws may be amended after submission of the proposed amendment at any regular or special meeting of the Medical Staff. A proposed amendment shall be referred to a special committee which shall report on it at the next regular meeting of the Medical Staff or at a special meeting called for such purpose. To be adopted, an amendment shall require a two-thirds vote of the active medical staff present. Amendments so made shall be effective when approved by the governing body (April 79, House of Delegates).

It should be noted that while many hospitals may have adopted bylaws provisions and other physician assistant policies in order to comply with accreditation standards and state regulations, some such hospitals do not have physician assistants functioning in the hospital. A survey conducted by the author during 1982 covering all the larger hospitals in one state indicated an uneven pattern of use of physician assistants.

There are still other approaches which have been taken in hospitals permitting physician assistant services. Some have established categories entitled "allied health personnel," "physician extenders," "PA/NP," "paramedical personnel" or other titles, and included varying degrees of detail. For example, one hospital amended its medical staff bylaws as follows:

6.6   *PHYSICIAN EXTENDER*

6.6-1   *Definitions*

a. Physician Extender—An individual, other than a physician or dentist, certified by the North Carolina Board of Medical Examiners, who provides some type of medical care under the supervision of a physician member of the medical staff, but who is not

an employee of Durham County General Hospital (i.e., physician assistants, nurse practitioners, and nurse midwives).
b. Medical Sponsor — Physician member(s) in good standing of the medical staff of Durham County General Hospital who accepts responsibility for all activities of the physician extender and whose supervision meets the standards set by Durham County General Hospital and those required by the North Carolina Board of Medical Examiners.

6.6-2 *Appointment of a Physician Extender*
   a. Each application for appointment shall be in writing, submitted on the prescribed form and signed by the applicant.
   b. The application form shall include detailed information concerning the applicant's qualifications, his physical and mental health, and the name(s) of the sponsoring physician(s).
   c. Upon approval by the chairman of the department in which the sponsoring physician has privileges and by the Credentials Committee, privileges will be extended to the physician extender through the sponsoring physician. The medical staff, nursing units, and other appropriate areas of the hospital will be notified of the appointment.
   d. Appointments will be for one year and reappointments will be made on the basis of satisfactory performance and continued competence as judged by the medical sponsor, the chairman of the sponsor's department, and the Credentials Committee.

6.6-3 *Privileges*
   a. Upon appointment, physician extenders will be authorized, under supervision of the sponsoring physician, to take medical histories, do complete physician examinations, and order laboratory examinations.
   b. For a physician extender to initiate any treatment or alter any treatment, there must be a prior communication with the sponsoring physician.
   c. A sponsoring physician shall not delegate to a physician extender any duty which the physician himself is not authorized to perform by his delineation of privileges. (Medical Staff Bylaws Amendment, May 9, 1979, for Durham County General Hospital, Durham, North Carolina)

Regardless of the amount of detail desired, however, not all of the policies and procedures regarding physician assistants should or can be included in the bylaws. Besides medical staff rules and regulations, physician assistant rights and responsibilities may be contained in hospital personnel policies, directives, memoranda, manuals and guidelines.

One hospital administrator has described his hospital's policies with regard to physician assistants as follows:

> We do have a number of physicians assistants as well as nurse practitioners who have been granted privileges here at the hospital. Normally those privileges include (1) history and physical, (2) assessment of patient needs, (3) writing of orders, (4) assisting in procedures and/or surgery and (5) dictating discharge summaries.
>
> Additionally, we maintain a manual on allied health practitioners and their specific privileges as well as their sponsoring physicians throughout the hospital so that all hospital employees know precisely what their privileges might be on an individual basis. We have found that this kind of information source serves us very well.
>
> Additionally, we routinely perform peer review on an annual basis on all physician's assistants and other allied health practitioners who have been granted practice privileges here at the hospital. This review consists not only of their performance but also the level of supervision that is provided to them by their sponsoring physicians. Given the results of that review their privileges are either continued or modified in some form.
>
> (Private communication from Dennis R. Barry, President of Moses H. Cone Memorial Hospital, Greensboro, NC, dated March 2, 1982)

There may be particular, more detailed written policies about certain procedures for physician assistants. One very sensitive area is order writing. A separate policy in use at Duke University Hospital provides a special protocol for physician assistants:

> Procedure D. Under the provisions of standing orders, the job description of the Nonphysician, or other pre-arrangement authorized in advance by the responsible physicians, the Nonphysician (e.g., a PA) exercises some *discretion* in determining which specific orders to write for a particular patient. Under such orders, the Nonphysician signs his or her own name and title and states the name of the supervising physician as follows:
>
> (signature of writer)   ,   (title)   , for Dr.
>
> In the absence of a physician, a ward Staff Nurse may accept a dictated (verbal) order from a Physician's Associate (Assistant) if a list of standing orders of the responsible physician is available and the order is covered therein. Such orders are to be carried out when written and thus before the specific orders come to the attention of any physician. Within 24 hours such orders are countersigned by the supervising physician or other responsible physician. The purpose of the countersignature is to document physician accountability and medical supervision of the Nonphysician.
>
> (Duke University Medical Center, Durham, North Carolina)

In some states, hospitals are required by statute or regulation to promulgate written policies about certain physician assistant functions. For example,

North Carolina General Statutes 90–18.1(d) authorizes physician assistants to "order medications, tests and treatments in hospitals, clinics, nursing homes and other health facilities" if four conditions are met:

1. Board of Medical Examiner regulations are promulgated,
2. Physician assistant has current approval from the Board,
3. Supervising physician has provided physician assistant with written general instructions about orders and will review each order within a reasonable time (Note: the Board requires review within 24 hours), and
4. Hospital or other health facility has adopted "a written policy, approved by the medical staff after consultation with the nursing administration, about ordering medications, tests and treatments, including procedures for verification of the physician assistant's orders by nurses and other facility employees and such other procedures as are in the interest of patient health and safety."

One North Carolina hospital has responded to the statutory requirements with these guidelines:

GUIDELINES FOR NURSE PRACTITIONERS (NPs) AND PHYSICIAN ASSISTANTS (PAs)

1. NPs must be licensed by the North Carolina Board of Nursing and approved by the Board of Medical Examiners of the State of North Carolina. Physician assistants must be approved by the Board of Medical Examiners of the State of North Carolina.
2. Direction and supervision of a NP/PA must be by a physician member of the Visiting Medical and Dental Staff of Charlotte Memorial Hospital and Medical Center in good standing. The sponsoring physician must assume full responsibility for all actions of the NP/PA in the performance of his duties in the hospital.
3. Those duties that the sponsoring physician delegates to the NP/PA must be within the boundaries of the laws of the State of North Carolina governing NPs and PAs, specifically delineated, and the capabilities attested to by the sponsoring physician.
   a. The specific delineation of duties must be attached to the NP/PA's application for privileges at Charlotte Memorial Hospital and Medical Center. Privileges for NP/PA must be approved by the Credentials Committee upon recommendation of the respective Clinical Department.
   b. Before changing any specific duties, the sponsoring physician must submit and have revised duties approved by the Credentials Committee upon recommendation of the respective Clinical Department.

    c. The NP/PA will not be allowed to examine and/or treat patients in the Emergency Department except under the direct personal supervision of the sponsoring physician while the sponsoring physician is physically present on the hospital premises.

4. All orders and/or entries made to the chart by the NP/PA must be countersigned within 24 hours by the sponsoring physician or by the delegated physician associate where accorded by law. NP/PA may not write any orders other than those on the approved protocol from his sponsoring physician and only upon instruction from the sponsoring physician. Transmission of orders from sponsoring physician is permitted. Each NP/PA's individual protocol must be approved by the Credentials Committee upon recommendation of the respective Clinical Department.

5. NP/PA will not be permitted to perform procedures on hospital patients independent of his sponsoring physician unless he is in direct attendance and then only if the procedure has been approved by the Credentials Committee upon recommendation of the respective Clinical Department.

6. Name tag identification of the NP/PA must be such that he will not be confused with a physician.

7. Specific duties and privileges shall be regularly monitored and evaluated by the sponsoring physician to ensure that the NP/PA's duties are performed in a competent and professional manner. At the time of annual reapplication for privileges, the sponsoring physician must submit a written evaluation of NP/PA to the Chairman of the respective Clinical Department.

8. The performance of the NP/PA will be reviewed by the Credentials Committee when annual reapplication for privileges is submitted upon recommendation of the respective Clinical Department.

9. List of standing orders and specific duties and privileges and name of sponsoring physician will be filed by the Nursing Office as reference for the nursing staff who work with and carry out the orders of the NP/PA.

10. Any health care professional's questions about specific duties of the NP/PA should be discussed with the sponsoring physician.

11. The following privileges will not be granted to NP/PAs:
    a. Dictating or recording the admission history.
    b. Dictating or recording the admission physical examination.
    c. Dictating or recording the discharge summary.
    d. Dictating or recording the operative notes or summary of operative procedure.

12. Unfavorable actions affecting NP/PA privileges will be governed by those applicable provisions of the By-Laws Rules and Regulations of the Visiting Medical and Dental Staff and such other rules, regulations, or policies as the Hospital or the Visiting Medical and Dental Staff shall establish.
13. Further additions or deletions to the above requirements may be forthcoming in the future.
    (Charlotte Memorial Hospital and Medical Center, Charlotte, North Carolina)

It should be noted that in several states the hospital association or medical society has published guidelines to assist hospitals in developing bylaws provisions as well as other written policies. In addition to the Pennsylvania "Guide" referenced above, there is the Maryland Hospital Association's "Hosital Guidelines for Utilizing Physician's Assistants" dated November 1977. On a broader scale the American Hospital Association has issued two relevant documents: "Guidelines on the Physician's Assistant in the Hospital" (1975) and "Policy and Statement on Privileges and Quality Assurance for Health Practitioners Other Than Medical Staff Members and Employees" (1980).

To summarize the considerations involved in using physician assistant services in a hospital, the 1980 AHA "Policy and Statement . . ." contains this advice:

It should be the function of the medical staff of the hospital, after consultation with and through the administration of the hospital, to recommend to the governing body of the hospital the scope of clinical activities to be performed by these individuals. To carry out this obligation, the following procedures should be established and provided for pursuant to the medical staff bylaws:

1. Determination of the general qualifications to be required to these practitioners and the level of medical supervision needed.
2. Recommendations regarding the scope of activities for each practitioner, determined on the basis of an assessment of qualifications, such as educational background, licensure, certification, experience, and demonstrated current competence.
3. Recommendations regarding categories for appointment, performance review procedures, reappointments, disciplinary actions, and appeals procedures.

The privilege of performing activities in a hospital carries with it certain obligations to the hospital. These obligations include attendance at educational meetings and acceptance of appointments on appropriate committees, consistent with the bylaws and rules of the medical staff and the overall policies of the institutions. (American Hospital Association, Chicago, Illinois)

One further point should be made. While many hospitals have not acted favorably on physician assistant privileges, it is clear that physician assistants can legally be given the privilege of performing clinical activities in hospitals as dependent practitioners under the supervision of a physician. The policies of state and national organizations, as well as the standards of the JCAH support this principle. There is no reason to expect the courts to rule otherwise nor any present trend for state legislatures to enact restrictions on hospital physician assistant policies.

However, reports about unreliable physician assistant quality assurance, or the occurrence of malpractice lawsuits involving physician assistants, or inappropriate functions being performed by physician assistants in hospitals — any of these could trigger, or perhaps reinforce, restrictive and cautious attitudes on the part of medical staff members or hospital governing board members who together with the medical staff have the ultimate legal responsibility for determining who shall have privileges in each individual institution.

REFERENCES

1. Appointments and Clinical Privileges: Role and Responsibilities of the Board of Trustees. *QRB/Quality Review Bulletin* (May 1980).
2. Fisher, Ron: Hospital Utilization of PAs. *Physician Assistant & Health Practitioner*, p. 102 (Sep. 1981).
3. Friedman, E: Staff Privileges for Nonphysicians. *The Hospital Medical Staff, 7:*3, pp. 22–28 (Mar. 1978).
4. Grad, John D., Jr.: Allied Health Professionals and Hospital Privileges: An Introduction to the Issues. *Law, Medicine & Health Care, 10:*4, pp. 165–167 (Sep. 1982).
5. Health Professionals Access to Hospitals: A Retrospective and Prospective Analysis. *Vanderbilt Law Review, 34:*1161 (1981).
6. Heinrich, J. Jeffrey, *et al.:* The Physician's Assistant as Resident on Surgical Service. *Archives of Surgery, 115:*310–314 (Mar. 1980).
7. Medical Staff. *1982 Accreditation Manual for Hospitals.* Joint Commission on Accreditation of Hospitals, Chicago (1981).
8. Morris, C., and R. Deen: Hospital Provides Rules for Assistants' Privileges. *Hospitals, J.A.H.A., 49:*56–57 (Oct. 1, 1975).
9. Privileges and Quality Assurance Mechanisms for Nonphysicians. *Hospital Medical Staff, 9:*34 (1980).

Chapter 44

REIMBURSEMENT POLICY AND NONPHYSICIAN HEALTH CARE PROVIDERS

C. EMIL FASSER, PA-C
QUENTIN W. SMITH, M.S.
PETER L. ANDRUS, M.D.

Among the most complex features of the health care system in the United States are the variety of mechanisms through which health care services are financed. While health services are generally purchased by individual consumers, payment mechanisms often call for an exchange of dollars between the health care provider and a "third party," such as an insurance company or a governmental agency. In order to provide for some degree of quality control, promote cost containment, and reduce the potential for fraud or abuse, third party payors have developed regulations governing reimbursement for health care services which are quite specific with respect to the types of services for which reimbursement will be made, the level at which reimbursement will occur, and the types of providers who are eligible to receive reimbursement.

While the reimbursement policies of private insurers were in existence for many years prior to the advent of the new category of health professionals generically referred to as physician extenders, they became codified in 1965 with the passage of the Medicare/Medicaid legislation. According to the wording which appears in the Medicare legislation, payment for services can be made only when they are ". . . furnished as an incident to the physician's professional service, of kinds which are commonly furnished in physicians' offices, and are commonly either rendered without charge or included in the physician's bills" (1). These provisions were intended to allow for coverage of ancillary services, such as those typically provided by a nurse, therapist or technician. Thus, in the absence of clarification to the contrary, the "incident to" wording has been interpreted to exclude coverage of services "typically and characteristically rendered by physicians" (2) if those services are rendered by a nonphysician. Since private insurers have tended to follow the lead of the federal programs, one result has been that nonphysician providers, such as physician assistants, who render legitimate health care services in a responsible fashion have found it difficult or impossible to receive payment for those services.

While recognizing that restrictive reimbursement policies were developed to protect the public from unqualified practitioners and to maintain a degree of control over aggregate health care costs, it can also be argued that these policies have created barriers to innovative approaches to health care delivery and restricted the effective utilization of some categories of health care providers (3). As relative newcomers to the health care industry, physician assistants have been influenced by restrictive reimbursement policies more than any other category of provider. While it is difficult to quantify the effects of these reimbursement policies exactly, one can analyze their influence with respect to task delegation to the physician assistant, underutilization costs, and impact on employment opportunities and physician assistant incomes. All of these factors will be considered as each of five generic components—quality of services, productivity, costs, interprofessional politics, and payment mechanisms —of the reimbursement issue are discussed below.

QUALITY OF SERVICES

During their relatively short history as a professional group, perhaps no other type of health care provider has been more intensively studied than have physician assistants. As a new and controversial entity in health care delivery, physician assistants have come under intense scrutiny by a variety of research disciplines. Much of the research has focused on comparative studies of the quality of medical services provided by physician assistants and those provided by physicians. From the literature published on this subject, it can be generally concluded that, within the scope of the physician assistant's role, services which he/she provides are equal in quality to those provided by a physician (4, 5, 6). This appears to be true not only for ancillary tasks which traditionally had been delegated to nonphysicians prior to the advent of physician assistants but also for those tasks, such as history taking and physical examination, that traditionally have been exclusively within the domain of the physician.

The implications of this research, as it relates to reimbursement for physician assistant services, would appear to be that (1) patients who receive appropriate services rendered by physician assistants rather than by physicians are at no greater risk of harm, and (2) that the quality of services rendered is comparable for both the physician assistants and the physicians. Based on these two points, there appears to be little rationale for withholding reimbursement for services provided by a physician assistant.

PROVIDER PRODUCTIVITY

A second component of the reimbursement issue concerns the productivity of physician assistants in delivering health care. Two key questions with respect to reimbursement for physician assistant services are involved. First, can physician assistants provide services in sufficient volume to warrant their inclusion in health care delivery? And, in a related way, does employing a physician assistant in the practice significantly increase the productivity of the physician employer's practice?

The first of these two questions deserves careful analysis. One justification for the use of physician assistants in medical practice settings has been the physician assistant's purported ability to improve practice productivity while providing patient education and counseling services that the physician may not always have time to provide. Since these tasks are time consuming yet delegable, they may, in fact, account for a significant portion of the physician assistant's working time, thereby limiting the number of patients actually seen by the physician assistant. A number of comparative studies on physician assistant and physician productivity have been carried out. In a comprehensive review of the literature on productivity, a study group of the Graduate Medical Education National Advisory Committee (GMENAC) concluded that ". . . nonphysicians were substitutable for physicians at a ratio of .5-.75 to 1, when the number of visits was used as the output measure" (7). These ratios are important as they suggest that the content of care given by nonphysicians may be different from that provided by physicians; i.e., the nonphysician visit may be longer because the physician extender is providing other services. Data from a study on experimental reimbursement supports this notion, as physician assistants spent more time with the patient and provided services that were preventive in nature (8).

The research reports which address the second question posed above are somewhat mixed. The Physician Extender Reimbursement Study found that total patient volume for solo practices employing physician assistants increased by 46 percent over solo practices not employing physician assistants (9). The study further reported that 63 percent of the increase appears to be attributable to increased physician productivity (10). While other studies (11, 12, 13) claim that physician productivity increases significantly with the employment of a physician assistant in the practice, others show that the positive gains reported may be overstated (14, 15, 16). These differences in reported productivity gains due to physician assistant utilization suggests that this is an area requiring additional study. It should be noted, however, that any additional research on practice productivity related to employing physician assistants, should examine factors which limit physician assistant productivity, i.e., supervision requirements, availability of support personnel, as well as quantity and mix of services provided (17).

INDIVIDUAL AND SOCIETAL COSTS

The original perception of the physician assistant's role in health service delivery was framed in terms of controlling rapidly escalating health care expenditures while addressing an identified shortage of primary care physicians (18). Because of its complexities the cost issue must be examined not only from the point of view of expenditures by the patient, but also from the perspectives of costs for education, costs for supervision, costs arising from differential uses in support services and resources, and cost variations resulting from better or poorer health care services being delivered to the population.

Costs to the patient have generally been viewed in terms of the potential savings to be derived from use of a less expensive care provider (19). The Physician Extender Reimbursement Study showed that per patient visit practice expenses were 29 percent lower in solo practices employing physician assistants than within comparable solo practices not employing physician assistants (20). Other evidence suggests that practices employing a physician extender (PE) may charge patients less than those practices which do not employ physician extenders. "Average charges per visit to the patient or third party payor were lower in practices with PEs than in non-PE practices. . . ." (21). Depsite these optimistic findings, there is to date limited evidence suggesting that patient costs have been significantly reduced as a result of having services delivered by a physician assistant. Several explanations may be offered as to why savings to the consumer have not been realized as anticipated. First, physician assistants generally spend more time with patients than do physicians. The productivity studies previously cited indicate a substitutability ratio of .50-.75 to 1 (22). Thus a physician assistant will see one half to three quarters as many patients as the physician in a given period of time. Some of this extra time spent with patients may be attributable to more patient education and counseling than would be carried out in a physician only practice (23).

A second factor to be considered, as it relates to the physician assistant's ability to lower costs to patients, is that of responsible physician supervision. Early estimates of supervisory and consultative time required of the physician placed this time commitment as high as 20% of total working time (24). One well designed research study, conducted within a large health maintenance organization (HMO) which employed physician assistants, estimated that such employment resulted in 8% of a physician's time being devoted to general supervision (25). More recent studies have estimated supervision and consultation time at between 5 and 8 percent of the physician's time (26). Incorporating the use of complex computer modeling, another study determined that the effect of adding only 4 minutes of supervision per patient visit would undoubtedly reduce practice productivity (27). The effect of supervision as dictated by codifying state legislation, on the degrees of maximum substitutability must therefore be considered in computing cost estimates associated with the employment of physician assistants.

Another factor which may influence consumer costs relates to differences in the use of support services and resources. The employment of a physician assistant may necessitate the purchase of new office equipment, addition of examining rooms, or hiring additional support staff. These costs, when added to the overall expenses of operating a practice, may offset, in part, the savings realized through the employment of a provider whose costs of training and annual salary are less than the physician.

An often overlooked aspect of physician assistant cost effectiveness derives from differences between the physician assistant and the physician in patterns of ordering diagnostic tests and procedures. The literature, again, presents conflicting viewpoints. Morris and Smith found that physician assistants ordered 16 to 21 percent more diagnostic procedures than physicians (28). Other studies have found smaller differences between the ordering practices of physician assistants and physicians. Goldberg and Jolly have concluded that in the absence of ". . . unwarranted ordering of tests, procedures, or therapies" there was no evidence to "demonstrate unnecessary utilization on the part of physician assistants . . . as compared with physicians" (29).

The final component with respect to costs to consumers and society relates to the potential benefit that might be realized as a result of better quality health care being delivered to the public. There are no reliable estimates of potential dollar savings that might be realized from the utilization of physician assistants in medical practice settings. Any research study undertaken to examine long-term benefits should scrutinize both practices using physician assistants and those not using physician assistants in patient care. These studies must include carefully developed indices to document the quality of care delivered and any cost savings resulting from reduced incidence of disease and subsequent decreases in mortality and morbidity rates.

INTERPROFESSIONAL POLITICS

The issue of reimbursement for health services rendered by nonphysician health care providers involves very complex interprofessional political concerns. The concerned parties include physician assistants themselves, organized medicine, other nonphysician providers, legislative bodies and regulatory agencies, and the private and governmental insurers which are responsible for the payment of fees to health care providers. All of these groups have a substantial interest in how reimbursement issues are ultimately resolved.

The relationship between the physician assistant and the physician has been based on the concept of the physician assistant's dependence on physician supervision in the practice setting. Physician acceptance of the notion of non-physician medical care providers has been based, for the most part, on a mutual understanding of the physician assistant's dependent role. Under such circumstances, reimbursement for services provided by the assistant goes directly to the medical practice or to the physician. With very few exceptions, such as in the case of certain rural health clinics, reimbursement for services provided by the physician assistant is not distinguished from reimbursement for services provided by the physician.

By way of contrast, other nonphysicians have lobbied for direct reimbursement for services provided. The best known examples are nurse practitioners and nurse midwives. Their arguments have been based on the premise that nursing services are different from the medical services provided by the physician. This, they argue, removes them from the jurisdiction of state medical practice acts and effectively eliminate the interdependent relationship between the nurse and physician (30). Because this approach has put organized medicine on alert with respect to reimbursement issues, one can postulate that any additional efforts by physician assistants to obtain reimbursement for services may be interpreted by the medical community as a move toward greater independence in practice. Given present concerns about the impact of a physician surplus on future health care expenditures, organized medicine could understandably view the adoption of policies that might further fragment the delivery of health care with disfavor.

The proliferation of providers covered under reimbursement policies has been cause for concern both to legislative bodies and regulatory agencies. Uncertain about the economic impact and extent to which third party payment would intensify inflation in medical care expenditures by increasing both the price of services and the quantity of services delivered, Congress amended the Social Security Act in 1972 by charging the Social Security Administration to study the costs and benefits of employing physician assistants. In authorizing the Physician Extender Reimbursement Study, Congress also expressed the opinion that the rate of experimental reimbursement for physician extender services should be lower than the rate for physician services. Pending the outcome of this study, the Health Care Financing Administration (HCFA) maintained the strict interpretation originally applied to the "incident to" wording of Medicare legislation. This was done to lessen the likelihood of excessive profits accruing to physicians employing numerous physician extenders. Key findings of the study support assertions that the use of physician extenders increases practice productivity and decreases average per visit charges to the patient or third party payor (31). These findings were cited in support of the enactment of P.L. 95-210, the Rural Health Clinic Services Act, allowing for rural health clinics to obtain reimbursement for services that are provided by a physician extender in areas with an identified shortage of health care personnel. HCFA has only recently taken steps to examine performance of physician extenders in these clinics and, with current efforts aimed at the containment of federal expenditures, it is unlikely that HCFA will administratively redefine services incident to the physician's services to include those provided by physician assistants who are not working in designated rural health clinics. Thus, the only apparent alternative available for changing reimbursement policy is legislative, requiring amendment to Titles XVIII and XIX of the Social Security Act.

The impact of legislation at the state level on reimbursement for nonphysician health care services has been significant. With the passage of physician assistant enabling legislation, individual states have included language in opposition to direct reimbursement for services provided by nonphysician providers. Only in those states where enabling legislation has allowed for implementation of the previously mentioned Rural Health Clinic Services Act (P.L. 95-210), has reimbursement for physician assistant services been provided independent of the physician's allowed services. This act was originally viewed as a vehicle for facilitating the delivery of health care services in medically underserved communities. But, as the GMENAC report observed, "For a variety of reasons, the Rural Health Clinic Services Act, which authorized Medicaid and Medicare reimbursement to certified clinics for nonphysician services, has not had a high level of participation and it, therefore, has not served as the catalyst in this area that some had hoped" (32).

Finally, reimbursement issues must be examined from the perspective of the third party payor. There are several major sources of third party dollars for health care services, including Medicare, Medicaid, Blue Cross-Blue Shield plans, commercial insurance companies, and prepaid plans. The Medicare perspective, based on the "incident to" wording, has been discussed in some detail above. The Medicare program is currently willing to reimburse physician assistant services which are *not* normally provided by the physician. Under Part A, Medicare will also reimburse for services provided by physician assistants in institutional settings when those services are included in the overall billing for institutional services. Similarly, the Medicaid program provides for reimbursement of physician assistant services if it appears that the physician provided the service (33). As of 1978, 21 states had explicit policies which provided for Medicaid reimbursement for ". . . NP and/or physician assistant services in at least some outpatient settings" (34). Some states have specific restrictions on the type of nonphysician provider eligible for reimbursement, i.e. ". . . three states will only reimburse PAs and not NPs, while one state only recognizes NPs" (35).

The private health insurance industry has generally followed the lead of the Federally financed programs: private insurers will pay for physician assistant services in the institutional setting when they are included in the overall billing. They also appear willing to pay for physician assistant services if they appear to have been delivered by the physician (36). As one author put it, "It would be reasonably safe to assume that in most instances where the physician certifies that a service has been provided, the carrier generally does not 'look behind the bill' to see who actually provided it" (37). This position has undergone review since passage of P.L. 95–210. With the absence of specific language addressing reimbursement of physician assistant-provided services to Medicare recipients in office-based settings, the intent of Congress was interpreted as disallowing such payments. Subsequently, all intermediaries were instructed by HCFA to notify physicians that physician services rendered by physician assistants are not covered under Part B of Medicare. Moreover, recent challenges by private payors to providers billing for services in this fashion appear to indicate that the practice of "not looking behind the bill" has changed: closer scrutiny may become more commonplace as aggregate health care expenditures continue to rise.

PAYMENT MECHANISMS

Under a system allowing for full reimbursement of physician assistant-provided services under the name of the physician at "usual and customary" rates, the addition of the physician assistant to a medical care practice would not appear to offer any opportunity for savings to either the patient or the third party payor. This premise has been used to encourage the containment of expenditures for health care through the reimbursement of physician assistant-provided services at some rate less than usual, customary, and reasonable charges paid to the physician for similar services. However, the current stance of the medical community is one of supporting reimbursement at existing rates regardless of who provides the service. While this position may facilitate greater utilization of physician assistants, it also offers the potential for considerably greater income to be realized through employment of a physician assistant. The American Academy of Physician Assistants (AAPA) has taken a position favoring reimbursement at a "non-inflationary rate under (i.e., less than) the usual, customary, and reasonable fee for service system" (38). The 1981–1982 *APAP Policy Manual* states that, "Whereas physicians receive reimbursement at 80% of the usual, customary, and reasonable charges for services rendered, that physician assistant services be reimbursed at not less than 70% of the usual, customary, and reasonable charges" (39). These statements have been interpreted to indicate that the physician assistant community favors "fractional reimbursement" at a rate that can allow for profit to the physician, continued utilization of physician assistants, and cost savings to society.

A number of health care providers as well as health policy makers have suggested that the most cost-effective approach to reimbursement for health care services would be one in which a "fixed fee" system was established. They argue that this approach would encourage containment of health care expenditures while allowing for the reimbursement of additional health care providers. Under such a "fixed fee" system, the lowest reasonable charge for providing a particular health care service would be determined. The fee to be paid for that service would be fixed at this lowest cost, regardless of who provided the service. Thus, the "fixed fee" approach would encourage physicians to delegate more responsibility to less expensive providers and to seek more economical ways of delivering services. However, it might also reduce the economic incentives to the point where physicians chose to reduce their participation in publicly sponsored health care programs. This would clearly be an undesirable outcome.

IMPLICATIONS FOR PUBLIC POLICY

The combination of rising expenditures and the growing propensity of government to address this problem by reducing benefits compels examination of the appropriateness of adding physician assistant services to the Medicare and Medicaid benefit packages from two viewpoints: (a) is there a consumer need for additional health services? and (b) should participants in Federal programs be asked to accept services from less extensively trained providers?

Improvements in human life expectancy have created a situation in which chronic diseases now affect more people for longer periods of time. Thus, the expenditures for current and future illness care can be expected to pose an increasing financial problem for society. One strategy to help constrain these rising costs would be to place greater emphasis on health promotion and disease prevention. In this connection, physician assistants have a documented history in the delivery of services "that are . . . preventive and . . . oriented toward education and counseling of the patient" (40). The need for such services is evidenced by smoking, overindulgence in alcohol, overeating, and the lack of exercise as part of an accepted lifestyle in our society. In a delivery system designed to provide and reimburse for illness-oriented services, considerable inertia would have to be overcome to bring about a greater emphasis on preventive services and the recognition of such services as being an integral part of those provided by physicians and other health care providers.

With regard to the delivery of health services by lesser trained providers, we have previously noted that the quality of care provided by physician assistants and nurse practitioners is at least as high as the care rendered by physicians for that range of services and clinical skills for which these providers have been trained (41). Studies on levels of patient satisfaction provide further support for this conclusion (42). These studies suggest that physician assistants may present the most cost-efficient means of providing certain services to consumers in general (not only governmentally funded programs) without sacrificing the quality or quantity of services. However, additional research will be needed to determine the mix of physician assistant-provided health and illness services which offer the greatest potential savings to the health care industry and consumer alike — regardless of the approach to reimbursement.

SUMMARY

Considering the several aspects of the reimbursement issue discussed above, it appears that quality of care does not present a major impediment to reimbursement for physician assistant services. Numerous studies reported in the literature support the argument that physician assistants provide services of comparable quality when utilized appropriately. Conclusions concerning practice productivity are less clear cut. Some evidence indicates significant increases in productivity while other data suggests that the magnitude of the productivity gains may be overstated.

In terms of societal and individual patient costs, conclusions must again be tentative. While potential savings derived from reduced training expenses and lower annual physician assistant income may be important, there is only limited data to suggest that practices employing physician assistants actually charge patients less for comparable services than practices not employing physician assistants. Whether this is due to increased practice overhead costs of physician supervision or differences in the use of support services and resources is unclear. To adequately address this topic, further study is necessary.

Closely tied to reimbursement and productivity issues are the realities of interprofessional politics and the pattern of physician assistant dependence on the physician. There appears to be support within the physician community for payment to the practice at established physician reimbursement rates for services provided by the physician assistant. The support for full reimbursement (equal to that usually received by the physician) appears to provide economic incentives to use physician assistants while assuring recovery of costs related to physician supervision and the delivery of quality medical care services. On the other hand, discussions of reimbursement for services at a lower rate for nonphysician providers and the pursuit of direct reimbursement by certain nonphysician providers have tended to unify the medical profession in its opposition to such proposals.

State legislation has incorporated the idea of practice dependence within laws that codify the physician's right to delegate medical care activities to physician assistants. While states with such laws have redefined the content and extent of services "incident to" the physician's services, policies at both the national and state levels regarding reimbursement have not been progressive and at times have added to the confusion as to whether service provided by the physician assistant, nurse practitioner, or both would qualify for reimbursement under Medicare or Medicaid. Varying state requirements on supervision of the physician assistant further constrain opportunities for enhanced productivity and cost-effectiveness.

Finally, while savings may be possible through the use of a less costly provider of services, it has been suggested by Schweitzer and Record (43) that containment of expenditures for health care can be realized within a system where the fee for service is fixed at the lowest cost regardless of provider. While this might allow an incremental approach to the inclusion of physician assistant services under Medicare and Medicaid as well as setting the stage for a more rational distribution of labor between the physician and physician assistant, the degree of profit to the practice might be reduced to a point where physicians might decrease their level of participation in publicly sponsored health care programs. A further outcome of such an approach could be that beneficiaries of these programs might be placed in the situation of having to absorb a greater portion of their personal health care expenditures through increased rates of coinsurance.

Whether the status quo is maintained, fractional reimbursement is adopted, or a fixed fee system is established remains to be determined. However, the issue of reimbursement for nonphysician provided medical care services has forced us to examine closely the kinds and amounts of health care we are buying, how much, and the manner in which we pay for them. This cannot be anything but a healthy development.

REFERENCES

1. U.S. Department of Health, Education, and Welfare, Social Security Administration, Office of Research and Statistics: personal communication to C.E. Fasser on April 25, 1975, p. 1.
2. *Ibid.*, p. 1.
3. McKibbin, R.: Cost Effectiveness of Physician Assistants: A Review of Recent Evidence. *The PA Journal* (8) 2:110–115, Summer, 1978.
4. Sox, H.: Quality of Patient Care by Nurse Practitioners and Physician's Assistants: A Ten Year Perspective. *Annals of Internal Medicine, 91* (3): 459–468, September 1979.

5. Rushing, W., and Miles, B.: Physicians' Assistants, and the Social Characteristics of Patients in Southern Appalachia. *Medical Care, 15*(12): 1004–1013, December 1977.

6. U.S. Department of Health, Education, and Welfare, Public Health Service, Health Resources Administration: *Report of the Physician Extender Workgroup:* June 1977, pp. 43–53.

7. U.S. Department of Health and Human Services, Public Health Service, Health Resources Administration: Report of the Graduate Medical Education National Advisory Committee (GMENAC) to the Secretary, Department of Health and Human Services, *Volume VI: Nonphysician Health Care Provider Technical Panel,* 1980, p. 9.

8. Mendenhall, R., and Repicky, P.: *Collection and Processing of Baseline Data for the Physician Extender Reimbursement Study: Executive Summary,* Contract HEW-05-100-75-0034, University of Southern California, 1978.

9. System Sciences, Inc.: *Survey and Evaluation of the Physician Extender Reimbursement Experiment,* Final Report. Prepared under Contract SSA-600-76-0167. DHEW, Health Care Financing Administration, Office of Policy, Planning and Research. March 1978.

10. System Sciences, Inc.: *Ibid.,* see note 9.

11. Mendenhall, R., and Repicky, P.: *Ibid.,* see note 8.

12. Golladay, F., Miller, M., and Smith, K.: Allied Health Manpower Strategies: Estimates of the Potential Gains from Efficient Task Delegation. *Medical Care, 11*(6): 457–469, November-December 1973.

13. Nelson, E., Jacobs, A., Breer, P., and Johnson, K.: Impact of Physician's Assistants on Patient Visits in Ambulatory Care Practices. *Annals of Internal Medicine, 82:*608–612, May 1975.

14. Hershey, J., and Kropp, D.: A Re-Appraisal of the Productivity Potential and Economic Benefits of Physician's Assistants. Working Paper.

15. Major, E.: A Comment on 'Re-Appraisal of the Productivity Potential and Economic Benefits of Physician's Assistants.' *Medical Care, 18*(6):686–690, June 1980.

16. Office of Technology Assessment: Case study #16: The costs and effectiveness of nurse practitioners. In *The Implications of Cost-Effective Analysis of Medical Technology,* Washington DC, United States Congress, July 1981, p. 4.

17. Hershey, J. and Kropp, D.: supra, note 13.

18. Congress of the United States, Congressional Budget Office: *Physician Extenders: Their Current and Future Role in Medical Care Delivery,* Background Paper, April 1979, p. ix.

19. Congress of the United States: Congressional Budget Office, ibid., p. xi.

20. System Sciences, Inc.: supra, note 9.

21. System Sciences, Inc.: supra, note 9.

22. GMENAC: supra, note 8, p. 7.

23. Mendenhall, R., and Repicky, P.: supra, note 8.

24. Congress of the United States: Congressional Budget Office, supra, note 18.

25. Record, J., O'Bannon, J., and Mullooly, J.P.: *Cost Effectiveness of Physician's Assistants in a Large HMO.* Final Report, Contract N01-MB-44173(P), Kaiser Foundation Health Services Research Center, November 1975, p. 21.

26. Goldberg, G., and Jolly, D.: *Quality of Care Provided by Physician's Extenders in Air Force Primary Medicine Clinics.* Contract F49620-77-C-0023, The Rand Corporation, January 1980, p. 33.

27. Hershey, J., and Kropp, D.: supra, note 13, p. 602.

28. Congress of the United States: Congressional Budget Office, supra, note 17, p. 17.

29. Goldberg, G., and Jolly, D.: supra, note 26, p. 28.

30. Zimmerman, A.: Comments and Recommendations before the Subcommittee on Rural Development, Committee on Agriculture, Nutrition, and Forestry, Unites States Senate, March 29, 1977.
31. System Sciences, Inc., supra, note 9.
32. GMENAC: supra, note 8, p. 46.
33. Robyn, D., and Hadley, J.: New Health Occupations: Nurse Practitioners and Physicians' Assistants, *National Health Insurance: Conflicting Goals and Policy Choices,* The Urban Institute, Washington, D.C., 1980, pp. 269–299.
34. GMENAC: supra, note 8, p. 45.
35. GMENAC: supra, note 8, p. 46.
36. Weston, J.: Distribution of Nurse Practitioners and Physician Assistants: Implications of Legal Constraints and Reimbursement. *Public Health Reports,* Vol. 95, No. 3, 253–258, May–June 1980.
37. Hanft, R.: Reimbursement for the Services of Physician's Assistants Under Federal and Private Insurance, *Intermediate Level Health Practitioners* (Lippard, V. and Purcell, E., eds.). Josia Macy Foundation, New York, 1973, p. 157.
38. American Academy of Physician Assistants: 1981¢1982 Policy Manual, 307.01.02b., p. 7.
39. American Academy of Physician Assistants: Ibid., 307.01.01.
40. Mendenhall, R., and Repicky, P.: supra, note 8.
41. Cohen, E.: *An Evaluation of Policy Related Research on New and Expanded Roles of Health Workers.* Office of Regional Activitis and Continuing Education, Yale University School of Medicine, October 1974, pp. 97–107.
42. Robyn, D., and Hadley, J.: supra, note 33, p. 274.
43. Schweitzer, S., and Record, J.: Third-Party Payments for New Health Professionals: An Alternative to Fractional Reimbursement in Outpatient Care. *Public Health Reports,* 92(6):518–526, November-December 1977.

Addendum/Author's Note
Office of Technology Assessment: Case study #16: The costs and effectiveness of nurse practitioners. In: *The Implications of Cost-Effective Analysis of Medical Technology,* Washington DC, United States Congress, July 1981, p. 4.

Chapter 45

FACTORS ENCOURAGING THE CONTINUED UTILIZATION OF PRIMARY CARE PHYSICIAN ASSISTANTS,

HENRY B. PERRY, M.D.
JERRY L. WESTON, Sc.D.

The possible negative impact of the growing supply of physicians on the utilization of physician assistants in primary care settings cannot be ignored. A surplus of physicians has been predicted by the Graduate Medical Education National Advisory Committee (GMENAC) by 1990 (see Table 45.1). While a significant surplus of primary care physicians is not envisioned by GMENAC in the near future, a recent RAND study shows that non-primary physicians are going to less-urbanized areas for practice (Newhouse, 1982). There are reports of primary care physician assistants in small communities being displaced by physicians entering practice (Brooks, et al., 1981). Certainly, there will continue to be small communities that cannot support a physician. These will benefit by having a physician assistant.

TABLE 45.1

ESTIMATED NEED AND SUPPLY OF PRIMARY CARE PHYSICIANS IN 1990

Specialty	Estimated Need in 1990	Estimated Supply	Difference (Supply Minus Need)
Family Practice	61,300	64,400	+ 3,100
General Internal	70,250	73,800	+ 3,550
General Medicine	30,250	37,750	+ 7,500
Total	161,800	175,950	+ 14,150

Source: GMENAC, Vol. 1, 1980.

There are a number of populations in dire need of primary care that are not usually considered in such a discussion. The primary care needs of these populations are frequently written off as subsidiary to their principal problems. Prisons, nursing homes, and institutions for the chronically physically and mentally ill are practice settings to which physicians are not usually attracted. The primary care for these types of patients can be provided by physician assistants. In his study of physicians in correctional institutions, Lichenstein concludes that "physician retention should become a secondary goal of correctional health administrators with quality and efficiency of care being primary goals" (1981). He notes that continuity of care could best be accomplished by the use of non-physician providers, with a moderate physician turnover as a built-in constraint. Schultz (1977) in analyzing primary health care needs of the elderly, has pointed out how closely integrated are their physical, mental, and social needs and how these needs could be met by non-physician providers.

Institutional providers of primary health care such as hospitals, industries, health maintenance organizations, community-based clinics, and government operated health programs (e.g., the Indian Health Service, military health care programs) incur significant financial advantages by employing physician assistants or other nonphysician health care providers in place of primary care physicians. Third party reimbursement is usually more readily received by institutional providers than by private practitioners for services provided by nonphysician health care providers. In contrast to private practice settings, there is no significant financial risk to the institutional employer of nonphysician health care providers. The cost-savings generated by salary differentials between the physician assistant and the physician (the former's being usually less than half of the latter) are readily apparent to the institutional providers of primary health care and should result in a continued demand for physician assistants in primary care (Record and O'Bannon, 1976).

Another factor which could very likely influence positively the demand for physician assistants and other nonphysician providers in primary care is the runaway inflation of health care costs and the greatly heightened appreciation of the need to develop policies which lower medical costs. Such policies will undoubtedly encourage the expanded use of nonphysician providers in primary care settings. It is even more likely that such policies could even result in the authorization of a more independent form of practice for properly certified nonphysician primary care providers. Such a policy could lead to an improved geographic distribution of primary care providers and, more importantly, to greater economic competition among providers and consequently lower prices for consumers of primary care services. Current efforts by the Federal Trade Commission to deregulate the practice of medicine and "demonopolize" the medical profession are consistent with this approach, although staunch opposition of the American Medical Association and other medical professional organizations has been incurred.

In many states, physician assistants have been given authorization to write prescriptions for non-narcotic medications (Perry and Breitner, 1982). The approval of policies by third party payors to reimburse nonphysician health providers directly rather than to employing physicians or institutions will be the next major hurdle to be overcome in making financially independent practice feasible. Should such arrangements become feasible, opportunities for physician assistants in primary care will certainly grow considerably.

BEYOND 2000—THE LONGER RANGE VIEW

The current basis for utilizing physician assistants in the delivery of primary care services is clear. But the more important question is what will be the eventual role of physician assistants and other nonphysician health care providers? Stated another way, how will policy decisions regarding the long-term need for physicians in our society be affected by our experience with nonphysician providers of primary care?

This is a most critical question which will, we hope, receive considerable attention over the next two decades. At stake, in part, is a decision on how much our society is willing to spend for health care services.

As Record and O'Bannon (1976) have shown, 75% of adult medical ambulatory visits and 90% of pediatric ambulatory visits can safely be delegated to nonphysician assistants and nurse practitioners. They have estimated that the total cost of primary care services could be reduced by 45% if these theoretical levels of delegation were actually achieved. An implementation of such a policy, however, would require the education and training of far fewer primary care physicians than currently envisioned.

Given the current concern of medical care costs, such a long-term policy does not seem as far fetched as it once might have. Economists have frequently depicted physicians as gate keepers to medical expenses ("supplier induced demand") and furthermore that, in order to earn a reasonable income, physicians encourage medical expenditures for their patients in diagnostic studies, hospitalizations, and so forth (Evans, 1974). Taking this perspective and calculating average health expenditures per physician, Ginzberg (1977) estimated that each physician in 1976 was responsible for $250,000 in health care expenses.

With this perhaps overly simplistic economic concept in mind, it is readily conceivable that long-term manpower projections for physicians can have major implications for society's health care expenditures if physicians maintain their "gate keeper" status. The GMENAC (Vol. 1, 1980) Summary Report recommended a 10% reduction in medical school class size by 1984 and a severe restriction in the number of foreign medical graduates entering the United States yearly. If a full delegation of primary care services to nonphysician providers were seriously envisioned, then considerable reductions beyond 10% in medical school class sizes would be feasible.

A major reliance upon nonphysicians as providers of primary care is indeed unorthodox and almost heretical to many physicians. In a recent editorial addressing the issue of who would give primary care (Rogers, 1981), a major role for physician assistants and nurse practitioners was not given serious consideration. As cost of care issues continue to grow in importance, we believe that support for a strong role of nonphysician providers in primary care will increase over the next several decades. The following evidence supports this line of reasoning:

a) Under appropriate supervision (which is assumed under the full delegation model of Record and O'Bannon described above), the quality of primary care services is just as high as if physicians alone had provided the services.

b) The current need in health care policy today is felt by many to be in identifying strategies of cutting health care costs without sacrificing quality. An expanded role for nonphysician providers in primary health care represents such a policy.

c) Consumer satisfaction, accessibility and availability of services, and costs for services are likely to be optimized by a full delegation of primary care services to nonphysician providers.

d) A decreased reliance upon physicians in providing primary care services would limit their "gate keeper" function as well, thereby reducing medical costs further. Nonphysician providers could more readily than physicians work within clearly stated protocols aimed at keeping costs down without sacrificing quality.

As we look beyond the year 2000, our society will have to decide what role we envision for the primary care physician in the future. Will the emphasis on traditional values lead us to continue to place the physician in the center as the provider of primary care or will an emphasis on reducing costs without sacrificing quality lead us to expand the role of nonphysician providers and cut back significantly in our training of physicians? The policy debate is only now beginning, but the stakes are quite high.

According to one health policy analyst:

The government, by compelling medical schools through the lure of public subsidies to expand their enrollments, has dramatically increased the physician pool. As Washington now reduces its support, the schools will be forced to decide how to respond. The responses to this set of questions are bound to influence how much money the United States ultimately spends on medical care in the future (Inglehart, 1981).

The concept of physician assistants and nurse practitioners as properly trained health professionals capable of providing primary health care *interdependently* rather than *dependently* with physicians has not yet achieved full acceptance, hence the resistance to recognizing those nonphysicians providers as fiscally autonomous providers. The notion of the nurse-midwife as a legitimate provider of uncomplicated maternity care is now finally, after years of struggle and conflict, achieving widespread acceptance (Perry, 1980). This is exhibited by the attitude of the GMENAC Nonphysical Technical Panel toward nurse-midwifery:

> Nurse-midwives should practice interdependently in a health care delivery system and with a formal written alliance with an obstetrician, or another physician or a group of physicians who has/have a formal consultation arrangement with an obstetrician-gynecologist. In some cases, the agreement may be with a hospital which is then responsible for providing obstetrical backup (GMENAC, Vol. 6, 1980).

The appropriateness of properly trained nurse-midwives to perform uncomplicated deliveries is no longer being questioned, and third party payors are recognizing the right of nurse-midwives to receive reimbursement directly partly because of the considerably lower costs involved.

Although the final verdict is far from delivered, we can envision a similar process evolving for nurse practitioners and physician assistants in primary care. As such individuals receive proper training and certification, they will be able to carve out interdependent niches for themselves in primary care settings with formal backup and referral arrangements which allow them to function as semi-autonomous providers of primary care with the capacity to receive payments directly for their services. Such a development should expand consumer choice, lower prices, and expand accessibility without lowering quality. Such a development should provide a secure, important role for the physician assistant in the provision of primary care services in the United States.

*The views presented here are solely the authors' and not necessarily those of the National Center for Health Services Research.

REFERENCES

1. Brooks, E.F., P.A. Guild, and Jane S. Stein: The Future-If-Any-Of New Health Practitioners in Rural Primary Care. Paper presented at the Annual Meeting of the American Public Health Association, 1981.
2. Carter, R.D., and J.F. Gifford: The Emergence of the Physician Assistant Profession. In, Perry, HB and Breitner, B.: *Physician Assistants: Their Contribution to Health Care.* New York, Human Sciences Press, 1982, pp. 19-50.
3. Evans, R.G.: Supplier-Induced Demand—Some Empirical Evidence and Implications. In, M. Perlman (ed.). *The Economics of Health and Medical Care.* New York, N.Y., Halstead Press, 1974.

4. Ginsberg, E.: Paradoxes and Trends: An Economist looks at Health Care. *New England Journal of Medicine, 296:*814-816, 1977.
5. GMENAC (Graduate Medical Education National Advisory Committee) Vol. 1: GMENAC *Summary Report to the Secretary, Department, of Health and Human Services,* 1980, DHHS Publication No. (HRA) 81-651.
6. GMENAC (Graduate Medical Education National Advisory Committee) Vol. 6: *Nonphysician Health Care Provider Technical Panel,* 1980, DHHS Publication No. (HRA) 81-656.
7. Inglehart, J.C.: Shrinking Federal Support Brings New Era to Education in the Health Professions, *New England Journal of Medicine, 305:*1027-1032, 1981.
8. Lichtenstein, R.: *Physician Job Satisfaction and Retention in Correctional Health Programs.* Final report to National Center for Health Services Research (HS 04127). 1981 National Technical Information Service, Springfield, Va., Access No 82-146101.
9. Nelson, E.C., A.R. Jacobs, K. Cordino, and K.G. Johnson: Financial Impact of Physician Assistants on Medical Practice. *New England Journal of Medicine, 293:*527-530, 1975.
10. Newhouse, J.P., *et al.*: Where Have All the Doctors Gone? *Journal of the American Medical Association, 247:*17:2392-2396.
11. Perry, H.B.: Role of the Nurse-Midwife in Contemporary Maternity Care. In D.D. Youngs and A.A. Erhardt (eds.), *Psychosometic Obstetrics and Gynecology,* New York, Appleton-Century-Crofts, 190.
12. Perry, H.B., and B. Breitner: *Physician Assistants: Their Contribution to Health Care.* New York, Human Sciences Press, 1982.
13. Record, J.C., and J.E. O'Bannon: *Cost Effectiveness of Physician Assistants.* HEMIA Contract No 1-MB-44173 (P). Bethesda, Md., Bureau of Health Manpower, 1976.
14. Rogers, D.F.: Who Should Give Primary Care? The Confirming Debate. *New England Journal of Medicine, 305:*577-578, 1981.
15. Schultz, P.R.: *Primary Health Care to the Elderly: An Evaluation of Two Manpower Patterns.* Final report to Medical Care and Research Foundation, Denver, Colorado, 1977.
16. Systems Sciences, Inc.: *Survey and Evaluation of the Physician Extender Reimbursement Program.* Department of Health, Education and Welfare, Contract No SSA-600-76-0167, Bethesda, MD, 1978.
17. Tompkins, R.K., R.W. Wood, B.W. Wolcott, and B.T. Walsh: The Effectiveness and Cost of Acute Requiratory Illness Medical Care Provided by Physicians and Alogorithm-Assisted Physician's Assistants. *Medical Care, 15:*991-1003, 1977.
18. Wright, D.D., R.L. Kane, G.F. Snell, and F.R. Wooley: Costs and Outcomes for Different Primary Care Providers. *Journal of The American Medical Association, 238:*46-50, 1977.

Chapter 46

THE FUTURE FOR THE PRIMARY CARE PHYSICIAN ASSISTANT

JAMES F. CAWLEY, MPH, PA-C
JOHN E. OTT, M.D.

It is now well established that PAs are competent providers of primary care health services. Studies performed over the last ten years show that PAs can manage the majority of patient problems encountered in primary care. Also, the quality of care provided by PAs is comparable to that of physicians. Since the introduction of PAs, major changes have taken place in American health manpower and health care delivery. With the clinical performance of PAs no longer at issue, the question becomes to what extent their capabilities will be used in future delivery of health care services.

THE MANDATE OF PRIMARY CARE

During the 1970's, PA education and deployment focused on solving the major perceived health manpower need of the time—a shortage of primary care providers. Medical educators and health policy makers viewed the PA as a quick and effective way of improving public access to primary care. Although this conceptualization of the PA role as a primary care provider departed from Stead's original views (1), the political momentum for primary care, as well as the acceptance of the assistant concept by organized medicine, created the climate for PAs to emerge as primary care providers.

The political impetus for PAs to enter primary care stemmed largely from the interest of federal policy makers. Based on the success of early (1965) pilot PA educational programs, the National Advisory Commission on Health Manpower in 1967 recommended that the government give "high priority to the training of new categories of health professionals" (2). Among the stipulations attached to financial support for new programs was that PAs be educated as primary care providers, and that emphasis be given to their deployment in medically underserved areas. With passage of the 1971 Comprehensive Manpower Act, the federal mandate for PAs was clearly established in primary care. Over 50 primary care PA programs became operational by 1975. These programs developed a variety of innovative approaches to define relevant curriculums which delineated the specific tasks required of PAs in primary care.

Co-option of PAs by federal policy-makers to primary care was a direct response to counter the growing number of subspecialist who dominated American medicine in the 1960's. PAs were seen as a way to revive some attributes of medical practice that were lost with the demise of general practice. As conceptualized, PAs would reintroduce a humanistic approach to patient care eroded by technology and specialization. By possessing enough medical capabilities to recognize and treat most common patient problems, PAs would also be equipped to re-engender effective patient rapport, to establish continuity of care, and to incorporate the lost attributes of caring, empathy, and provider availability into medical practice.

The practicalities of using PAs as physician extenders was another important reason for the movement toward primary care. Since the medical profession is well known for its conservatism and traditionalism, the founders of the PA concept found it challenging to introduce a new health professional whose role substantially overlapped that of established physicians. PAs would not assume tasks emanating from new technologic advances, like other allied health occupations, but would rather engage in medical practice by performing traditional functions reserved before 1965 only for physicians. Obviously, the political climate and strong federal interest in PAs put organized medicine on the defensive and led to their acceptance of the concept. Even so, the endorsement of PAs by organized medicine was a crucial step in the establishment of the PA profession which represented a dramatic change in the division of medical labor in the United States.

The endorsement of the PA concept by organized medicine has been fully recounted elsewhere (3). A key step was adoption by the AMA House of Delegates in 1971 of guidelines to accredit programs. Entitled "Essential for an Educational Program for the Assistant to the Primary Care Physician" (4), these guidelines represented the AMA's response to growing political and social pressures to legitimize PAs, but carefully defined the expected role of graduates as assistants to physicians in primary care. By limiting the role of PAs to primary care, an area relatively neglected to this point, and by stipulating that PAs must practice under the supervision of their employing physician, the AMA theoretically defined how PAs would be used in medical practice. However, this theoretical plan neither precluded PAs from adapting to changes in demand for health manpower dictated by the medical marketplace nor constrained them from developing new roles outside of primary care.

Perception of the PA role differed amongst founders of the concept. Stead and others at Duke initially defined the PA role as being more technical and routine task oriented and less involved in diagnosis and treatment. On the other hand, Silver and colleagues at Colorado envisioned diagnosis and management as essential skills if Child Health Associates were to effectively expand primary health services. Gradually consensus emerged as PAs entered practice. As quoted by Eugene Schneller, Harvey Estes recalls that, "Those of us who were associated with the early development of the (Duke) PA program did not appreciate the true nature of primary care practice, nor did we understand the needs of the primary care practitioner. This practitioner found that the PA was sufficiently well trained to assume additional duties, and these duties were quickly assigned. Experience revealed that the PA could handle these functions, and they quickly became established as standard" (5). According to Schneller, the PA role evolved from assistant status (performing routine tasks, requiring close supervision) to associate status (performing diagnosis and treatment, requiring remote supervision) and become based on negotiated performance autonomy rather than on defined external standards.

As the PA role took shape within the framework of the primary care mandate, other forces in health manpower were simultaneously occurring that would impact on PAs and their usefulness. The health manpower legislation of the early 1970's not only requested support for education of primary care PAs, but also provided substantial funds to increase the number of physicians enrolled in medical schools. This latter step, along with continuing importation of foreign medical graduates, led to new dynamics affecting not only PAs, but the entire health manpower workforce.

FROM CRISIS TO SURPLUS IN PRIMARY CARE

Substantial progress has been made in resolving the primary care crisis of the late 1960's. Since 1970, the total number of physicians has risen from 323,000 to over 480,000. More physicians have entered primary care practice due to the growth of family practice residency programs and to increased emphasis on primary care education in general internal medical and pediatrics. Board-certified specialists are locating at greater rates in nonmetropolitan communities than in larger cities and in the process are assuming more primary care functions (6). The amount of primary care provided by specialists — a "hidden network" of primary care — may have caused an over-estimate of the original primary care provider deficit (7). Some authors project that, because of the increased number of physicians now enrolled in medical education, primary care physicians will be available for 85% of the population by 1985 and for 94% by 1990 (8).

Further evidence of rapid progress in primary care manpower is provided in the controversial 1980 report of the Graduate Medical Education National Advisory Committee (GMENAC). Based on needs projections in a number of medical specialties, the report suggests a surplus of 70,000 doctors by 1990. The committee acknowledges the substantial contributions of PAs to improvements in primary care delivery, and recommends continuation but not expansion of the number of PAs in training (9).

Some authors question methodology and the validity of GMENAC's projections (10). In many quarters, the report is regarded as inaccurate and alarmist. Moreover, very recent data from the Bureau of Health Professions suggests that some assumptions used by GMENAC were incorrect, and that recalculation shows a much smaller excess of physicians (11). Nonetheless, some view *any* excess of physicians as seriously jeopardizing the future for PAs. As more physicians enter primary care, with projected increased numbers of physicians in private practice, what happens to the rold of the PA in primary care?

One of the more controversial answers to this question has been put forth by Henry Perry. As one of the most notable scholars of the PA profession, Perry proposes that PAs in coming years be granted the opportunity to emerge as independent providers of primary care. Although this notion has been suggested by others, it is Perry who examines this prospect seriously. In his book *Physician Assistants: Their Contribution to Health Care,* Perry argues that "as experience in training these health professionals in primary care becomes more extensive, and as they obtain greater experience as primary care providers, we predict that their need for physician supervision will diminish, although there will continue to be a need for physician referral and consultation (12). Perry bases his rationale on cost-effectiveness data showing that PAs can manage anywhere from 60% to 75% of office visits in primary care at a much lower cost than physicians.

From the viewpoint of public policy in health, it is hard to refute Perry's suggestion. Until now, it has been the employers of PAs who have reaped the benefits of their cost-effectiveness and not the patients. Using PAs to deliver basic primary care services would have a favorable effect on the rising cost of health care delivery. Also, a more autonomous role would provide PAs greater personal and professional rewards.

Perry's idealism must be balanced however, with the practical realities of current day medical practice. Even he concludes that greater autonomy would place PAs in direct competition with primary care physicians in the fee-for-service sector and would no doubt be met by marked physician resistance. It is hard to believe that physicians who, on one hand, face the increasing economic constraints induced by the physician oversupply and who, on the other hand, hold extensive control over the educational, legal, and practice structure of the PA profession, would permit the emergence of PAs as direct competitors in primary care. We have already observed the forceful negative reaction of family physicians to the prospect of independent practice by nurse practitioners. Even Eugene Stead admits that "we can accept it as a given fact that if doctors have a dramatic fall in work load and income, they will combine to kill off all nurse practitioners and all other mid-level health workers . . . Doctors are, after all, human and nothing brings out our humanness more quickly than a threat to our pocketbooks" (13).

Since it is unrealistic to expect an independent role for PAs in primary care practice, what alternative prospects exists?

Much of this book is devoted to the delineation of many new roles for PAs. These roles, in specialty and subspecialty practice, mark a new transition in the use of PAs in medicine. These roles, in surgery, neonatology, geriatrics, occupational medicine, prison health, administration, and emergency medicine are growing, and represent a positive response on the part of PAs to the changing demands of the medical marketplace (14). In many ways, PAs have become true "utility persons" of health care services, fully capable of fulfilling their traditional roles in primary care, yet also able to enter specialty and subspecialty practice settings. Primary care roles for PAs will continue, particularly if one considers the institutional settings where such services are offered.

PRACTICE SETTING AND SPECIALTY

As the future roles expand for PAs, it is important to note the distinction between setting and specialty. Table 1 shows how the practice settings for PAs have shifted in recent years from private practice to institutional settings. The majority of PAs were employed by institutions in 1980. That is not to say however that most PAs are working in non-primary care practices.

TABLE 46.1
MAJOR PRACTICE SETTINGS OF PHYSICIAN ASSISTANTS

	1974 (N = 902) (%)	1978 (N = 3416) (%)	1981 (N = 4496) (%)
Private Solo Practice	23.8	17.9	19.3
Private Group Practice	33.3	16.8	16.5
Total Private Practice	57.1	34.7	35.8
Hospital	14.0	23.7	29.5
Ambulatory Clinic	13.9	23.4	24.9
Military	15.1	18.2	9.4
Total Institutional Practice	43	65.3	63.8

Data from: National Longitudinal Survey of Physician Assistants, Association of Physician Assistant Programs.

A clear majority of PAs indicate that they practice in primary care specialties of family practice, general internal medicine, pediatrics, obstetrics and gynecology (Table 2). Collectively, these figures show that, nearly 70% of PAs work in primary care. Since almost 64% of PAs are employed by institutions, it is obvious that many institutions employ PAs as primary care providers. Thus, while it may be true that the forecasted surplus of physicians, many of whom will probably enter the private practice sector, may curtail some employment possibilities for PAs in private practice, many opportunities will still exist for PAs in primary care institutionally-based settings. The use of PAs by nursing homes, multi-specialty fee for service group practices, HMOs, prison systems, and hospital ambulatory clinics are good examples of this trend.

TABLE 46.2
SPECIALTY DISTRIBUTION OF PHYSICIAN ASSISTANTS

Specialty	*1978 (N = 3416)*	*1981 (N = 4496)*
Family Practice	52.0	53.5
Internal Medicine	12.0	9.6
Surgical Subspecialties	6.2	8.5
General Surgery	5.5	4.9
Emergency Medicine	4.9	4.8
Medical Subspecialties	6.3	2.9
Pediatrics	3.3	3.7
Occupational Medicine	2.7	3.2
Obstetrics and Gynecology	2.0	2.6
Other Specialties	5.1	6.5

Data from: National Longitudinal Survey of Physician Assistants, Association of Physician Assistant Programs.

FUTURE ROLES IN PRIMARY CARE

Despite the anxiety raised by the forecasts of an excess of physicians, the future need for primary care manpower is not likely to abate in the near future. Steinwach and colleagues recently analyzed trends in graduate medical education and found that the number of physicians entering primary care residency training programs has leveled off. Their data show that an increasing percentage of MDs entered primary care specialties from 1970 to 1976 due largely to the growth of family practice. But from 1976 to 1980, there was no increase in percentages of physicians pursuing primary care training. Also, they note that the growth of family practice has now stabilized, and that increases in the primary care health providers are likely to be needed to meet demand (15).

Even so, it is still difficult to predict an unlimited future for PAs in private practice settings offering primary care services. Increasing competition between primary care providers, physician concern over independent practice by nurse midwives and nurse practitioners, and the ready availability of newly graduated physicians are all likely to constrain the employment prospects of PAs in private practice. Nevertheless, opportunities in primary care in other settings will continue.

One cannot underestimate the importance of the cost effectiveness of PAs, particularly to institutions. Hospitals and other health care facilities have been forced recently to operate within increasingly constrained budgets. As health care dollars become less readily available, many institutions will seek solutions that will allow them to maintain the quality and quantity of existing primary care services, but at a lower cost. Many of these institutions will consider new approaches to manpower staffing patterns, and the use of PAs in such approaches seems logical and beneficial.

Other settings that may benefit from the use of primary care PAs are free-standing clinics. The growing trend toward corporate involvement in health care delivery has led to the opening of many free-standing health clinics, often known as surgi-centers, emergi-centers, and so forth. The benefits of using PAs in such clinics has not been formally studied, but it would appear from studies on PA use by HMOs that PAs would be cost-effective and improve access to care in these facilities as well.

The future for PAs in primary care, as well as in all other areas, is intimately linked to the physicians who employ or will employ them. As we have indicated, the PA profession has undergone a considerable transformation since it was founded, a transformation characterized by an ability to meet the changing demands for medical manpower throughout a wide spectrum of settings. Certainly, a marked increase in physician population by 1990 will have an effect on PAs just as it will on physicians. And it may be that we will see a return of the PA role to that of "true assistant" as predicted by Schneller. The PA, instead of becoming the primary care provider of the 1990s, may become more closely aligned in their roles to physicians, be it in primary or specialty care (5).

The role of the PA in primary care will undoubtedly change during the 1980's. Many tasks in primary care will remain with the PA and could possibly expand if increasing emphasis continues in the area of preventive services and health education. These practice areas continue to be avoided by physicians and represent services that complement rather than duplicate the activities of physicians. Should public demand for preventive services increase, the need for primary care PAs will most certainly grow.

In examining the PA profession, many authors have described it as the single most dramatic innovation in health manpower of the last 25 years. Such a description is apt. Given the contributions and accomplishments of PAs thus far, the innovation will continue to grow and evolve in the next 25 years as dramatically as it has in the last.

REFERENCES

1. Stead, E.A. The Duke Plan for Physician Assistant. *Med Times,* 1967, *95:*40-48.
2. National Advisory Commission on Health Manpower. *Report of the National Advisory Commission on Health Manpower (Vols. I and II).* Washington, D.C., U.S. Government Printing Office. November, 1967.
3. Carter, R.R., Gifford, J.F. The Emergence of the Physician Assistant Profession. *PAs: Their Contribution to Health Care.* Henry B. Perry and Bina Breitner. New York: Human Science Press, 1981.
4. American Medical Association Council on Medical Education. *Essentials of an Accredited Educational Program for the Assistant of the Primary Care Physician* Chicago: AMA, 1971.
5. Schneller, E.S. *The Physician Assistant—Innovation in the Medical Division of Labor.* Lexington, MA: D.C. Heath Co., 1978.
6. Schwartz, W.B., Newhouse, J.P., Bennett, B., Williams, A.P. The Changing Geographic Distribution of Board Certified Physicians. *New England Journal of Medicine,* 1980, *303:*1032-1038.
7. Aiken, L.H., Lewis, C.E., Craig, L., Mendenhall, R.C., Blendon, R.J., Rogers, D.E. The Contribution of Specialists to the Delivery of Primary Care. *New England Journal of Medicine* 1979, *300:*1363-1370.
8. Aiken, L.H. Physicians: How Many Do We Need? *Ann Int Med,* 1980, *93:*135-136.
9. U.S. Department of Health and Human Services. *Report of the Graduate Medical Education National Advisory Committee.* Hyattsville, MD: Department of Health and Human Services, 1980, DHHS Pub. No. 81-651.
10. Reinhardt, U. The GMENAC Forecast: An Alternative View. *Am Journal of Public Health,* 1981, *71:*1149-1157.
11. U.S. Department of Health and Human Services. *Third Report to the President and Congress on the Status of Health Profession Personnel in the United States, January 1982.* Hyattsville, MD: Department of Health and Human Services, 1982; DHHS Pub. No. 82-2.
12. Perry, H.B., Breitner, B. *Physician Assistants: Their Contribution to Health Care.* New York: Human Science Press, 1981.
13. Stead, E.A. Physician Assistants and Internal Medicine. *Am Journal of Medicine,* 1981, *70:*1161-1162.
14. Cawley, J.F., Ott, J.E., DeAtley, C.A. The Future for Physician Assistants. *Annals of Internal Medicine,* 1983, *98:*993-997.
15. Steinwachs, D.M., Levine, D.M., Elizinga, D.J., Salkever, D.S., Parker, R.D., Weissman, C.S. Changing Patterns of Graduate Medical Education. *New England Journal of Medicine,* 1982, *396:*10-14.

Chapter 47

ISSUES REGARDING THE DEVELOPMENT OF COMPETENCY EVALUATION OF PHYSICIAN ASSISTANTS IN NON-PRIMARY CARE SPECIALTIES

HENRY R. DATELLE, ED.D.
DON E. DETMER, M.D.

The title, "Physician Assistant," as interpreted by the National Commission on Certification of Physician Assistants, is a generic term referring to a type of mid-level health practitioner who performs tasks traditionally within the purview of physicians and under the supervision of a clearly identified physician. In many instances, those people who qualify as physician assistants may perform under different titles such as: physician's associate, child health associate, Medex, nurse practitioner, nurse clinician, surgeon's assistant, surgical physician assistant, and so forth. Although the major training emphasis has been in primary care, physician assistants function in a wide variety of specialty settings (1, 2).

Historically, physician assistants perform an evaluative function; they are capable of eliciting a complete history and performing routine physical examinations on all types and ages of patients and across all body systems. Additionally, physician assistants can order and/or perform non-life-threatening diagnostic procedures and can interpret results and isolate abnormalities. They are also trained to carry out specific management regimens under physician direction and to take necessary, immediate action to preserve life in emergency situations. They often perform minor surgical services (e.g., removal of foreign objects from eyes, minor sutures, and so forth). Physician assistants may perform other isolated functions specific to the specialty setting in which they work. It is important to emphasize that *physician assistants are not independent;* they must work under physician supervision, and the identified physician supervisor is clearly responsible for the physician assistants professional activity.

Physician assistant programs developed and proliferated in the late 1960's and early 1970's with major emphasis in one specialty area: primary care. The efforts of organizations including the American Academy of Family Physicians, American Academy of Pediatrics, American College of Physicians, American College of Surgeons, American Medical Association, and American Society of Internal Medicine brought focus to the need that mechanisms and formal sets of essentials were necessary to accredit training programs in order to assure the quality of the education processes. Consequently, the above listed organizations developed the *Essentials of an Approved Educational Program for the Assistant to the Primary Care Physician,* which was charged with the responsibility of reviewing and recommending accreditation of programs to the AMA Council on Medical Education through its Advisory Committee on Allied Health. It was understood that surgeon's assistants programs would be accredited by the American College of Surgeons, which subsequently generated appropriate essentials for surgeon's assistant training programs. The AMA adopted these essentials and in an effort to provide generic accreditation. The two processes were then merged in 1976 to form the Joint Review Committee on Educational Programs for Physician Assistants (JRC-PA), which now functions under the aegis of the Committee on Allied Health Education and Accreditation (CAHEA). CAHEA accredits both primary care and surgical care programs as physician assistant programs. Accreditation is awarded to programs preparing assistants to the primary care physician and surgeon's assistants when they conform with the appropriate essentials.

Such accreditation mechanisms, however, only evaluate the educational processes and not the products of the training programs. The next step, under the auspices of the federal government and private foundations and with the endorsement of the physician assistant profession, was to develop a mechanism to assess the competency of the products of the training programs. The National Board of Medical Examiners (NBME) developed and first administered the Certifying Examination for Primary Care Physician Assistants in December, 1973. At the same time, nurse practitioner, nurse clinician, and child health associate programs were gaining momentum. Graduates of these programs were also eligible to take the examination, as were informally trained primary care physician assistants who had met specific, stringent eligibility criteria as attested to by supervising physicians. Since the examination was in primary care, graduates of surgeon assistant programs were not eligible.

The responsibilities for establishing eligibility criteria for the examination and for subsequently certifying those who passed the examination were new and uncomfortable roles for NBME. Consequently, NBME, together with representatives of 13 other professional groups (see Table 47.1), agreed in late 1973 to form a free-standing, independent commission to assure the physician assistant profession, employers, state licensing boards and, most importantly, the patients, of the competency of this new class of health professional. In February, 1975, after being formally structured, organized, and funded by the Department of Health, Education, and Welfare (Division of Associated Health Professions), and the Robert Wood Johnson Foundation, the National Commission on Certification of Physician Assistants (NCCPA) opened its national offices in Atlanta, Georgia.

TABLE 47.1
NCCPA BOARD OF DIRECTORS

American Academy of Family Physicians
American Academy of Pediatrics
American Academy of Physician Assistants
American College of Physicians
American College of Surgeons
American Hospital Association
American Medical Association
American Nurses' Association
American Society of Internal Medicine
Association of American Medical Colleges
Association of Physician Assistant Programs
Federation of State Medical Boards of the United States
National Board of Medical Examiners
Department of Defense

The major charge of NCCPA has been directed toward the specialty area of largest physician assistant concentration—primary care. DHEW (now DHHS) has previously funded, with a few exceptions, only training programs in this specialty. Consequently, the certifying examination was developed for administration to those people who had been trained and were functioning in the primary care role.

The rapid growth of the physician assistant concept and the resulting state rules and regulations enabling physician assistant practice have created a dilemma for the physician assistant who has graduated from or works in a non-primary care setting. This is particularly true for surgeon's assistants. In many states, a physician assistant is not allowed to practice until he is certified by NCCPA. However, the current examination is designed to measure competency in primary care only. Currently, there is not an appropriate mechanism available to evaluate the competencies of those individuals trained in specialty settings other than primary care. In order to prevent disenfranchising the surgeon's assistant, and only as an interim solution, graduates of accredited surgeon's assistant programs have been eligible to sit for the NCCPA examination since 1976.

This paper will discuss the position of NCCPA with reference to the current dilemma now facing the specialty physician assistant with emphasis on the surgeon's assistant. Emphasis will be given to identifying the problem, discussing the need, reviewing ways to measure specialty competency, identifying the eventually desired solution, and specifying evolutionary steps to attain that solution.

STATEMENT OF THE ISSUE

The substantial amount of public and private money expended to support programs training assistants to the primary care physician testifies to the degree of interest in the physician assistant concept, notably to relieve primary care manpower shortages in medically underserved areas. There was a concern that physician assistants would follow the trend in medicine, and gravitate to secondary and tertiary care centers in the suburbs. The data thus far shows that this has largely not occurred, although certainly there are physician assistants working in such settings (1, 2). A substantial percentage of physician assistants may be found in areas of health care scarcity, and most are involved in primary care. Further, most physician assistants seem to be remaining in primary care as their careers.

Some surgeons have suggested that qualified surgeon's assistants work in teaching centers, replacing interns and junior residents. This would allow the system to decrease the production of excess numbers of surgeons. A substitution of surgeon's assistants performing some of the functions usually performed by surgical residents would also produce economies which are sorely needed. Surgical utilization data suggests that an increase in the number of surgeons *increases* the total volume of surgery performed (3). This argument for training surgeon's assistants is most compelling from a public policy perspective. However, it is also possible that surgeon's assistant training programs will develop in excess numbers relative to need, since it is possible to pay a student in training far less than one would pay a fully fledged surgeon's assistant in such a situation. After producing too many surgeon's assistants for teaching center needs, the market might then become over-supplied, causing surgeon's assistants to move into suburban practice settings in order to secure employment. NCCPA is concerned that programs carefully monitor demand for manpower and only train surgeon's assistants in appropriate numbers.

The issues surrounding the certification of any and all types of specialty physician assistants are complex. At this time, the principal need is for a competency examination in the surgical specialty. The arguments in favor of the development of a surgical examination are most compelling, but since the physician assistant concept is still a relatively recent one, it is important that due caution be exercised. Undue haste in developing an independent surgical examination may, if not integrated into a sensible overall strategy, lead to excessive specialization of physician assistants similar to that seen in medicine generally. The NCCPA intends to approach the surgical examination in a manner consistent with an orderly evolution of this important new profession.

At present, there is no nationally acceptable, clearly defined role for any specialty physician assistant other than in primary care. A careful review of the surgical field will provide a good model for generalizing to all other physician assistant specialties. Currently, surgical physician assistants seem to fall into five categories:

1. graduates of accredited surgeon's assistant programs;
2. graduates of primary care programs who have taken a surgical track;
3. graduates of primary care programs who are employed by surgeons;
4. informally trained surgeon's assistants;
5. graduates of unaccredited surgeon's assistant programs.

Surgical physician assistants are not only trained in a variety of different settings, but they are also functioning in a variety of roles. The challenge of measuring competency in a relevant manner is, therefore, a matter of identifying the role of the physician assistant in surgery and assuring that surgical physician assistants and surgeons are willing to accept the identified role as being appropriate place. A statement of the American College of Surgeon's position regarding Surgeon's Assistants may be found in the April, 1977 (Vol. 62, No. 4) and December, 1977 (Vol. 62, No. 12) Bulletin of the American College of Surgeons Journal.

NCCPA has struggled with this issue for three years, and has actively pursued meeting the needs of this population. During this period, many recommended solutions have evolved. First, the Specialty Physician Assistant and Eligibility Committees have allowed graduates of AMA-approved Surgeon's Assistant Programs to sit for the primary care certifying examination beginning in 1976. It was decided that, although this examination is decidedly not a measure of the surgical competencies needed by a surgeon's assistant, eligibility offered a reasonable short term solution. This approach does not solve the basic problem, however. It requires surgeon's assistants to possess what *may* be irrelevant knowledge and skills and does not measure competency specific to surgery. However, a number of Fellows of the American College of Surgeons have voiced the opinion that surgeon's assistants do need to possess primary care competencies.

Second, in 1977 NCCPA's Eligibility Committee recommended re-evaluating the eligibility criteria for the informally trained physician assistant. It was decided that an individual who was performing primary care functions in the employment of a surgeon and met certain eligibility criteria would be allowed to sit for the examination. This decision allowed some additional surgeon's assistants to sit for the examination beginning in 1978. The issue of eligibility is still being actively examined by the appropriate committees within the Commission and it is feasible that further changes will occur in the future.

Third, NCCPA has looked at different alternatives to assessing the competence of the specialty physician assistant. One alternative considered was to develop a separate examination for each specialty. This method would examine a highly specific knowledge base, a very favorable quality. However, it would be a very costly method. It might also create market imbalances, making it difficult for some physician assistants to find work. This method would also confuse the already muddy legal issue of state regulations.

A second alternative considered was to administer a "core" primary care examination with specialty add-ons. This would be an easy examination to administer, but the specialty physician assistant would be required to be knowledgeable in some areas that may not be relevant to his specialty role. Also, this method leaves one with the impression that primary care does not require special expertise.

A final alternative would require the separation of primary care from core, an activity that NCCPA has already attempted once, without success. While this type of an examination might be easy to administer, it is very difficult to develop.

The nature of any certifying examination requires that development of test items be very thorough. The test must possess reliability and internal validity and must provide a broad spectrum sample of knowledge and skills necessary to perform in the professional role. One must first know the role of the population being examined. Prior to the development of the National Certifying Examination for Primary Care Physician Assistants, detailed surveys were provided to over 800 physician assistants and were then reduced to a malleable manner. Examination test questions were then developed on the basis of skills and knowledge necessary to perform the tasks depicted in the task statements. NCCPA has already accomplished the development of an interim surgical examination.

After considerable discussion, NCCPA has decided to continue to strive for the development of an examination that will measure the core competencies required of a generic physician assistant while simultaneously evaluating the specialty areas in question.

Preliminary steps taken toward the Surgical Examination are representative of approaches to other specialty areas. A survey form was developed and mailed to 225 known surgeon's assistants, and a similar form was sent to their employing surgeons. Based on the distribution of response, a Test Committee utilized the information provided from the questionnaires to develop test items. The Test Committee is composed of surgeon's assistants, surgeon's assistant training program personnel, and surgeons acceptable to the American College of Surgeons. The surgical examination component emphasized general surgery but allowed for those with emphasis in a surgical sub-specialty. Graduates of accredited surgical sub-specialty programs might eventually be eligible for the examination. To pass, one would have to have sufficient knowledge in general specialties. For example, an orthopedic assistant would be expected to do well in the general surgical questions, extremely well in the orthopedic questions, and perhaps not so well in the urological questions. This is the philosophy behind the primary care examination which has worked so extraordinarily well. It allows for a general examination while still permitting considerable latitude in training emphasis. The examination has been administered twice with statistically reliable results. Currently, if a physician assistant successfully completes both the primary care examination and surgery add-on, certification is granted as a physician assistant with Special Recognition in Surgery. NCCPA is continuing to review this process and is considering a request from the American College of Surgeons regarding full certification as a surgeon's assistant. However, NCCPA still remains committed to generic certification and that position remains the current policy.

POSITION OF NCCPA

At a recent NCCPA Board of Directors meeting, a decision was reached which places NCCPA in the position of accepting the responsibility for the certification of all physician assistants regardless of their specialty training. In concert with this, the decision was made that examinations would be developed as soon as appropriate participating organizations requested such development and funding is arranged to support such examinations.

The major goal of NCCPA is to provide a generic core examination that all physician assistants would have to pass. This core examination would be supplemented by additional specialty sub-parts that would be optional choices for examination candidates. NCCPA may use an interim surgical examination as an initial step toward this ultimate goal. The results of this examination could be studied with the intent of identifying those items most appropriate for measuring the competency of surgeon's assistants, as well as identifying those items most appropriate for developing the "core" examination.

If NCCPA pursues this option, it anticipates gaining knowledge that will enable it to develop future examinations that will not only evaluate core knowledge and skills, but will also provide a mechanism for evaluating specialty areas that an individual physician assistant may choose. We anticipate that three to five years of experience will be needed to achieve the ultimate objective.

NCCPA has a unique responsibility as a national certifying body with its diverse representation from the health professions and the public. At this time, the Commission is uncertain about the immediacy for development of any specialty examination beyond that for Surgeon's Assistants. However, looking toward the future, NCCPA will seek to address the needs of both the public and the physician assistant profession. To achieve this end, the Commission will periodically review professional realities and adjust its positions as circumstances warrant.

REFERENCES

1. Light, J.A., Crain, M.J., and Fisher, D.W.: Physician Assistant: A Profile of the Profession, 1976. *The P.A. Journal,* Vol. 7, No. 3, 1977.
2. Perry, H.B., and Fisher, D.W.: The Physician's Assistant Profession: Results of a 1978 Survey of Graduates. *Journal of Medical Education, 56*:839–845, 1981.
3. Detmer, Don E., and Tyson, Timothy, J.: Regional Differences in Surgical Care Based Upon Uniform Physician and Hospital Discharge Abstract Data. *Annals of Surgery,* Vol. 187, No. 2, February, 1978, J.B. Lippincott Company, page 166.

Chapter 48

THE ROLE OF SURGICAL PHYSICIAN ASSISTANTS IN CORRECTING THE OVERPRODUCTION OF SURGEONS

HENRY B. PERRY, M.D.
DON E. DETMER, M.D.

The Graduate Medical Education National Advisory Committee's (GMENAC) 1980 report on physician manpower dramatically argued that at current rates of production, the number of general surgeons projected for 1990 would exceed by 11,800 the estimated reasonable need. This was the largest "surplus" projected for any single specialty, although the *total* projected surplus of all physicians in 1990 was 70,000.

Our own calculations lead us to project a considerably smaller surplus of general surgeons in 2000 of approximately 2,500 (Perry and Detmer, 1983). Nevertheless, there is widespread agreement that too many general surgical specialists are now being trained and that a reduction in the number of surgical residents is now in order. Major influences on the development of this point of view were the Study on Surgical Services for the United States (SOSSUS), which documented an alarming increase in the numbers of surgeons being trained in the mid-1970's (Zuidema, 1982), studies which have documented very low operative work loads of general surgeons in the United States (Hauck *et al.*, 1979; Hughes *et al.*, 1976), and studies showing that the number of general surgeons per capita in England and in prepaid group practices in the United States is almost half that for the U.S. in general (Bunker, 1970; Boardman, 1971; Hughes *et al.*, 1974; Watkins *et al.*, 1976).

CAUSE OF THE SURPLUS OF GENERAL SURGEONS

Although the number of medical students in the U.S. virtually doubled in the period from 1965–1975, this was not the cause of the overproduction of general surgeons. Rather it had to do with local manpower needs within hospitals for surgical housestaff. Immediately after World War II, a number of residency programs in all specialties were instituted around the United States. The war had created a "backlog" of U.S. physicians wanting to pursue residency training since at that time the virtues of specialization were becoming widely appreciated. As this "backlog" completed their training in newly established residency programs in the early 1950's, the supply of new medical graduates was not sufficient to fill all the available slots for residency training (Creditor and Creditor, 1975). By this time, hospitals had learned that residents were useful and valuable. Neither the hospitals as institutions nor their physician attending staff wanted to terminate residency training, particularly in surgery, because of the valuable services they performed: managing emergencies at all hours, providing continuous and close care of critically ill patients, performing routine patient care duties for private patients including admission history and physical examinations and postoperative care, providing care for indigent patients, and providing assistance to private surgeons in the operating room.

An appreciation for the services provided by residents led to an expansion of residency training programs. Available training positions soon far outstripped the available supply of U.S. medical graduates. Thus, the two decades following the mid 1950's demonstrated a marked continuous growth in numbers of residency positions, numbers of residents *and* numbers of foreign medical graduates entering residency training in the U.S. (see Figure 48.1). It was this post-World War II development which provided a major stimulus for the specialty maldistribution, which is only now beginning to be corrected, of too few primary care physicians and too many non-primary care physicians. The incentives to teaching hospitals to develop and expand training programs in primary care were not as great as the incentives to do so in non-primary care specialties.

In surgery, the number of residents being trained was not based on total projected need in the region or in the area of the institution but rather on the local *intrainstitutional* manpower needs for physician housestaff. Thus, by 1974 the rate of increase in the production of general surgeons was seven times the rate of increase of the U.S. population (Moore, 1976).

RECENT EFFORTS TO REDUCE THE NUMBER OF GENERAL SURGEONS BEING TRAINED

Because the projected surplus of surgeons has been recognized by the surgical profession and by the public, there have been serious efforts to reduce the number of general surgeons being trained. The number of general surgical residency *programs* has decreased from 536 in 1970-1971 to 352 in 1980-1981 (Zuidema, 1982). Nevertheless, the total number of surgical

residents has remained relatively constant. Since 1981, however, the number
of first year residency positions in general surgery has declined substantially
from 2,746 in 1978-1979 to 2,100 in 1982-1983 (American Medical Association, 1978 and 1982).

Nevertheless, there is an ever growing appreciation that high quality patient
care, especially in surgery, requires the round-the-clock close support that
housestaff can provide. As the care of surgical patients becomes increasingly
complex and labor intensive, the need is for *increasing* numbers of housestaff,
not a diminishing number.

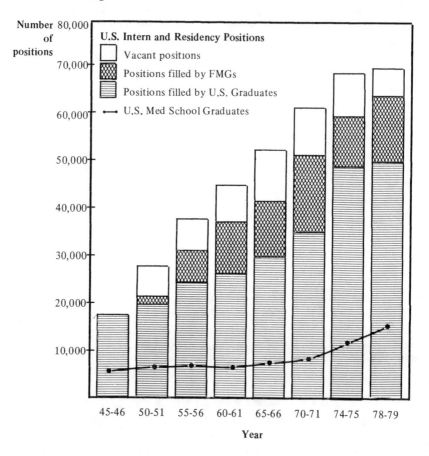

Figure 48.1. Internship and Residency Training Positions since World War II

Reprinted by permission from *Physician Assistants: Their Contribution To Health Care.* By
H.B. Perry and B. Breitner. Human Sciences Press, Inc., New York, N.Y.

THE ROLE OF THE SURGICAL PHYSICIAN ASSISTANT

The only meaningful way to solve the dilemma of reducing the number of housestaff because of a surplus of surgeons and at the same time to provide increasing numbers of support personnel for patient care responsibilities is to use housestaff who will not become practicing surgeons. While it is conceivable that such a role could be carried out by physicians willing to serve in a housestaff position as a permanent job rather than as an educational experience, we feel that this would be an unwise policy. Physicians would be relatively costly to employ. Considerably greater salaries would be required compared to those received by residents-in-training. Furthermore, the possibility of professional frustration would be quite high. Stated in other terms, a physician would be overtrained for the position, especially after functioning with the same set of responsibilities for several years.

Our bias is strongly in favor of using surgical physician assistants in this type of role (Detmer and Perry, 1982). The basis for our attitude lies in the very positive experiences of many institutions in employing physician assistants to function in this manner (Heinrich *et al*, 1980). It should be clearly stated that such persons would not actually perform surgery, as physician surgical residents do under supervision. Surgical physician assistants working in housestaff positions would serve as a supporting member of a surgical team functioning under the direction and authority of a fully trained general surgeon or, in some cases, under the direction of a senior resident.

Although nurses could possibly be trained to function in these kinds of roles if appropriate training were provided, we are reluctant to promote this option. For the surgical physician assistant concept to work effectively, it must be crystal clear that the team approach to patient care under the leadership of a fully trained surgeon or senior surgical resident is fully accepted. Physician assistants are trained with these team concepts in mind.

The general trend of professional independence in nursing, on the other hand, would easily become counterproductive to the close supervision and teamwork which surgical residency programs require for effective patient care. Nurses working in expanded roles in hospital settings typically remain under the administrative control of nursing departments.

NUMBERS OF SURGICAL PHYSICIAN ASSISTANTS REQUIRED TO REPLACE SURGICAL RESIDENTS

We have reported elsewhere an estimate of the reduction in the number of general surgical residents being trained which would be required if the surplus of general surgeons now projected for the year 2000 were to be avoided (Perry,

Detmer, and Redmond, 1983). We calculated that the number of first year residents in general surgery should be reduced from 2,100 in 1982-1983 to 1,690 in 1984-1985 and maintained at that level thereafter until the year 2000 in order for the number of general surgeons in the year 2000 to correspond to the anticipated need. It is readily acknowledged that determining the antici-pated need for general surgeons requires making a number of assumptions which could be subject to criticism (See Perry, Detmer, and Redmond, 1983, for more details).

Nevertheless, assuming such a reduction were made and surgical physician assistants were employed to replace the "lost" physician surgical residents, we estimate that approximately 300 physician assistants per year for five years beginning in 1984 would need to be employed to provide the services now be-ing provided by those physician residents. It has been the experience at the University of Alabama at Birmingham that three surgeon's assistants perform the patient care responsibilities of two surgical residents (Laws *et al.*, 1978).

There are sufficient numbers of physician assistants now being trained to make this feasible — 1,500 per year. Furthermore, it is quite possible that some physician assistants now working in primary care positions could be attracted into surgical employment, particularly if jobs in primary care become harder to find as a result of a rapidly growing physician population.

We anticipate that surgical physician assistants will become increasingly used in hospitals as surgical housestaff even if the number of general surgical residents is not reduced. The need for surgical housestaff is growing, and it is very clear that for the foreseeable future there will be no increase in physician surgical housestaff. This will be especially so in surgical specialties such as orthopedics or cardiac surgery where the number of operations per capita is growing rapidly. This is in contrast to general surgery where the number of operations per capita is remaining constant or declining (Rutkow and Zuidema, 1981, Rutkow, 1982). Surgical physician assistants can provide very helpful support in institutions in which the number of junior physician surgical residents rotating on these subspecialty services is not adequate to

A national survey of surgical department chairmen in hospitals of 400 or more beds in 1979 demonstrated a use of surgical physician assistants in one-third of these institutions, a very positive attitude toward surgical physician assistants among department chairmen in institutions in which surgical physi-cian assistants were working, and a major expansion in the utilization of surgical physician assistants envisioned over the next five years (Perry, Detmer and Redmond, 1981). Thus, the stage for implementing a policy of replacing a selected number of general surgical residents and even possibly residents in surgical subspecialties with surgical physician assistants now seems to be set.

CONCLUSION

The days during which a university or community based teaching hospital could determine the need for surgical housestaff on the basis of intrainstitutional demands for patient care has now passed. As we look toward the future, we can project an ongoing need for high level support personnel who function in a manner similar to physician housestaff. This is also true for medical subspecialties whose growth during the past decade in many ways parallels the growth of surgical specialties.

The growth of the non-primary care specialties for which future surpluses are now predicted can be readily brought under control by replacing physician trainees with physician assistants in the housestaff role. Some may criticize the growing employment of physician assistants in these non-primary care fields since the original vision for the physician assistant movement was to provide assistance to overworked primary care physicians in rural areas. Nevertheless, it should be recognized that the utilization of physician assistants as housestaff in non-primary care specialties gives hospitals the policy option of reducing the number of physicians being trained in specialties for which a significant surplus is now envisioned. This is now possible because the patient care responsibilities assigned to these physician housestaff can, in large measure, be turned over to physician assistants. Thus, physician assistants provide, for the first time, a leverage which makes it possible to readjust more appropriately a mix of primary care and non-primary care physicians without sacrificing the quality of care for hospitalized patients or overly inconveniencing their supervising physicians.

REFERENCES

1. American Medical Association: Directory of residency training programs (All volumes). Chicago, American Medical Association, 1972-1981.
2. Boardman J: Utilization data and the planning process: In: Somers A., ed.: The Kaiser-Permanente Medical Care Program: a symposium. New York, The Commonwealth Fund, 1971; 61-70.
3. Bunker, JP: Surgical manpower: a comparison of operations and surgeons in the United States, and in England and Wales. *N. Engl J Med, 282*(3):135-177, 1970.
4. Creditor, MC, and Creditor, UK: Residency: The Fallacy of need. *N. Engl J Med., 293*:1202-1203, 1975.
5. Crowley AE: Graduate medical education in the United States. JAMA, *246*(25):2938-2944, 1981.
6. Goodman LF: Physician distribution and medical licensure in the U.S., 1976. Chicago, American Medical Association, 1977.
7. Graduate Medical Education National Advisory Committee: Summary report of the Graduate Medical Education National Advisory Committee to the Secretary, Department of Health and Human Services; Volume I.

8. Griffen WO: American Board of Surgery: Annual Report. *Bull Am Coll Surg,* *65*(12):36-38, 1980.

9. Hauck WW, Nickerson RJ, Bloom BS, and Peterson, OL: General surgeons and their surgical practices. *Surgery, 85*(3):303-310, 1979.

10. Haug, JN and Kuntzman K: Socio-economic factbook for surgery 1980. Chicago, IL, American College of Surgeons, 1980.

11. Heinrich JJ, Fichlander, BC, Beinfield M, Frazier W, Krizek TJ, and Baue AE: The physician's assistant as resident on surgical service. *Arch Surg, 115*(3):310-314, 1980.

12. Hughes EFX, Fuchs VR, Jacoby JE, and Lewit EM: Surgical work loads in a community practice. *Surgery, 71*(3):315-327, 1972.

13. Hughes EFX, Lewit EM, Watkins RN, and Handschin R: Utilization of surgical manpower in a prepaid group practice. *N. Engl J Med, 291*(15):759-763, 1974.

14. Hughes EFX, Lewit EM, and Lorenze FV: Time utilization of a population of general surgeons in community practice. *Surgery, 77*(3):371-383, 1975.

15. Laws HL, Kirklin MK, Diethelm AG, Hall J, and Kirklin JW: Training and use of surgeon's assistants. *Surgery, 83*(4):445-450, 1978.

16. Moore FD: Manpower goals in American surgery. *Ann Surg, 184*(2):125-144, 1976.

17. Nicherson RJ, Colton T, Peterson OL, Bloom BS, and Hauck WW: Doctors who perform operations: a study on in-hospital surgery in four diverse geographic areas. *N. Engl J Med, 295*(18):982-989, 1976.

18. Perry HB, and Breitner B: *Physician assistants; their contribution to health care.* New York, Human Sciences Press, 1982.

19. Detmer, DE, and Perry, HB: The Utilization of surgical physician assistants: Policy Implications for the Future. *Surg. Clinics of N. Amer., 62*(4):669-675, 1982.

20. Perry, HB, Detmer DE, and Redmond EL: The current and future role of the surgical physician assistants: report of a national survey of surgical chairmen in large U.S. hospitals. *Ann Surg, 193*(2):132-137, 1981.

21. Perry HB, Detmer DE, and Redmond EL: A policy proposal for correcting the imbalance in general surgical manpower. *Surgery* (in press), 1983.

22. Rutkow IM: Rates of surgery in the United States. *Surg. Clinics of N. Amer., 62:*559-578, 1982.

23. Rutkow IM, Zuidema GD: Surgical rates in the United States: 1966 to 1978. *Surgery, 89*(2):151-162, 1981.

24. Wunderman LE: Physician distribution and medical licensure in the U.S., 1979. Chicago, IL, American Medical Association, 1980.

25. Zuidema GD: The study on surgical services for the United States (SOSSUS) and its impact on American surgery. *Surg. Clinics of N. Amer., 62:*603-612, 1982.

Chapter 49

THE VIEWPOINT OF THE
AMERICAN COLLEGE OF SURGEONS
TOWARDS THE SURGEON'S ASSISTANT

HAROLD A. ZINTEL, M.D., F.A.C.S.

The vigorous and sustained approval of the Surgeon's Assistant (SA) by the American College of Surgeons is best documented by a brief review of the College's role in the development of the surgeon's assistant and the assistant to the primary care physician, hereafter referred to as the primary care assistant. These two categories of allied health personnel are subdivisions — or species — of the genus Physician Assistant.

College policy supports the concept that the surgeon's assistant should ideally be fully certified as a surgeon's assistant and can function in all settings in which the surgeon functions. The interest of the College in the surgeon's assistant began when physician assistants were being graduated from recognized schools and were working for physicians who performed surgical operations. Some of these physicians had surgical training. Others had no formal surgical training. Since the primary purpose of the College is to assure high standards of care to the surgical patient, the College recognized its duty to help assure high standards of educational physician assistant programs and high standards of certification for both the surgeon's assistant and the primary care assistant who worked for surgeons. This is part of a broader College commitment "to keep abreast of governmental and socio-economic developments and help formulate College policies so as to exert as constructive an effect as possible toward the improvement of the care of the surgical patient."

In 1968, the Board of Governors of the College investigated the development of paramedical personnel and recommended that the College be represented on the agencies approving these personnel and their educational programs — certification of the individual and accreditation of schools. The Regents of the College in 1969 appointed the Committee on Allied Health Personnel (CAHP).

The purpose of CAHP was to "investigate paramedical personnel." At the first meeting of CAHP on September 11, 1970, the following recommendations were made: (1) That the American College of Surgeons approve the principle of its Fellows utilizing the services of properly trained and accredited allied health personnel. (2) That such allied health personnel work in a dependent relationship under the direction and responsibility of a qualified physician. (3) That the College collaborate with the Council on Medical Education (CME) and Council on Health Manpower (CHM) of the American Medical Association (AMA) in developing guidelines and essentials for acceptable programs in surgery. (4) That the College position be that of encouraging experimentation, innovation and continued study. These recommendations were made so the College could exert as constructive an effort as possible toward the improvement of the care of the surgical patient. Studies were to be made not only of the role of the assistant to the surgeon in the operating room, but the role of the physician assistant who, among other things, was trained to obtain patient histories and to perform physical examinations. Prior to this time, the combination of these two activities — as is now embodied in the activities of the surgeon's assistant — had not been recorded by the College.

In 1970, 8,000 Fellows of the College in response to a questionnaire indicated that they would hire a trained, non-M.D. surgeon's assistant if such were available (1). An additional number indicated that they would hire such individuals within the next five years.

In 1971, representatives of the American Academy of Family Physicians (AAFP), the American Academy of Pediatrics (AAP), the American College of Physicians (ACP) and the American Society of Internal Medicine (ASIM) worked with the Council on Medical Education of the American Medical Association (CME of AMA) to prepare the Essentials of an Educational Program for the Assistant to the Primary Care Physician and to have the Essentials approved by their respective organizations. The collaborating organizations suggested the completed document might later be altered to included the surgeon's assistant.

With the assistance of several staff members of AMA, the College prepared the "Essentials of an Approved Educational Program for the Surgeon's Assistant" (Surgeon's Assistant Essentials). These Surgeon's Assistant Essentials were approved by the Board of Regents of the College in February 1972. Subsequently, they were approved by the Council on Medical Education of the AMA. The College and the Council on Medical Education anticipated at that time the Surgeon's Assistant Essentials would be published jointly by the College and AMA. However, the Council on Medical Education could not proceed further because the Advisory Committee on Education for the Council on Allied Health Professions and Services of the Council on Health Manpower of the AMA failed to approve of the Surgeon's Assistant Essentials indicating that the Council on Health Manpower had inadequate evidence to justify such an additional allied health category. A letter dated January 9, 1973 from Dr. Malcolm C. Todd, Chairman of the AMA Council on Health Manpower, indicated that "evidence was lacking for a completely new occupation to perform these functions" and the Council "did not endorse the need for a new occupation per se." In February of that year, the College withdrew the Surgeon's Assistant Essentials from consideration by the AMA.

The College, restating its beliefs, resubmitted the Surgeon's Assistant Essentials to the AMA for discussion by representatives of the College and the AMA in May 1973. That discussion ended with the Council on Health Manpower of the AMA neither approving nor disapproving the Essentials.

In June 1973, the Regents of the College approved of the unilateral publication of the Surgeon's Assistant Essentials in the Bulletin of the American College of Surgeons pointing out that during the three years of negotiations, additional education programs had been and were being established. These programs were graduating surgeon's assistants as well as physician assistants who had participated in surgery without adequate supervision and control of the surgeon's assistant educational programs and without any provision in the immediate future for certification, registration or certification maintenance of the surgeon's assistant graduate. The Surgeon's Assistant Essentials were published in the College Bulletin in August 1973 (2).

It is of interest to note that in 1973 the Office of Education of the Department of Health, Education and Welfare "requested that generic accreditation of Physician Assistants be seriously considered to eliminate the duplication of man hours and other costs which would be involved in separate accreditation procedures for each of the two types of Physician Assistants . . . —the SA (surgeon's assistant) and PCA (primary care assistant). The above would involve eight medical organizations and the American Medical Association. The Essentials and guidelines for each special type of assistant (the SA or the PCA) would be retained." It was also recommended there be a common core educational program for both surgeon's assistant and physician assistant.

Meanwhile, in early 1974, the College was asked to join and did join with the AMA and 26 other collaborating organizations in a Joint Council for the Accreditation for Allied Health Education which, through several modifications, became the current Committee on Allied Health Education and Accreditation (CAHEA). CAHEA is a Committee of the AMA, however, it functions as *one of forty-seven collaborating organizations in accrediting twenty-six Allied Health occupations independently of councils* and *committees of the AMA and of the House of Delegates* of the AMA. This body is therefore, independent in judgment in accreditation matters and its decisions are final. Establishment of CAHEA as an autonomous body meant that the AMA was no longer the accrediting body but was one among 47 that collaborated with the new committee in accrediting allied health programs.

In 1974, the National Commission on Certification of Physician's Assistants (NCCPA) was formed with fourteen member organizations including the College. These organizations are now represented by one NCCPA Director each, except for the American Academy of Physician Assistants (AAPA) which has five directors and three members-at-large, one of which is a physician. NCCPA was separated from the AMA and established in its Atlanta, Georgia headquarters in February, 1975.

The College was invited, in 1975, to join with the Joint Review Committee on Educational Programs for the *Assistant to the Primary Care Physician* (JRC/APCP). The JRC/APCP changed its name in 1976 by substituting the words *Physician's Assistant* for the words *Assistant to the Primary Care Physician*. Thus, the resulting Joint Review Committee on Educational Programs for the Physician's Assistant (JRC/PA) recognized in its title the agreement to the generic concept of the physician assistant which included both the primary care assistant and the surgeon's assistant. This generic concept was approved by each of the original collaborating sponsors: American Academy of Family Practice, American Association of Pediatrics, American College of Physicians, American Society for Internal Medicine and American Academy of Physician's Assistants and by the College. In fact, the governing bodies of these organizations had originally recommended that one body "review both the educational programs for assistants to primary care physicians and for surgeon's assistants." Acceptance of the generic concept made it possible for the College to become a collaborating sponsor. On October 19, 1975, the NCCPA also approved of this type of generic concept in relation to certification of surgeon's assistants and physician assistants. The Association of Physician Assistant Programs (APAP) later petitioned to become a sponsor and was admitted as such in 1978. The function of the JRC/PA is to receive applications for accreditation of educational programs, to survey educational programs, and to make recommendations for accreditation to be considered by CAHEA for final action. Revised Surgeon's Assistant Essentials have been prepared by the collaborating sponsors and CAHEA for publication early in 1983.

At about this time, there were some 50 educational programs for the training of primary care physician assistants graduating 1200 individuals a year. Most of these programs were accredited. There were three accredited educational programs producing 53 surgeon's assistants a year and two unaccredited programs producing an unknown number of surgeon's assistants. Estimates of the number of primary care assistants who worked as surgeon's assistants for surgeons or for physicians who had no surgical training but performed surgery varied up to about ⅓ of the total number of primary care assistant and surgeon's assistant graduates. It is generally regarded that about a third of the graduates of the oldest program, the Physician Assistant Program of Duke University, has practiced with surgeons or with physicians who do surgery (3).

The surgeon's assistant in no way conflicted with or overlapped the activities of the Operating Room Technician for which the College had collaborated with the American Hospital Association (AHA), the AMA, the Association of Operating Room Nurses and the Association of Operating Room Technicians in producing Essentials for Educational Programs for the Operating Room Technician as published in 1972 (4). Several years ago, the Operating Room Technicians changed their name to Surgical Technologists and that of the organization to the Association of Surgical Technologists.

The first surgeon's assistant educational program to be surveyed by the College's *Joint Review Committee on the Surgeon's Assistant* was the Surgeon's Assistant Program at Cornell University on December 4, 1974. The AMA Council on Medical Education gave accreditation status to this program early in 1975 when the AMA agreed to collaborate in this effort. In September 1975, the Surgeon's Assistant Program of the University of Alabama in Birmingham was accredited by the AMA Council on Medical Education upon recommendation of the JRC/PA.

It was soon agreed that the surgeon's assistant could function in any area in which the surgeon functioned. He could work in the surgeon's office, in the hospital helping to establish the diagnosis and preparing the patient for operation, in the operating room, during the postoperative period in the hospital and in the follow-up period in the office.

In October of 1977, the Regents approved of the policy statement on the surgeon's assistant which read as follows:

"The Surgeon's Assistant, one of several categories of Physician Assistants, is supported by the College. The College was the first to describe the category and publish *Essentials* for the educational training programs. College representatives participate in the national certification and accreditation processes for this category of allied medical personnel.

"The Surgeon's Assistant, one of several categories of the generic Physician's Assistant, is a skilled person qualified by academic and clinical training to provide patient services under the direction, supervision, and responsibility of a licensed surgeon as defined in the ACS Statement on Qualifications for Surgical Privileges in Approved Hospitals (5). The assistant is capable of collecting historical and physical data, organizing these data, and presenting these in such a way that the physician can visualize the patient's problem and determine appropriate diagnostic or therapeutic procedures. He functions in any setting in which the surgeon functions. He is distinguished by his ability to integrate and interpret findings on the basis of general medical knowledge and to exercise the degree of independent judgment approved by his responsible surgeon.

"A College representative is a director of the National Commission on Certification of Physician's Assistants, and the College provides three representatives to the 21-man Joint Review Committee on Educational Programs for the Physician's Assistant which approved the educational programs for accreditation."

The policy statement on qualifications of surgical assistants in the operating room which is defined in section II of the ACS Statement on Qualifications for Surgical Privileges in Approved Hospitals (5) is as follows:

In the absence of specifically trained and readily available surgical operating room assistants for a great number of the many operating rooms in this country, the assistant's role has traditionally been filled by a variety of individuals with quite diverse backgrounds as indicated by the following:

(1) A qualified surgeon as identified above.

(2) An MD in a recognized surgical training program.

(3) An MD without complete surgical training.

(4) Certified physician or surgeon's assistants who are not authorized to operate independently.

(5) A registered nurse or OR technician trained as "scrub nurse" without formal assistant surgical training other than "on the job" or "at the table" experience.

The American College of Surgeons supports the concept that, ideally, the first assistant at the operating table should be a qualified surgeon or a resident in an approved surgical training program. Attainment of this ideal in all hospitals is recognized as impracticable, and certain individuals without complete surgical training are currently necessary to serve as assistants to qualified surgeons in a number of hospitals. Certified physician assistants or surgeon's assistants must make application to the hospital outlining their qualifications and stipulating their requests to assist at the operating table. They shall be responsible to the surgical staff and their performance shall be subject to periodic review.

The College has been aware of a number of programs for surgeon's assistant graduate education for certified physician assistants and for registered nurses. These have been referred to as surgeon's assistant postgraduate courses for graduate physician assistants and nurses. The CAHP has been asked several times by representatives of these educational programs for assistance in developing accreditation for the schools and certification for graduates of the schools. Since no other medical organizations had expressed an active interest in these proposed activities, and especially since no ready sources of funds to develop these activities were available, the CAHP decided their development must await greater interest and financial support. In 1979, the College provided a grant in the amount of $21,481 to NCCPA for exploratory work in the development of a certifying examination for the surgeon's assistant.

The exact number of surgeon's assistants and physician assistants who work as surgeon's assistants is unknown. The number would include those who work for physicians trained and certified in surgery, for physicians trained but uncertified in surgery, or for physicians without surgical training. Several studies do give some indication as to the possible numbers, however none of the studies were designed to provide specific answers for all elements of the above statement. In using figures from any study, it must be borne in mind that only about 60% of the operations in this country are performed by physicians trained in surgery and that, in general, all graduates of medical schools, when licensed, are licensed to practice medicine and surgery.

Using the figures of the 1978 National Survey (6) of 11.7% indicating the proportion of physician assistants working in surgery and using the total physician assistant population of 15,000 as projected by the AAPA for 1981, would suggest that the surgeon's assistants currently would number 1,755. Using an earlier figure 15.1% from a similar study by Light (7) in 1976 would suggest a total number of 2,265 surgeon's assistants. It should be emphasized that neither of the above mentioned studies (6, 7) included physician assistant activities in surgical operations of obstetrician gynecologists or those performed by the 42.5% of the supervising physicians whose practice was family practice. In a more recent study published in 1981 by Perry *et al* (8), 775 surgeon's assistants were found to be working in 552 hospitals of 400 beds or more. Extrapolating the documented number of 755 surgeon's assistants to the possible number for the country as a whole by using the ratio of the total number of patient admissions of all acute care hospitals in the United States indicates that 3,400 surgeon's assistants might be working in hospitals of the United States.

Regardless of the exact numbers, the number of surgeon's assistants is growing. Frequently, in the published physician assistant job listings, the number of positions offered for surgeon's assistants represents one-third of all positions offered physician assistants of all types.

The growth of the surgeon's assistant has lead to a national organization established in 1970, the American Association of Surgeon's Assistants. It has now held five national annual meetings and supports a journal and a newsletter. There are several state organizations of surgeon's assistants and several subsections of surgeon's assistants of constituent state physician assistant chapters.

The College for more than a decade has strongly endorsed the concept of the surgeon's assistant as a trained individual, graduated from an accredited educational program, working dependently to a surgeon in all areas where the surgeon functions. The College and its fellows have not altered this position. At the same time, the College has been well aware that many of the members of several of the organizations that have participated in allied health activities similar to those of the College documented in this chapter recently have had second thoughts about the movement. No such general reactions have been expressed to either chapters, governors, or the headquarters of the College.

The College has consistently maintained that the surgeon's assistant certification process should parallel that of the physician assistant in the generic sense as has been repeatedly emphasized by several sources over more than a decade. Such a process is referred to several times in this brief review. On many occasions, the College has been assured that full certification for the surgeon's assistant was promptly forthcoming, yet at the time of this writing there is no assurance of a specific date for full certification of the surgeon's assistant. In June of 1981, the College urged NCCPA and AAPA in the strongest of terms to expedite the administration of a surgeon's assistant certifying examination without further delay and suggested it be made available in 1982. The College has constantly and actively demonstrated its support of the surgeon's assistant by its contributions and participation in the agencies approving these personnel and their educational programs—certification of the individual and accreditation of school.

REFERENCES

1. American College of Surgeons: Results of the Fellowship Questionnaire. *Bulletin of the American College of Surgeons, 56:*10; 11-12, 1971.
2. American College of Surgeons: Essentials of an Approved Educational Program for the Surgeon's Assistant. *Bulletin of the American College of Surgeons 58:*8; 58-61, August 1973.
3. Toth, P., Pickrell, K., and Thompson, L.: Role of the Physician Assistant and the Plastic Surgeon. *Southern Medical Journal, 71–4:*430-431, April 1978.
4. Essentials of an Approved Educational Program for the Operating Room Technician. American Medical Association, December 1972.
5. Statement on Qualifications for Surgical Privileges in Approved Hospitals. *Bulletin of American College of Surgeons, 62:*4; 12-13, April 1977.
6. Perry, H.B., and Fisher, D.W.: The Physician's Assistant Profession: Results of the 1978 Survey of Graduates. *Journal of Medical Education, 56:*10; 839-845, October 1981.
7. Light, J.A., Crain, M.J., and Fisher, D.W.: Physician Assistant: A Profile of the Profession. *The P.A. Journal, 7:*3, 1976.
8. Perry, H.B., Detmer, D., and Redmond, E.: The Current and Future Role of Surgical Physician Assistants. *Annals of Surgery, 193:*1; 132-137, January 1981.

Chapter 50

THE FUTURE FOR SURGEON'S ASSISTANTS AS VIEWED BY THE AMERICAN ACADEMY OF PHYSICIAN ASSISTANTS,

PETER D. ROSENSTEIN
SUSAN ANDERSON

The concept of the physician assistant was born in 1961, when Charles Hudson, MD, called for an advanced medical assistant with special training between that of a technician and a physician who would be able to handle many technical procedures, and in addition, take some degree of medical responsibility. Four years later, in 1965, Dr. Eugene Stead launched the first physician assistant program at Duke University with the admission of four ex-military corpsmen to be trained as assistants to the primary care physician. With the start of this new profession, an organization was needed to represent their collective needs. In 1968, the American Academy of Physician Assistants was founded to serve the interests of physician assistants, who at that time were employed mainly in the area of primary care. By 1972, 12 physician assistant programs were in operation, and since that time, with impetus from the Comprehensive Health Manpower Training Act of 1971, the number of programs has risen to over 50 and at this time graduate nearly 1,500 physician assistants annually. In addition to an expansion in the number of programs, the type of programs offered has changed over the years. There are now programs in many specialty areas including surgery. Many physician assistants have moved out of the area of primary care and work in these specialty areas.

In 1973, the joint national office of the American Academy of Physician Assistants and the Association of Physician Assistant Programs was established with funding from the Robert Wood Johnson Foundation, the Ittleson Family Foundation, and the van Amerigen Foundation in the form of three-year grants. At that time, approximately 500 physician assistants were Academy members. The Association included 45 training programs for the assistant to the primary care physician. Today, there are over 7,000 members of the

Academy, including both graduate physician assistants and student physician assistants, located in the 50 states of the United States, the District of Columbia and several foreign countries. The Association of Physician Assistant Programs membership includes more than 52 programs. Though the exact number of practicing physician assistants in the country is difficult to determine, the Academy maintains a mailing list of over 16,000 practicing physician assistants and students.

Since 1965, the history of the physician assistant has been one of steady progress. The physician assistant has been generally well accepted by both the medical community and the public, though certain skeptics remain. There are those who maintain, as they have for years, that only the physician can provide medical care to the public, and only the physician, with his or her training, can be responsible to the public to provide the kind of care that they believe is necessary. But these feelings are slowly changing. Part of the reason they are changing is because the cost of health care in this country has skyrocketed dramatically over the last few years. These inflated costs have created the kind of problems that people did not realize would exist. We now have a situation where neither the private sector nor the public sector can continue to pay the costs that are being generated by the health care used in this country.

Since its inception, the physician assistant profession has been supported to varying degrees by the medical community. Statements of support have been issued by the American Medical Association, the American Academy of Family Physicians, the American Society of Internal Medicine and the American College of Surgeons, among others. The Academy has worked closely with these groups to insure that the kind of quality care that we believe physician assistants can deliver will continue to be used to its maximum. As the role of the physician assistant moves and shifts, the Academy has also tried to maintain its representation of all physician assistants. As more and more physician assistants move from the primary care field into the field of surgery, the Academy has moved along and developed close relationships with the American College of Surgeons. The Academy has fostered the development of special interest groups in the AAPA and worked with groups on the outside to make sure that we meet the needs of all physician assistants. The development of a surgery add-on exam to the primary care examination administered by the National Commission for Certification of Physician Assistants is an indication of the Academy's support for this specialty group.

The certifying examination for primary care physician assistants was developed by the National Board of Medical Examiners and first administered in December 1973. Graduates of nurse practitioner, nurse clinician and child health associate programs were eligible to take the exam, as were informally trained primary care physician assistants who had met stringent eligibility criteria. Since the examination was in primary care, graduates of surgeon's assistant programs were not eligible.

The growth of the physician assistant profession and the resulting state rules and regulations that often required certification by the NCCPA created a serious problem for specialty physician assistants. As an interim solution, beginning in 1976, graduates of accredited surgeon's assistant programs have been eligible to sit for the examination. However, the American College of Surgeons and the House of Delegates of the AAPA have been on record since the first NCCPA examination urging the development of relevant examinations for specialty physician assistants.

The American College of Surgeons contributed the necessary funds to support the NCCPA's efforts in exam development. A Specialty Physician's Assistant Committee and a test committee jointly developed the surgery exam first given in 1979 to a test audience. The audience which also took the exam in two subsequent years was composed of a mix of graduate and undergraduate primary care physician assistants and surgeon's assistants. The goal is the development by 1983 of a core examination with specialty exams in primary care and surgery. Successful completion of the exam will give certification as a physician assistant or as a surgeon's assistant.

Originally, it was thought the inequities of access to health care and service provision resulted from shortages of physician manpower. Persistent consumer dissatisfaction, despite the substantial increase in overall physician supply, indicated that these inequities are related to disparities in physician distribution by specialty and geography. A more important aspect of physician supply is the actual productivity of physician specialists and the quantity of medical and surgical services rendered by them. Provision of health care services is not divided easily into distinct categories of medical versus surgical care. Without doubt, medical care is provided to patients whose primary pathology requires surgical treatment and vice versa. Therefore, it is not surprising to find that primary care, as an evolving concept in health services in the United States, means different things to different people. The problem with the definition is further complicated in view of the ongoing evolution of our health system. Unanimously, the opinion as to the definition of primary care is elusive. However, the Health Profession's Educational Assistance Act of 1976, Public Law 94-484, considered family medicine, internal medicine and general pediatrics as primary care specialties. It is almost unanimously agreed now that the physician assistant should have a basic medical knowledge, which would allow them to move into the specialty of primary care or the specialty of surgery.

In its recent report, the Graduate Medical Education National Advisory Committee (GMENAC) recommended that research be undertaken to determine the extent and nature of present physician assistant involvement in surgical care and the potential for increased delegation in these specialties, meaning general surgery and other surgical specialties. They went further in their *Recommendation 19* to say that consideration should be given to using physician assistants and nurse practitioners to provide some of the services which residents provide, should a decrease in the number of surgical residents occur. The Academy strongly supports the concept of using physician assistants in this area. Programs such as the graduate programs for surgical assistants at Montefiore Hospital in New York, Franklin Square Hopsital in Baltimore, and Norwalk Hospital/Yale in Connecticut, have proven the effectiveness of using surgeon's assistants. More and more community hospitals are seeing the value in surgeon's assistants, as are surgeons themselves. There are presently four CAHEA accredited surgeon assistant programs in operation. In addition there are postgraduate surgeon assistant programs offered to physician assistants who have graduated from a primary care program. These programs are being opened because of the demand for graduates that exist despite GMENAC's projected oversupply in most areas of surgery by 1990.

GMENAC recommended that the class size in allopathic and osteopathic medical schools be reduced by a minimum of 10 percent as well as severely restricting the number of graduates of foreign medical schools allowed to enter the United States. Thus, the need has arisen for personnel to fill the spots of surgical residents. There has been strong support for this position from the American College of Surgeons. Naturally, some of this has to do with their own pocketbooks. Over the years it has been seen that an excess of surgeons tends to produce an excess of operations, as more operations are performed to increase income. It is believed that if the level of surgeons trained was kept at the level of need, affordable surgeon's assistants could be used to take up the slack and assist in surgery. Since physician assistants cannot practice independently, they are not perceived to be in direct competition with surgeons presently practicing.

The Academy support for the concept of the surgeon's assistant and our belief that they are very effective in providing services to patients, comes in part from a number of studies surveying the attitute toward surgeon's assistants among health professionals in teaching and in community hospitals. These studies have indicated that community hospitals show the most positive attitude toward surgeon's assistants. Among professional groups, nurses and administrators demonstrated the most positive attitudes. Surprisingly, in some cases, allied health workers held the least positive attitudes toward the surgeon's assistant. Among hospital-based physicians, the surgical specialist exhibited the most favorable attitude toward surgeon's assistants. Studies done on the use of physician assistants in the community practice of general surgery reported that in a small rural community hospital emergency room, quality of care and acceptance of surgeon's assistants by patients and paraprofessionals was excellent. Studies have noted the improvement of patient care with comprehensive and continuous monitoring of patient's needs through the use of physician assistants.

One study showed that in a small community, utilization of a physician assistant did not appreciably increase the income of a practice; however, it estimated that four or five surgeons, utilizing physician assistants as surgeon's assistants, could have done the same work as eight surgeons. These studies show that physician assistants in non-primary care settings are as effective as those in primary care settings with regard to patient satisfaction, quality of care and acceptance by physicians and paraprofessional personnel. In addition, since according to the National Center for Health Services research, it costs approximately 25 percent of the total cost of preparing graduate physicians to prepare a graduate physician assistant, the cost effectiveness projections of physician assistants remain in effect, irrespective of physician assistant practice settings or specialty interest.

One of the stumbling blocks for total utilization of physician assistants and surgeon's assistants has been federal reimbursement policies. Traditionally, health care service payors have been very conservative with regard to new service providers. These payors oppose changes because they may increase costs that they believe are already too high. However, this is myopic, as the use of allied health providers will, in the long run, cut costs per patient, though they may increase costs initially through expanded access to care. Traditional reimbursement barriers have been extremely difficult to surmount for new modes of service delivery such as the free-standing surgical facility. As an example, Medicare will reimburse primary care physicians for their services as a first assistant in surgery, but will not reimburse for a physician assistant who would provide the same service under the same circumstances. The restrictions on reimbursement until now, have not been critical in the expansion of the number of physician assistants used because they are widely used in settings where funding is assured: HMOs, hospitals, and federally funded clinics. However, the full deployment of physician assistants as providers of care will require changes in the approach to reimbursement. The Academy is taking a leading role, and has noted as its top priority, the securing of reimbursement under Medicare, Part B. This is the area that covers third-party reimbursement. This reimbursement policy, if changed, would allow the surgeon's assistant to be hired directly by the surgeon to work closely with that surgeon and that surgeon's patients. The Academy strongly believes that this would help to insure quality care for the patient and reduce overall health care costs.

Another area that the Academy is working on is the concept of gaining staff privileges for physician assistants who work for private physicians. We have worked with individual hospital boards as well as the American Hospital Association, to disseminate information on the role of the physician assistant. It is important for the surgeon's assistant to have hospital privileges if he or she is to follow patients postoperatively. The Academy will support, and continue to support, the training and employment of surgeon's assistants. However, there are issues involved which will have to be monitored.

One of these is the inherent salary differential between primary care physician assistants and surgeon's assistants. It is likely that all individuals trained in CAHEA approved programs will continue to function under the generic name of physician assistants — that all will continue to be required to take a core examination for certification with a specialty exam in either surgery, primary care or other new specialties physician assistants will want to go into. The Academy believes that in the long run, the continued production and training of surgeon's assistants will be of value in facilitating policies that are designed to significantly reduce the total surgical manpower pool. Surgeon's assistants could increase the productivity of an area surgeon, not only by assisting at operations, but also by performing delegated surgical tasks. They could substitute for surgical residents in assisting and performing other service tasks in teaching hospitals which are seeking to reduce the number of their residents. Such substitutions would enable these hospitals to meet surgical service needs without having to train additional surgeons.

The Academy will continue to encourage the formation of special interest groups and caucuses in the areas of surgery so that people with the same needs and problems will have a chance to communicate with each other directly and will be able to communicate those needs to the Academy. At the Academy, we realize that the specialty area of surgery will be one of the fastest growing physician assistant specialties, and we will do all we can to encourage that and to insure the training of surgeon's assistants meets established standards and that job opportunities are available for the graduates of surgeon's assistant programs in as many diverse settings as possible.

APPENDICES

Appendix A

ESSENTIALS AND GUIDELINES OF AN ACCREDITED EDUCATIONAL PROGRAM FOR THE ASSISTANT TO THE PRIMARY CARE PHYSICIAN

Initially adopted 1971; revised and adopted 1978 by the
AMERICAN ACADEMY OF FAMILY PHYSICIANS
AMERICAN ACADEMY OF PEDIATRICS
AMERICAN ACADEMY OF PHYSICIAN ASSISTANTS
AMERICAN COLLEGE OF PHYSICIANS
AMERICAN COLLEGE OF SURGEONS
AMERICAN MEDICAL ASSOCIATION
ASSOCIATION OF PHYSICIAN ASSISTANT PROGRAMS

Program Review Committee
JOINT REVIEW COMMITTEE ON EDUCATIONAL PROGRAMS
FOR PHYSICIAN'S ASSISTANTS

Essentials, which present the minimum accreditation standards for an educational program, are printed in regular typeface. The extent to which a program complies with these standards determines its accreditation status; the *Essentials* therefore include all requirements for which an accredited program is held accountable. Guidelines, explanatory documents which clarify the *Essentials,* are printed in italic typeface. Guidelines provide examples, etc., to assist in interpreting the *Essentials.*

PREAMBLE

Objective

The education and health professions cooperate to establish and maintain minimum standards of appropriate quality for educational programs for the assistant to the primary care physician and to provide recognition for those programs which meet or exceed the standards outlined in these *Essentials*.

These *Essentials* are to be employed as minimal standards for the development and self-evaluation of programs educating the assistant to the primary care physician. Lists of accredited programs are published for the information of potential students, employers, and the public. Students enrolled in programs are taught to work with and under the direction of licensed registered physicians in providing health care services to patients.

Description of the occupation

The assistant to the primary care physician* is a skilled person, qualified by academic and clinical training, to provide patient services with and under the supervision of a doctor of medicine or osteopathy who is responsible for the performance of that assistant. The physician's assistant is also responsible for his/her own actions. The assistant may be involved with the patients of the physician in any medical setting in which the physician participates.

The functions of the assistant to the primary care physician include performing diagnostic, therapeutic and preventive activities and services to allow more effective use of the physician's knowledge, skills and abilities. While the physician remains responsible for the decisions relating to individual patient management, the assistant to the primary care physician is involved in the processes necessary to reach decisions and in the implementation of the therapeutic plan.

Intelligence, the ability to relate with people, capacity for calm and reasoned judgement in meeting emergencies, and a demonstration of commitment to the patient are qualities essential for the assistant to the primary care physician. An attitude of respect for the patient and confidentiality of the patient's record is necessary.

Since the function of the primary care physician is interdisciplinary in nature such as family medicine, internal medicine, surgery, pediatrics, psychiatry, obstetrics/gynecology, and others, the assistant to the primary care physician should be educated to assist the physician in providing those varied medical services.

The ultimate role of the assistant to the primary care physician cannot be rigidly defined because of the variations in practice requirements due to geographic, political, economic, and sociologic factors. The high degree of responsibility an assistant to the primary care physician assumes requires that at the conclusion of the formal education process, the assistant possess the knowledge, skills and abilities necessary to providing those services appropriate for a primary care setting. These services should include, but need not be limited to the following:

1. Initially approaching a patient of any age group in any setting to elicit a detailed and accurate history, perform an appropriate physician examination, identify problems, and record and present pertinent data;
2. Performing and/or interpreting routine diagnostic studies including common laboratory procedures, common radiologic studies, electrocardiographic tracings, obtaining pap smears, and others;
3. Performing therapeutic procedures including but not limited to injections, immunizations, suturing and wound care, incision and drainage of superficial infections, cast application, and followup of simple fractures;
4. Instructing and counseling patients regarding physical and mental health including information relating to diet, disease prevention and therapy, normal growth and development, family planning, situational adjustment reactions, and others;
5. Assisting the physician in in-patient settings by conducting patient rounds, recording patient progress notes, determining and implementing therapeutic plans jointly with the supervising physician and compiling and recording pertinent narrative case summaries;
6. Assisting in the delivery of services to patients requiring continuing care (home, nursing home, extended care facilities, etc.) including reviewing and monitoring treatment and therapy plans;
7. Independently performing evaluation and therapeutic procedures when responding to life threatening situations; and
8. Facilitating the referral of patients and maintaining awareness of the community's health facilities, agencies, and resources.

REQUIREMENTS FOR ACCREDITATION

I. Sponsorship
Educational programs may be established in
A. Medical schools;
B. Colleges and universities in affiliation with an accredited teaching hospital, which together are capable of providing the clinically oriented basic science education and the necessary clinical teaching and experience;
C. Medical education facilities of the federal government and of other institutions with the ability to provide necessary clinically oriented basic science teaching and which have an active and defined affiliation with institutions

actively engaged in providing the appropriate clinical teaching and experience.

All institutions must be accredited and have sufficient teaching faculty to insure adequate pre-clinical preparation for the assistant to the primary care physician.

The Essentials *recognize that educational programs of basic quality may be established and operated successfully under a variety of administrative auspices. Among the optional organizational bases are:*

Medical Schools and academic centers;

Senior colleges and universities in affiliation with an accredited teaching hospital;

Medical education facilities of the federal government such as Veteran's Administration hospitals, U.S. Public Health Services hospitals and agencies, U.S. Public Health Service hospitals and agencies, and the military services; and

Other institutions with clinical facilities, which are acceptable to the Council on Medical Education of the American Medical Association. (These include junior and community colleges in affiliation with accredited teaching hospitals, and accredited teaching hospitals in affiliation with an accredited educational institution.)

The institution should be accredited or otherwise acceptable to the Council on Medical Education. Senior colleges and universities must have the necessary clinical affiliations. (Essentials I)

The acceptability of these organizational bases may be suggested or attested to by other accrediting bodies such as the Liaison Committee on Medical Education or regional education accreditation bodies.

Experience to date suggests the following general observations, each of which is subject to exception in existing practice:

Academic medical centers, medical schools, and larger academic institutions, by nature of their size, often have a broader range and greater depth of resources with consequent potential for contribution to the didactic and practical education of physician's assistants. This is true not only of the usual faculty resources associated with clinical medicine, but often includes as well more faculty who are knowledgeable in communication skills such as listening, interviewing, and counseling, and those faculty knowledgeable in the behavioral sciences.

Traditionally primary care has not been a major focus of the academic medical center, although exceptions to this generalization are increasingly apparent. The emphasis of institutional activities in the academic medical center has traditionally been on secondary and tertiary care. As a consequence, some believe that extra efforts have to be taken to insure that physician's assistant students become imprinted with a primary care orientation, when the institutional priorities and faculty interest are likely to be on the evaluation and management of acute care problems arising from less common manifestations of disease and illness. Students have to receive a substantial body of instruction and supervised clinical experience in the evaluation and management of patients who have degenerative diseases and health maintenance problems that are characteristic of primary care.

It is a program's duty to assure students of adequate direct access to patients. Through coordinated scheduling with medical school and other health sciences faculty, several programs have arranged to minimize the competition among medical students, junior house staff, student physician's assistants, and other students for clinical contacts with patients. There can be, and reportedly often develops, complementary tutorial relationships among medical and physician's assistant students by virtue of a quid pro quo that exists as a result of differing educational and clinical experience backgrounds.

Affiliations with community hospitals often increase student access to patients, due to the absence of medical students and fewer, if any, house officers. These affiliations are valuable also, in that students receive greater concentration of clinical experience in the care and management needs of patients with the more ordinary manifestations of an acute illness.

When smaller institutions, agencies, and clinics develop a special education program like that for the physician's assistant, special attention and effort are required in obtaining the scope and quality of clinical affiliations necessary for the practical instruction of students. Such organizations may have a strong understanding and concern for the delivery of primary personal health services and through creative efforts develop an educational program which produces competent physician's assistants.

It is important that any program, regardless of organizational sponsorship, prepare assistants to the primary care physician with those attitudes, skills, and knowledge which are fundamental to caring for persons in need of primary health care services. The commitment of the program administration and faculty to such a primary care orientation is fundamental to the success of any program.

II. Curriculum

A. The length of educational programs for the assistant to the primary care physician may vary. The length of time individuals spend in training may also vary on the basis of the student's background based on previously acquired education, experience, knowledge, skills and ability, and ability to perform the processes, tasks, functions and duties implied in the "Description of the Occupation."

The length of the educational program is determined largely by its objectives and complementing student selection criteria. Although they are not restricted to this time frame, programs are commonly 24 months in length with principal, if not total, focus on clinical didactic and clinical practicum instruction.

B. General courses and topics of study, both preclinical and clinical should include the following:

   1. General courses and topics of study must be directed toward providing the graduates with necessary knowledge, skills, and abilities to accurately and reliably perform tasks, functions, processes, and duties implied in the "Description of the Occupation."

Both the clinical didactic and clinical practicum components of the curriculum should focus on the knowledge, skills, and attitudes related to the health care needs and concerns that adults of all ages, teenagers, and children commonly bring to the primary care setting.

Both components of the curriculum should include the preparation of assistants to primary care physicians who can make knowledgeable and skilled life-saving responses to life-threatening situations: e.g., trauma, acute coronary distress, precipitous delivery, suicidal risk, et cetera.

Skill development in interviewing, listening, and counseling are recognized as important components of clinical competence in primary care, not only in relation to eliciting a personal health history, but in helping individuals arrive at practical approaches to the maintenance of their own health, and in responding to those who express concerns about other than health-related problems.

Clarity in definition of program objectives is fundamental. Preferably, the objectives of each course, and ultimately each class session may be defined so that there is full understanding among faculty and students of what is to be taught and what is to be learned in any given session of instruction. Evaluation processes should be developed to assure the student that he obtains the level of understanding and performance that are basic to the assistant to the primary care physician.

A program cannot evaluate the knowledge and proficiency which students have acquired unless it has first defined the specific functions and tasks they are expected to learn. As a consequence, a program must define course objectives in such a way that the students, faculty, and evaluator can recognize the level of proficiency and knowledge students are expected to attain from various courses and the program as a whole. For example, objectives might be differentiated in varying levels according to those that require a high level of knowledge and proficiency in the performance of given functions or tasks, those requiring a working knowledge and skill level upon which proficiency could later be developed and those requiring only an awareness of the function of a given level of knowledge and/or skill.

Programs should examine carefully the prior educational and vocational experience of each student in order to reduce the redundance of instructional efforts and the length of time spent by students in the curriculum. Use of proficiency measures should be developed for appropriate placement of students and to give credit for previous accomplishments of learning.

2. Instruction should be sufficiently comprehensive to provide the student with understanding of physical and mental problems experienced both by the ambulatory and institutionalized patient. Attention should be given to preventive medicine and principles of public health as well as to social and economic aspects of health care.

   Instruction should stress the role of the assistant to the primary care physician as it relates to health maintenance and comprehensive health and medical care. Throughout, the student should be encouraged to develop basic intellectual, ethical and moral attitudes and principles essential for gaining and maintaining the trust of professional associates, the support of the community, and the confidence of the patient.

Primary care by its nature deals principally with ambulatory patients, and consequently requires that the clinical practicums of a curriculum have major orientation to ambulatory care as characterized by mild or degenerative disease processes. However, primary care physicians also manage the care of many patients through an acute phase which requires hospitalization. It is in this context that instruction of physician's assistants should include clinical didactic and clinical practicum components dealing with the usual features of the care and management needs of hospitalized patients. It is desirable that students receive similar instruction relating to patients in extended care facilities and in home health services to acquire an appreciation of the value of the care of the patient in his own environment.

It is desirable that graduates have a functional understanding of personality development and of normative human behavior. Courses incorporating content regarding psychosomatic manifestations of illness and injury; child development; normative psychological and physiological responses to stress in daily living; human sexuality; and the social responses to dying, death, and the surviving spouse are illustrative of behavioral science content which has a strong practical relation to the substance of primary care.

Through his clinical education the student should receive a thorough orientation to the range of responsibilities and functions expected of the assistant to the primary care physician as well as to how to work with the physician and other health service personnel in a variety of patient care settings.

Attention should be given to preventive medicine and principles of public health as well as to social and economic aspects of health care.

It is in the context of preventive medicine that skill development in counseling has significant potential for helping patients follow prescribed treatment regimens or to modify their attitudes and behaviors to more healthful patterns. These skills are fundamental also in making health hazard appraisals for individual patients.

There is need also for graduates to have an understanding of the personal, social and economic consequences of decisions relating to options in the management of personal health, both in its maintenance and in its restoration. A survey course descriptive of the variety of organizational approaches to the delivery of personal health services and to the impact of social and economic factors on physical and emotional well-being is desirable.

Throughout, the student should be encouraged to develop basic intellectual, ethical and moral attitudes and principles essential for gaining and maintaining the trust of professional associates, the support of the community, and the confidence of the patient.

3. An ambulatory care teaching facility such as the family practice centers used by family practice residency programs should be incorporated where feasible so medical students, house staff, and student assistants to the primary care physician can jointly share educational experiences in an atmosphere that reflects and encourages the actual practice of primary medical care.

It is preferred that the physician's assistant student receives exposures to staff who are experienced primary care physicians, graduate physician's assistants, nurses, and the various other health personnel who function within a model practice setting. Scheduling of staff and patients should assure that the student has sufficient access to patients in order to develop his skills in identifying their health status and in assessing their health care needs.

It is helpful to students to receive a portion of their practical clinical experience in one of a number of settings recognized as models for the delivery of primary care when such a unit is accessible to the program as a clinical affiliate. For example, the following definition is exemplary of a model unit of primary medical care and is from the 1971 edition of a Guide for Residency Programs in Family Practice, *published by the Residency Review Committee for Family Practice.*

A model unit of primary medical care is a facility used in the education of resident physicians in family medicine. Such a facility is characteristic of family practice offices, with enough rooms to provide each resident the use of a private consultation room, an examination and treatment room or a minor operating room at almost any time he needs them. In addi-

tion, there is an attractive and comfortable reception room, a nurses' sta-tion, a receptionist and/or secretary's area, and a conference room and/or a library used for teaching purposes. If laboratory and x-ray facil-ities are not within the unit, they are readily available to the patients. Whether in or out of the hospital, the unit is a distinct entity. The unit is reasonably near the parent hospital in which the resident cares for most of his hospitalized patients.

C. Instruction, tailored to meet the student's needs, should follow a planned outline and should include
   1. Assignment of appropriate instructional materials
   2. Classroom and laboratory presentations, discussion and demonstrations
   3. Supervised practice discussion
   4. Examinations, tests, quizzes — practical, written and oral — for the pre-clinical and clinical portions of the educational program.

As mentioned earlier, evaluation protocols should be established to insure that the student develops command of the knowledge and skills required of an assistant to the primary care physician. This allows the faculty to identify specific areas of weakness, and to strengthen the student's knowledge of a sub-ject or clinical skills.

Preceptorships Programs commonly require students to spend a portion of their advanced training in one or more preceptorships.[2] These range from one to several months in duration, depending upon program objectives for the preceptorship. Principally, they are intended to accelerate the development of the student's clinical knowledge and skills and his ability to respond to in-dividual patients and their clinical problems and situations.

The purpose and objectives of preceptorships should be committed to writing in clearly stated language in order to minimize the opportunity for misunderstanding among program administration, preceptors, and students; to provide a basis for evaluation of the relevance of the objectives to the devel-opment of student's knowledge and skills; to evaluate the student's achieve-ment resulting from the preceptorship; and to evaluate the degree to which the preceptor and his practice serve and meet the objectives.

This should be supported by evaluation protocols that provide for measure-ment of the extent of the intended learning which the student experiences as a result of the preceptorship and the extent to which the preceptor meets or ex-ceeds his teaching responsibility to the student.

Evaluation protocols may be more effective when their purpose and methods are understood and supported by preceptors and students.

The time required to administer preceptorships varies in relation to class size, the geographic accessibility of preceptors, the size of the preceptor pool to

serve the long-term needs of the program, and the character of physician attitudes regarding physician's assistants.

Evaluation *Although it is recognized that in many respects contemporary
evaluation methodologies are not fully adequate, within the best means available, educational programs must develop and implement evaluation of all
components of the program. In addition, the program should assume responsibility for evaluating the graduates' performance as an indication of the adequacy and appropriateness of the curriculum, student selection criteria, and
other elements of the educational process.*

*Programs should be encouraged to develop behavioral objectives for the
supervised clinical practice components of the curriculum as well as for the
courses offered in the didactic phase of the program. Any effort to assess student performance should be made in relation to stated objectives.*

*It is recommended that, where possible, the evaluation be undertaken on a
collaborative basis with similar programs in order to enlarge the numerical size
of the sample population.*

III. Resources

Resources must be adequate to support the number of students admitted to
the program.

A. **Program Officials**
  1. Program Director
     a. The program director should meet all requirements specified by the
        institution responsible for providing the didactic portion of the edu-
        cational program and maintaining the operation of the overall
        program.
     b. The program director should be responsible for the organization,
        administration, periodic review, continued development, and
        general effectiveness of the program.
  2. Medical Director
     a. The medical director should provide continuous competent medical
        direction for the clinical instruction and for clinical relationships
        with other educational programs. The medical director should ac-
        tively elicit the understanding and support of practicing physicians.
     b. The medical director should be a physician experienced in the de-
        livery of the type of health care services for which the student is
        being trained.
     c. The medical director may also be the program director.
     d. If there is a change in the program or medical director, prompt
        notification should be sent to the Department of Allied Health
        Education and Accreditation of the AMA. The curriculum vitae of
        the new director, including details pertinent to the individual's

training, education, and experience must be submitted. The Department of Allied Health Education and Accreditation should be similarly notified about any acting director serving on an interim basis before identification of a permanent director.

3. Administrative Staff

The program must have an adequate administrative staff.

Obviously, a program administration functions most effectively when it has the wholehearted support, both attitudinal and financial, of senior administrative offices as well as the enthusiastic support of its staff.

Within the administrative leaders of the program, there should be a body of work experience in the delivery of primary care services with full understanding and respect for the individuality of the person seeking primary care services. Effective administration requires an ability to work within the medicopolitical and legal milieu that accompany the change in attitudes and practices within the health services culture which are brought about by the education of physician's assistants.

The general effectiveness of a program is enhanced by the degree to which the administration and faculty subscribe to and actively pursue a process of self-analysis prior to an accreditation on-site evaluation. Such a process involves a critical review of program objectives, the appropriateness of curriculum content in view of those objectives; the effectiveness of the instruction; the adequacy of the resources and facilities devoted to the program; an analysis of the strengths and limitations of the program; and a plan for program improvement. Evidence of a process of program self-analysis is required of the Council on Medical Education by the U.S. Office of Education.

B. **Instructional Faculty**

1. The faculty must be qualified through academic preparation and experience, to teach assigned subjects. This necessitates teaching ability as well as clinical experience. There must be adequate numbers of faculty to teach assigned subjects.

2. Faculty for the supervised clinical practice portion of the educational program must include physicians and may include assistants to the primary care physician and other health professionals who are experienced in the provision of patient care services. Because of the unique characteristics of the assistant to the primary care physician, it is necessary that the preponderance of clinical teaching be conducted by physicians experienced in practice.

It is imperative that the faculty have an appreciation for teaching with a strong orientation toward clinical problems common to primary care. Instructional faculty may include house staff, medical center clinical staff, and practicing physicians other than medical center-based faculty such as family physicians, internists, obstetrician-gynecologists, pediatricians, surgeons, psychiatrists, orthopaedists, et cetera. The specialists who are usually considered referral consultants in secondary care may be key faculty members by virtue of their specific knowledge in primary care: for example, a psychiatrist who is experienced in primary care such as that provided through a community mental health center. Instruction in the clinical practicum should be provided by faculty members who are experienced in primary care; programs should not rely chiefly on resident physicians who are still in the formative stages of their development and who usually have only limited experience in the management of primary health care problems.

In addition, students should receive some of their clinical practice instruction from clinical preceptors as discussed earlier. (See "Preceptorships")

Representative criteria for the selection of preceptors commonly include evidence of interest in teaching; ability to teach; the primary care focus in the given medical practice; understanding and commitment to the use of physician's assistants in the primary care setting; and the availability of physical space for the student to interview and examine patients.

Faculty and preceptor understanding and support for the role of the physician's assistant are critical to the students' development of confidence in this role. Otherwise, students may experience significant stress in grasping their identity as physician's assistants, inasmuch as they are frequently asked by others within the clinical setting to define who and what they are as physician's assistants. Nursing students, medical students, and others seldom are subject to similar inquiry because of the wide variety of nurse and physician role models found within the school and affiliated clinical facilities. Because of the limited number of physician's assistants, it is the exception rather than the rule for physician's assistant students to learn in settings where graduate physician's assistants are working.

C. **Financial Resources**
  1. Financial resources for continued operation of the educational program should be assured for each class of students enrolled.
  2. The institution shall charge student fees commensurate with the setting. Cost to the student shall be accurately stated and published. Also, policies and procedures for refunds of tuitions and fees shall be fair, published and made known to all applicants.
  3. Announcements and advertising must accurately reflect the program offered and be appropriate to an educational institution.
  4. Students shall use their scheduled time for educational experience. The program shall not substitute students for paid personnel to conduct the operation of clinical facility.

D. **Physical Resources**
1. Adequate classrooms, laboratories, and administrative offices should be provided.
2. Appropriate modern equipment and supplies for practical experiences should be available in sufficient quantities.
3. A library should be readily accessible and should contain an adequate supply of current medical and other scientific books, periodicals and other reference material related to the curriculum.

In addition to the above resources, and to the extent feasible, students should have free access to teaching/learning resources during evening, night, and weekend hours to foster maximum opportunity for study and self-instruction. Accessibility is perceived in terms of economy of time as it relates to students' movements from classroom to laboratory to clinical care settings to the library.[3]

4. Records
Satisfactory records should be maintained for all assignments undertaken by the student while enrolled in the program. The academic institution should be responsible for all records.
a. Curriculum
(1) A synopsis of the current curriculum should be kept on file.
(2) The synopsis should include the rotation of assignments, the outline of the instructions supplied, and lists of multimedia instructional aids used to augment the experience of the student.
(3) Written objectives of each course should be maintained and available to the students and instructors.

A brief yet descriptive statement of content of each course should be maintained including a diagramatic description of the given or random sequence of the clinical practicums students receive. Each course description should be complemented with an outline of the student learning that is expected to result from the course instruction. It is best that this expected learning be stated in definitive, behavioral terms.

A listing of multi-media resources should be maintained, identifying those which are available for instructor and student use. Their location, availability and a description of the processes to be followed in obtaining them should be available to help students and faculty gain access to these useful teaching/learning resources.

b. Student Records
Credentials used for admission, reports of medical examination upon admission and records of any subsequent illness during training, records of class and laboratory participation, and academic and clinical achievements of each student should be maintained in accordance with the requirements of the institution.

All student records should be maintained with full respect for their confidential nature. It is likely that these student records may be kept in differing locations with one or more offices sharing responsibility for their maintenance, safe-keeping, and the preservation of their confidential nature.

    c. Activity
        (1) A satisfactory record system shall be provided for all student performance.
        (2) Practical and written examinations should be continually evaluated.
        (3) The records should be reviewed periodically with the student.
        (4) The program should document an effective self-evaluation process.

A quality record system must be maintained to assure each student and graduate of the availability of the records of his academic performance to future interested parties, such as state regulating agencies, certifying bodies, academic institutions in which one may wish to pursue further studies, and potential employers.

Programs are ethically obligated to insure proper administration of these records in active and archive repositories.

E. Clinical Affiliations
    1. The clinical phase of the educational program must be under competent medical direction. It should be conducted in part in a setting where primary care services are provided on a regular on-going basis.
    2. In programs where the academic instruction and clinical teaching are not provided by the same institution, accreditation shall be given to the institution responsible for the academic preparation (student selection, curriculum, academic credit, etc.), and the educational administrators shall be responsible for assuring that the activities assigned to the students in the clinical setting are educational.
    3. In the clinical teaching environment an effective ratio of students to physician instructors who are experienced in practice shall be maintained.

In obtaining clinical education, students should have access to patients in adequate volume and in appropriate distributions by sex and age who present the common problems encountered in the delivery of primary care. Students ready access to patients in order to develop skills in clinical assessment and management; and in related counseling in regard to (1) the common injuries and pathophysiologies presented by hospitalized patients, (2) family-oriented ambulatory primary care needs, and (3) the crisis intervention in life-threatening situations.

Clinical affiliations should be established only with those settings under competent clinical direction, to assure that the student receives a constant assessment of his work.

Clinical education must occur within bona fide *clinical settings under competent clinical direction; however, faculty should take advantage of simulated clinical experiences in introducing students to applied clinical knowledge and in the structured development of clinical skills through the use of instructional models or programmed patients.*

F. **Advisory Committee**

An advisory committee should be appointed to advise the program in continuing program development and evaluation. For maximum effectiveness, the advisory committee should include representation from the primary institutions involved, the program administration, organized medicine, community based physicians, assistants to the primary care physician, students, the public and other appropriate groups.

It is strongly suggested that an Advisory Committee include diverse orientations that bring a breadth of perspective from the program administration and faculty, local primary care physicians, students, graduates, nurses, preceptors, faculty from other departments, representation from the state medical society and the like. Appointments of local primary care physicians to the Committee are considered especially helpful.

By definition, the advisory Committee advises, and as such serves as a sounding board for program plans, for modifications, and for evaluating the purpose and objectives of the program, as well as alternative approaches to resolving certain problems in program operation or progress.

Advisors promote understanding of program objectives among their constituent bodies and provide a means of maintaining a higher level of awareness and support for the program among significant groups within the professional community and the community at large.

IV. Students
A. Selection

1. Selection of students should be made by a designated admissions committee of which the members include adequate representation of those responsible for the various phases of the program. All admissions data should be on file in the institution responsible for the administration of the program.

2. Selection procedures must include an analysis of previous performance and experience and should accommodate candidates with a health related background and should give credit to the knowledge, skills, and abilities they possess. Potential to develop the interpersonal skills neces-

sary to perform the role as defined by the "Description of the Occupation" should be considered in the selection process.

Student selection criteria should be developed in consultation with the advisory and admissions committees. An admission committee should include a variety of perspectives, including those of student and graduate physician's assistants. Selection criteria should be evaluated periodically to determine what effect, if any, they may have had on student performance, attrition or graduate location and choice of practice setting.

Selection criteria may vary, but commonly include such factors as the prospective student's concept of the physician's assistant role, emotional and intellectual maturity, ability to communicate, financial stability, evidence of study skills necessary to handle the curriculum, and indication of the ability to obtain career satisfaction within the profession.

Programs of shorter duration commonly select only those students who have had previous education, training, and/or work experience in the health sciences. (See "Length of Program.")

B. **Number**

The number of students enrolled in each class should be commensurate with effective learning and teaching opportunities, should be consistent with acceptable student-teacher ratios, and should be compatible with demonstrated instructional needs.

Student/teacher ratios should vary according to the learning objectives and teaching methods used in any given instructional period. The appropriate ratio of students to teachers varies according to the instructional objectives of the various components of clinical instruction. Of principal concern is that the students receive not only the individualized or group instruction required to accomplish defined learning objectives, but that tutorial assistance be readily available for clarification and reinforcement, as required by one's individual learning patterns.

C. **Health**

Students should be required to submit evidence of good health essential to participating in the program, so that they will not endanger other students or the public, including patients.

D. **Counseling**

An active student guidance and placement service should be available.

Students should have ready access to faculty for counsel regarding their academic concerns and to professionally qualified staff for counsel about personal concerns and problems.

E. **Related Policy**

Criteria for completion of each segment of the curriculum and for graduation shall be given in advance to each student, as well as the policies and procedures for dismissal and withdrawal.

F. **Student Identification**
Students enrolled in the educational program must be clearly identified to distinguish them from physicians, medical students, and other health occupations students and graduates.

V. **Publication**
An official publication including a description of the program should be available. It should include information regarding the organization of the program, a brief description of the required courses, the names and academic ranks of principal faculty members, entrance requirements, tuition fees and other anticipated costs, and information pertaining to the hospitals and other facilities used in the course of training. It must reflect accurately the program offered and career expectations.

ADMINISTRATION OF ACCREDITATION

Accreditation
1. Application for accreditation of a program should be made to:
   Department of Allied Health Education and Accreditation
   American Medical Association
   535 N Dearborn St
   Chicago, IL 60610
2. The evaluation and accreditation of a program can be initiated only at the written request of the chief executive officer of the sponsoring institution or an officially designated representative.
3. A sponsoring institution may withdraw its request for initial accreditation at any time (even after the site visit) prior to final action.
4. The program being evaluated is given the opportunity to review the factual report of the visiting survey team and to comment on its accuracy before the final action is taken.
5. The Committee on Allied Health Education and Accreditation (CAHEA) and the cooperating review committees will periodically resurvey educational programs for continued accreditation.
6. The chief executive officer of the sponsoring institution may request that a return on-site evaluation be made in the event of significant deficiencies in the performance of an earlier evaluation team.
7. Adverse accreditation decisions may be appealed by writing to CAHEA. Due process will be followed.

Adopted by the Committee on Allied Health Education and Accreditation, October 1978

FURTHER INFORMATION

Applications for program approval and inquiries regarding program accreditation should be directed to the Department of Allied Medical Professions and Services, Division of Medical Education, American Medical Association, 535 North Dearborn Street, Chicago, IL 60610.

Additional information concerning education on physician's assistants may be obtained from the Association of Physician Assistant Programs, Suite 700, 2150 Pennsylvania Avenue, Washington DC 20037.

---

*The generic term "assistant to the primary care physician" is used to encompass such titles as the physician's assistant, physician associate, medex, and child health associate.

All direct quotations from the *Essentials of an Approved Educational Program for the Assistant to the Primary Care Physician* will hereafter be in italics.

---

[2]In this context, a preceptorship is an assigned clinical practicum under the tutelage of a physician who is experienced and knowledgeable in primary care.

---

[3]Norman S. Stearns, M.D. and Wendy W. Ratcliff, "A Core Medical Library for Practitioners in Community Hospitals," *The New England Journal of Medicine,* Vol. 280, No. 9, February 27, 1969.

Appendix B

ESSENTIALS OF AN ACCREDITED EDUCATIONAL PROGRAM FOR THE SURGEON'S ASSISTANT

Essentials initially adopted 1974; Revised 1982
Adopted by the
AMERICAN COLLEGE OF SURGEONS
AMERICAN MEDICAL ASSOCIATION

Program Review Committee
JOINT REVIEW COMMITTEE ON EDUCATIONAL PROGRAMS FOR PHYSICIAN'S ASSISTANTS
PREAMBLE

Objective

The education and health professions cooperate in this program to establish and maintain standards of appropriate quality for educational programs for surgeon's assistants, and to provide recognition for educational programs which meet or exceed the minimal standards outlined in these *Essentials.*

These standards are to be used as a guide for the development and self-evaluation of programs for the training and education of surgeon's assistants. A list of these approved programs is published for the information of employers and the public. Surgeon's assistants enrolled in the program are taught to work with and under the director of physicians in providing health care services to patients.

Description of the occupation

The assistant to the surgeon should be a skilled person qualified by academic and clinical training to provide patient services under the supervision and responsibility of a licensed physician who is in turn responsible for the performance of that assistant. The assistant may be involved with the patients of the surgeon in any medical setting.

The function of the assistant to the surgeon is to perform, under the responsibility and supervision of the surgeon, diagnostic and therapeutic tasks in order to enable the physician to extend his services through the more effective use of his knowledge, skills, and abilities. The assistant to the surgeon does not supplant the surgeon in the sphere of the decision making required to establish a diagnosis and plan therapy, but may assist in gathering the data necessary to reach the decision and in implementing the therapeutic plan for the patient.

Essential qualities for the assistant to the surgeon include the ability to relate with people, a capacity for calm and reasoned judgment in meeting emergencies, an awareness and understanding of one's professional role, an orientation toward service and a level of intelligence commensurate with the performance of one's professional skills. The assistant to the surgeon must maintain respect for the person and privacy of the patient.

The tasks performed by the assistant include transmission and execution of the surgeon's orders, performance of patient care tasks, and performance of diagnostic and therapeutic procedures as may be delegated by the surgeon.

The ultimate role of the assistant to the surgeon cannot be rigidly defined because of the variations in practice requirements due to geographic, economic and sociologic factors. The high degree of responsibility an assistant to the surgeon may assume requires that at the conclusion of his formal education he possesses the knowledge, skills and abilities necessary to provide those services appropriate to the surgical setting.

REQUIREMENTS FOR ACCREDITATION

I. Sponsorship

A. The clinical phase of the educational program must be conducted in a clinical setting and under competent clinical direction.

   In programs where the academic instruction and clinical teaching are not provided in the same institution, accreditation shall be awarded to the institution responsible for the academic preparation of students. The educational administrators will be responsible for assuring that assignments to students in the clinical setting are related to obtaining defined learning objectives.

B. Educational programs should be established in medical schools in conjunction with their department of surgery, or in other surgical facilities acceptable to the American Medical Association and the American College of Surgeons, in order to provide optimal conditions for the clinical training of the surgeon's assistant.

C. The sponsoring institution and affiliates, if any, must be accredited by recognized agencies or, in the judgement of the Committee on Allied Health Education and Accreditation, meet equivalent standards.

D. Responsibilities of the sponsor and each affiliate for program administration, instruction, supervision, and other administrative relationships must be clearly described in written documents such as affiliation agreements.

II. Curriculum

A. The length of the educational program for the surgeon's assistant may vary from program to program; however, the suggested program involves two full calendar years of integrated preclinical, clinical didactic and supervised practice instruction. The length of time an individual spends in the program may vary on the basis of the student's background and previously acquired education, experience, knowledge, skills and the person's ability to perform the tasks, functions and duties implied in "Description of the Occupation."

B. Instruction, tailored to meet the surgeon's assistant student's needs, shall follow a planned outline. It shall include:

1. Assignments of appropriate instructional materials, reading, and exercises.
2. Classroom and laboratory presentations, discussions, and demonstrations.
3. Supervised practice sessions.
4. Examinations, tests and quizzes — practical, written, and oral — for the preclinical and clinical portions of the educational program.

C. Preclinical and clinical didactic course content shall include the following:

1. Human anatomy, including neuroanatomy *at an advanced level with lectures, dissections, demonstrations and prosections.*
2. Medical physiology, *beginning at the cellular level and including all physiological systems, with special emphasis on the cardiovascular, respiratory, renal metabolic, gastrointestinal, endocrine, reproductive, and neurological systems.*
3. Fundamentals of clinical medicine, *including the pathophysiology clinical manifestations, diagnostic evaluation and therapeutic management of patients with commonly encountered medically related diseases and disorders.*
4. Medical terminology *which may use self-instructional texts as learning aids.*
5. Pharmacokinetics and pharmacodynamics *of frequently used groups of drugs, including their indications for use, beneficial and potential adverse effects, and interactions with other drugs.*
6. Fundamentals of general surgery, *including the pathophysiology, clinical manifestations, diagnostic evaluation and the non-opera-*

*tive, pre-operative, operative, and post-operative therapeutic
management of patients with commonly encountered surgically
related diseases and disorders, especially those of the peritoneum,
alimentary tract, liver, pancreas, spleen, head and neck, endocrine glands, breast, blood vessels, lung, and the common
surgically treated disorders of the heart and great vessels. Basic
fundamentals of surgical intervention for benign and malignant
tumors and basic immunology principles should be included also.*

7. Patient assessment *and the compilation of a complete patient data
base, including elicitation of a comprehensive patient history and
performance of a complete physical examination.*

8. Principles of surgical patient care, *including wound care, sterile
techniques, wound healing, systemic response to trauma and
multi-system injury, nutrition, fluid and electrolyte balance, low
output states, hemorrhage, appropriate use of blood and blood
component transfusions, post-operative infections and complications and the management of thermal injury.*

9. Surgically related patient care techniques, *including subcutaneous
and intro-muscular injections, arterial puncture, venipuncture,
intravenous catheterization, venous cutdowns, gastrointestinal
and tracheal intubation, urethral catheterization, removal of
pleural fluid accumulations, cardiopulmonary resuscitation and
suturing techniques.*

10. Introduction to interpretation of roentgenogram *with emphasis of
evaluation of the chest x-ray, abdominal x-rays especially in gastrointestinal obstruction and traumatic abdominal injury, evaluation of fracture of the extremities and the use of ultrasound and
computerized tomography in the evaluation of surgically related
diseases.*

11. Introduction to electrocardiographic recording techniques and
techniques and arrhythmia interpretations.

12. Respiratory function evaluation, support, and therapy, *including
techniques and appropriateness of ventilator support, precau-
tions, hazards, and the use of measured parameters of airway and
gas exchange, and safe administration of such care.*

13. Supervised clinical practice *instruction should be a minimum
equivalent of twelve calendar months. Students shall participate
in patient assessment, evaluation, and documentation of clinical
data, and shall participate in the pre-operative, operative, and
post-operative care of patients under the supervision of the responsible surgeon member of the program faculty. These clinical prac-*

tice experiences shall include but not be limited to general surgery, primary medical care, cardiothoracic, peripheral vascular, genitourinary, neurologic and orthopedic surgery, and the surgical care of acutely injured emergency patients.

III. Resources
A. Program Officials
The program must have an adequate administrative staff.
1. Program Director
   a. The program director shall be responsible for the organization, administration, periodic review, continued development and general effectiveness of the program.
   b. The program director should meet all requirements specified by the institution responsible for providing the didactic portion of the educational program and maintaining the operation of the overall program.
2. Medical/Surgical Director
   a. The medical/surgical director should provide continuous, competent direction for the clinical instruction and for clinical relationships with other educational programs. The medical/surgical director should actively elicit the understanding and support of practicing physicians.
   b. The medical/surgical director should be a physician experienced in the delivery of the type of health care services for which the student is being trained.
   c. The medical/surgical director may also be the program director.

B. Instructional Staff
1. Faculty for the clinical portion of the educational program must include general and specialty surgeons and may include surgeon's assistants and other health professionals who are experienced in the provision of patient care services. Because of the unique characteristics of the surgeon's assistant, it is necessary that the preponderance of clinical teaching be conducted by physicians experienced in surgical practice.
2. The faculty must be qualified through academic preparation and experience to teach assigned subjects. This necessitates teaching ability as well as clinical experience. There must be adequate numbers of faculty to teach assigned subjects.
3. Number — The number of students enrolled in each class should be commensurate with effective learning and teaching opportunities, should be consistent with acceptable student/teacher

ratios, and should be compatible with demonstrable instructional needs.

4. During any given course of instruction or supervised clinical practice rotation, students who are performing at a marginal or unsatisfactory level shall be counseled promptly.

C. **Financial Resources**

Financial resources for continued operation of the educational program shall be assured for each class of students enrolled.

D. **Physical Resources**

1. General—Adequate classrooms, laboratories, and administrative offices and other facilities shall be provided.
2. Laboratory—Appropriate modern equipment and supplies for directed experience shall be available in sufficient quantities for student participation.
3. Library—A library shall be readily accessible and shall contain an adequate supply of up-to-date and scientific books, periodicals, and other reference materials related to the curriculum.
4. Records

   Satisfactory records shall be kept on progress and accomplishments by the student in the training program. An annual report shall be prepared on the general operation of the program.

   a. Student Records

      Credentials used for admission, records of class and laboratory participation, and academic and clinical achievements of each student shall be maintained in accordance with the requirements of the institution.

   b. Curriculum

      1. A copy of the complete curriculum shall be kept on file.
      2. Copies of class schedules, course outlines, and teaching plans shall be on file and available for review.
      3. Copies of practical and written examinations shall be maintained and continually evaluated.

   c. Faculty

      A copy of the qualifications of each principal faculty member responsible for teaching each segment of the curriculum shall be maintained, with emphasis on their qualifications for that segment of the curriculum.

E. **Instructional Resources**

Instructional aids such as clinical material, reference materials, demonstration and other multimedia materials should be provided and accessible for classroom and independent study.

F. Advisory Committee

An advisory committee may be appointed to advise the program in continuing program development and evaluation. For maximum effectiveness, the advisory committee should include representation from the primary institutions involved, the program administration, organized medicine, community based physicians, surgeon's assistants, students, the public and other appropriate groups. Minutes should be maintained.

IV. Students

A. Program Description Students shall be provided with a clear description of the program and its content, including learning goals, course and competency objectives. Criteria for successful completion of each segment of the curriculum and for graduation shall be given in advance to each student.

B. Admission

1. Admission criteria shall be clearly defined, published, and presented to students upon filing for admission. Selection of students should be made by an admissions committee in cooperation with those responsible for the educational program.

2. Selection procedures should include an analysis of previous performance and experience to accommodate candidates with a health related background and give due credit for the knowledge, skills and abilities they possess.

3. Candidates for admission should have completed two years of college or the equivalent. Prior health related educational experience is desirable.

C. Health—Students must submit evidence of good health essential to participating in the program so that they will not endanger themselves, other students, or the public, including patients.

D. Student Identification—Students enrolled in the educational program must clearly be identified to distinguish them from physicians, medical students, and other health occupation students and graduates.

E. Student Guidance—An active student guidance and placement service should be available and reasonably accessible.

V. Operational policies

A. Catalog—An official publication including a description of the curriculum shall be issued. It should include information regarding the organization of the program, a brief description of required and elective courses, entrance requirements, tuition and fees, and information concerning hospitals and facilities used for clinical training. Announcements and advertising must accurately reflect the program offered and be appropriate to an educational institution.

B. Student matriculation practices and student and faculty recruitment shall be non-discriminatory with respect to race, color, creed, sex, age, handicap(s), or national origin.

C. Related Policy—Criteria for completion of each segment of the curriculum and for graduation shall be given in advance to each student, as well as the policies and procedures for dismissal and withdrawal and refunds of tuition and fees.

D. The institution shall charge student fees commensurate with the setting. Cost to the student shall be accurately stated and published. Also, policies and procedures for refunds of tuition and fees shall be fair, published and made known to all applicants before admission.

E. Students shall use their scheduled time for educational experience. The program shall not substitute students for paid personnel to conduct the operation of a clinical facility.

VI. Program evaluation processes

A. Accreditation—The evaluation of a program of study can be initiated only upon invitation by the chief administrator of the sponsoring institution or an officially designated representative. The evaluation shall be carried out through the Joint Review Committee on Educational Programs for Physician's Assistants (JRC/PA) and the Committee on Allied Health Education and Accreditation (CAHEA).

B. Program Self-Analysis—The program shall document an effective self-evaluation process.

VII. Maintaining accreditation

A. Reports—An annual report shall be made to CAHEA. A report form is provided and shall be completed, appropriately signed and returned promptly.

B. If there is a change in the program director or medical/surgical director, prompt notification shall be sent to the Department of Allied Health Education and Accreditation of the AMA. The curriculum vitae of the new director, including details pertinent to the individual's training, education and experience must be submitted. The Department of Allied Health Education and Accreditation shall be similarly notified about any acting director serving on an interim basis before identification of a permanent director.

C. Withdrawal—The institution may withdraw its request for initial accreditation at any time (even after an on-site evaluation) prior to

final action. CAHEA may withdraw accreditation whenever:
1. The educational program is not maintained in substantial compliance with the standards outlined above, or
2. There are no students in the program for two consecutive years.
D. Accreditation shall be withdrawn only after sufficient notice has been given to the chief executive officer of the institution that such action is contemplated, and the reasons therefore, to permit timely response and the use of established procedures for appeal and review.
E. Reevaluation
1. CAHEA will resurvey all educational programs at appropriate intervals.
2. Review — The head of the institution being evaluated is given the opportunity to become acquainted with the factual part of the report prepared by the on-site evaluators and to comment on its accuracy before final CAHEA action is taken.
3. Appeal — At the request of the head of the institution, a resurvey may be made. Accreditation decisions may be appealed by letter to CAHEA.

VIII. Administration of accreditation

Accreditation — Application and correspondence for accreditation of a program should be sent to:
Department of Allied Health Education and Accreditation
American Medical Association
535 North Dearborn Street
Chicago, Illinois 60610

Appendix C

IMPORTANT ADDRESSES
AND PHONE NUMBERS

American Academy Of Family Physicians   (800) 821-2512
1740 West 92nd Street
Kansas City, Missouri 64112

American Academy Of Physician Assistants   (703) 525-4200
National Office
1117 North 19th Street
Arlington, Virginia 22209

American College Of Surgeons   (312) 664-4050
55 East Erie Street
Chicago, Illinois 60611

American Medical Association   (312) 751-6280
Department of Allied Health
Education and Accreditation
535 North Dearborn Street
Chicago, Illinois 60610

Association Of Physician Assistant Programs (703) 525-4200
National Office
1117 North 19th Street
Arlington, Virginia 22209

National Commission On Certification   (404) 261-1261
Of Physician Assistants
3384 Peachtree Road, N.E., Suite 560
Atlanta, Georgia 30326

Appendix D

ASSOCIATION OF PHYSICIAN ASSISTANT PROGRAMS DIRECTORY
November 1982

ALABAMA
Surgeon's Assistant Program
University of Alabama
School of Medicine
Department of Surgery
University Station
Birmingham, AL 35294
(205) 934-4407

CALIFORNIA
Family Nurse Practitioner/
Physician Assistant Program
Department of Family Practice
2221 Stockton Blvd., Trailer 1532
Sacramento, CA 95817
(916) 453-3550

Primary Care Physician
Assistant Program
University of So. California
School of Medicine
2025 Zonal Ave.
Los Angeles, CA 90033
(213) 224-7101

MEDEX Physician Assistants Program
Charles R. Drew Postgraduate Med School
1621 E. 120th Street
Los Angeles, CA 90059
(213) 603-3051

Stanford-Foothill Primary Care
Associate Program
Stanford University Medical Center
Suite F-1 703 Welch Road
Palo Alto, CA 94304
(415) 497-6431

COLORADO
Child Health Associate Program
University of Colorado
Health Sciences Center
4200 East Ninth Ave.
Denver, CO 80262
(303) 394-7963

CONNECTICUT
Yale University
School of Medicine
Physician Associate Program
382 Congress Ave.
New Haven, CT 06510
(203) 785-4252

DISTRICT OF COLUMBIA
Physician Assistant Program
George Washington University
2300 Eye St. NW
Washington, D.C. 20037
(202) 676-4034

Howard University
Physician Assistant Program
6th & Bryand St., NW
Annex I, Room 312
Washington, D.C. 20059
(202) 636-7536

FLORIDA
Physician's Assistant Program
University of Florida
Coll of Health Related Professions
Box J-176, JHMHC
Gainesville, FL 32610
(904) 392-4326

GEORGIA
Physician Associate Program
Emory University School of Medicine
P.O. Box 22095
Atlanta, GA 30322
(404) 329-7825

Physician's Assistants Depart.
Medical College of Georgia
1120-15th Street
Augusta, GA 30912
(404) 828-3246

IOWA
University of Iowa
Physician's Assistant Program
College of Medicine
2333 Children's Hospital
Iowa City, IA 52242
(319) 353-5711 Office
(319) 353-6935 Director

KANSAS
Wichita State University
Physician's Assistant Program
5500 East Kellogg
Wichita, KS 67218
(316) 685-0249

KENTUCKY
Clinical Associate Program
University of Kentucky
Medical Center Annex #2, Room 110
Lexington, KY 40536
(606) 233-5743
     233-6344

MARYLAND
Essex Community College
Physician Assistant Program
7201 Rossville Blvd.
Baltimore, MD 21237
(301) 682-6000

MASSACHUSETTS
Northeastern University
Physician Assistant Program
202 Robinson Hall
360 Huntington Ave.
Boston, MA 02115
(617) 437-3195

MICHIGAN
Mercy College of Detroit
Physician's Assistant Program
8200 West Outer Drive
Detroit, MI 48219
(313) 592-6057

Western Michigan University
Physicians' Assistants Program
College of Health & Human Services
Kalamazoo, MI 49008
(616) 383-1636

MISSOURI
St. Louis University
Physician Assistant Program
School of Allied Health Professions
T504 South Grand Blvd.
St. Louis, MO 63104
(314) 664-9800 ext. 507

NEBRASKA
Physician Assistant Program
University of Nebraska
College of Medicine
42 Street and Dewey Ave.
Omaha, NE 68105
(402) 559-5266

NEW JERSEY
Physician's Assistant Program
Rutgers University
P.O. Box 101
Piscataway, NJ 08854
(201) 463-4444

NEW YORK
Albany-Hudson Valley
Physician's Assistant Program
Albany Medical College
Albany, NY 12208
(518) 445-5142 *or*
Hudson Valley Community College
Troy, NY 12180
(518) 283-1100 ext. 347

Cornell University Medical College
Surgeon's Assistants Program
1300 York Avenue
New York, NY 10021
(212) 734-3340

NEW YORK (cont.)

Long Island University/
The Brooklyn Hospital
Physician's Assistant Program
121 DeKalb Ave.
Brooklyn, NY 11201
(212) 270-4532

Stony Brook Physician's Asst. Prog
School of Allied Health Professions
Health Science Center
Suny at Stony Brook
Long Island, NY 11794
(516) 246-2517

Harlem Hospital PA Program
506 Lenox Ave., Room 6207
New York, NY 10037
(212) 491-8163

Touro College
Physician Assistant College
c/o Kingsbrook Jewish Med Center
East 49th Rutland Road
Brooklyn, NY 11203
(212) 493-6900
756-9700

Physician's Assistant Program
Bayley Seton Hospital
Bay Street & Vanderbilt Ave.
Staten Island, NY 10304
(212) 447-3010

NORTH CAROLINA
Duke University
Physician's Associate Program
Duke Medical Center, Box CFM 2914
Durham, NC 27710
(919) 684-6134 Admiss: 684-2506

Physician Assistant Training Prog
Bowman Gray School of Medicine of
Wake Forest University
1990 Beach Street
Winston-Salem, NC 27103
(919) 748-4356

NORTH DAKOTA
Family Nurse Practitioner Program
University of North Dakota
Department of Community Medicine
221 South 4th Street
Grand Forks, ND 58201
701/780-3114 or 3116
780-3111 (director)

OHIO
Kettering College of Medical Arts
Physician Assistant Program
3737 Southern Blvd.
Kettering, OH 45429
(513) 296-7201 ext. 5639
296-7238 (direct line)

Lake Erie College
Cleveland Clinic Foundation
Physician Assistant Program
391 West Washington St., Box 367
Painesville, OH 44077
(216) 352-3361 ext 380

Physician Assistant Program
Cuyahoga Community College
Western Campus
11000 West Pleasant Valley Road
Parma, OH 44130
(216) 845-4000

OKLAHOMA
Physician's Associate Program
University of Oklahoma
Health Sciences Center
P.O. Box 26901
Oklahoma City, OK 73190
(405) 271-2618 or 2619
271-2047 (assoc dir & dir)

PENNSYLVANIA
Gannon University
Physician Assistant Program
Perry Square
Erie, PA 16541
(814) 871-7340 or
(814) 871-7376

PENNSYLVANIA (cont.)

The Pennsylvania State University
Physician's Assistant Program
The Milton S. Hershey Medical Center
Hershey, PA 17033
(717) 534-8753

St. Francis College
Physician Assistant Program
Loretto, PA 15940
(814) 472-7000 ext. 276

Hahnemann Medical College & Hospital
Physician's Assistant Program
230 N. Broad Street, Room 412 CAHP
Philadelphia, PA 19102
(215) 448-7135

Assistant to the Primary Care
   Physician Program
Allegheny Campus
Community College of Allegheny County
808 Ridge Avenue
Pittsburgh, PA 15212
(412) 237-2570

Physician's Assistant Program
King's College
133 N. River St.
Wilkes-Barre, PA 18711
(717) 826-5853

TENNESSEE
Trevecca Nazarene College
Physician's Associate Program
333 Murfreesboro Road
Nashville, TN 37210
(615) 248-1225

TEXAS
The University of Texas
Health Science Center at Dallas
Physician Assistants Program
School of Allied Health Sciences
5323 Harry Hines Blvd.
Dallas, TX 75235
(214) 688-2830

Physician's Assistant Program
(Department of Health Care Sciences)
School of Allied Health Sciences
The University of TX Medical Branch
Galveston, TX 77550
(713) 765-3046 or 3047

Baylor College of Medicine
Physician Assistant Program
Center for Allied Manpower Dev.
1200 Moursund Avenue, Room 112-C
Houston, TX 77030
(713) 790-4619

UTAH
Utah MEDEX Project
University of Utah Medical Center
50 North Medical Dr., Build. 100
Salt Lake City, UT 84132
(801) 581-7764

VIRGINIA
Physician's Assistant Training Prog
Naval School of Health Sciences
Portsmouth, VA 23708
(804) 398-5056

WASHINGTON
MEDEX Northwest
802 Coach House
2309 NE 48th
Seattle, WA 98105
(206) 543-6483

WEST VIRGINIA
Alderson-Broaddus College
Physician's Assistant Program
College Hill
Myers Hall of Health Science
Philippi, WV 26416
(304) 457-1700

WISCONSIN
Physician Assistant Program
University of Wisconsin-Madison
1050 Medical Science Center
1300 University Avenue
Madison, WI 53706
(608) 263-5620
        263-6696 (director)

INDEX

DATE DUE